AF767550

Reconstructive Conundrums in Dermatologic Surgery

The Nose

Reconstructive Conundrums in Dermatologic Surgery

The Nose

EDITED BY

Désirée Ratner, MD
Director, Comprehensive Skin Cancer Program, Beth Israel Medical Center, Mount Sinai Health System, New York, NY, USA

Joel L. Cohen, MD
Director, AboutSkin Dermatology and DermSurgery, Englewood, CO, USA
Associate Professor, Department of Dermatology, University of Colorado, Aurora, CO, USA
Assistant Professor, Department of Dermatology, University of California, Irvine, CA, USA

David G. Brodland, MD
Co-Director, Z & B Skin Cancer Center, Pittsburgh, PA, USA
Assistant Professor, Departments of Dermatology and Otolaryngology, University of Pittsburgh, Pittsburgh, PA, USA

WILEY Blackwell

ASDS
American Society for Dermatologic Surgery

This edition first published 2014 © 2014 by American Society for Dermatologic Surgery

Registered office: John Wiley & Sons, Ltd, The Atrium, Southern Gate, Chichester, West Sussex, PO19 8SQ, UK

Editorial offices: 9600 Garsington Road, Oxford, OX4 2DQ, UK
The Atrium, Southern Gate, Chichester, West Sussex, PO19 8SQ, UK
111 River Street, Hoboken, NJ 07030-5774, USA

For details of our global editorial offices, for customer services and for information about how to apply for permission to reuse the copyright material in this book please see our website at www.wiley.com/wiley-blackwell

The right of the author to be identified as the author of this work has been asserted in accordance with the UK Copyright, Designs and Patents Act 1988.

All rights reserved. No part of this publication may be reproduced, stored in a retrieval system, or transmitted, in any form or by any means, electronic, mechanical, photocopying, recording or otherwise, except as permitted by the UK Copyright, Designs and Patents Act 1988, without the prior permission of the publisher.

Designations used by companies to distinguish their products are often claimed as trademarks. All brand names and product names used in this book are trade names, service marks, trademarks or registered trademarks of their respective owners. The publisher is not associated with any product or vendor mentioned in this book. It is sold on the understanding that the publisher is not engaged in rendering professional services. If professional advice or other expert assistance is required, the services of a competent professional should be sought.

The contents of this work are intended to further general scientific research, understanding, and discussion only and are not intended and should not be relied upon as recommending or promoting a specific method, diagnosis, or treatment by health science practitioners for any particular patient. The publisher and the author make no representations or warranties with respect to the accuracy or completeness of the contents of this work and specifically disclaim all warranties, including without limitation any implied warranties of fitness for a particular purpose. In view of ongoing research, equipment modifications, changes in governmental regulations, and the constant flow of information relating to the use of medicines, equipment, and devices, the reader is urged to review and evaluate the information provided in the package insert or instructions for each medicine, equipment, or device for, among other things, any changes in the instructions or indication of usage and for added warnings and precautions. Readers should consult with a specialist where appropriate. The fact that an organization or Website is referred to in this work as a citation and/or a potential source of further information does not mean that the author or the publisher endorses the information the organization or Website may provide or recommendations it may make. Further, readers should be aware that Internet Websites listed in this work may have changed or disappeared between when this work was written and when it is read. No warranty may be created or extended by any promotional statements for this work. Neither the publisher nor the author shall be liable for any damages arising herefrom.

Library of Congress Cataloging-in-Publication Data

Reconstructive conundrums in dermatologic surgery : the nose / edited by Desiree Ratner, Joel L. Cohen, David G. Brodland.
1 online resource.
Other title: Nose
Includes bibliographical references and index.
Description based on print version record and CIP data provided by publisher; resource not viewed.
ISBN 978-1-118-29498-7 (ePub) – ISBN 978-1-118-29499-4 (Adobe PDF) – ISBN 978-1-118-27232-9 (cloth)
I. Ratner, Desiree, editor of compilation. II. Cohen, Joel L. (Dermatologist), editor of compilation. III. Brodland, David G., editor of compilation. IV. American Society for Dermatologic Surgery, issuing body. V. Title: Nose.
[DNLM: 1. Nose – surgery – Case Reports. 2. Dermatologic Surgical Procedures – methods – Case Reports. WV 312]
RF350
617.523059 – dc23

2014002389

A catalogue record for this book is available from the British Library.

Wiley also publishes its books in a variety of electronic formats. Some content that appears in print may not be available in electronic books.

Cover images: © American Society for Dermatologic Surgery
Cover design by Andy Meaden

Set in 9/12 pt Minionpro by Laserwords Private Limited, Chennai, India

1 2014

MIX
Paper from responsible sources
FSC® C013604

Contents

Introduction

The Reconstructive Conundrum section of the journal *Dermatologic Surgery* first appeared in the year 2000. Edited by David Brodland, this section was intended to focus on teaching points related to closure type, defect site, and underlying anatomy. Photographs of the defect to be reconstructed, an immediate postreconstruction photograph, and two long-term follow-up views were required, and discussion of the closure specifically included the authors' thought process regarding the best option for repair, as well as possible alternative options and why they were not chosen. Historical details relevant to the case were often included in the presentation, and pearls relating to the specific closure or to reconstruction in general could be included in the discussion as well.

Over time, a wide variety of reconstructive conundrums have appeared in the journal exploring new directions with innovative repair options. Dermatologic surgeons in training, as well as more experienced practitioners, have found these manuscripts to be a valuable educational resource. The creativity of the surgeons authoring the conundrums, as well as the depth and breadth of their knowledge and experience, as demonstrated by the cases they present, is both impressive and inspiring.

Our trainees are always looking for texts and atlases illustrating reconstructive options for difficult defects. It occurred to us that a collection of the "best of the best" reconstructive conundrums might therefore be both interesting and useful as an educational resource to residents in dermatology, plastic surgery, otolaryngology, Mohs surgery fellows, and reconstructive surgeons still early in their careers. These physicians would most benefit from a book focusing on critical analysis of tissue defects and creative approaches to soft tissue reconstruction. Our intent in putting together such a text is to compile these cases for easy perusal as it is difficult at this point of time to view multiple conundrums consecutively and efficiently either electronically or in print, and it seemed to us that an "atlas-like" textbook would therefore be of value to these groups of readers. Because the nose is by far the site that tends to cause the most angst among reconstructive surgeons, as well as the most common site discussed in these conundrums, it made sense for the first group of cases to focus on complex nasal reconstruction.

While the reasoning and thought processes associated with the accomplishment of each closure are thoroughly discussed in each published conundrum, there are always alternative points of view which highlight additional points and "pearls". We therefore felt that commentaries by more experienced reconstructive surgeons would both complement and supplement the existing text.

To this end, we have compiled a series of 30 outstanding nasal reconstruction cases published in the Reconstructive Conundrum section over the past 10 years, grouped them by nasal subunits, and appended them to commentaries of our own. We have sought to include a diverse group of defects and reconstructions, and in some cases, we have included our own photographs of similar defects with contrasting closures to illustrate points relevant to a particular case.

We hope that you will find this compilation of nasal reconstructive conundrum cases both educational and inspirational and that you will enjoy reading them and thinking about them as much as we have.

Désirée Ratner, MD
Joel Cohen, MD
David Brodland, MD

I

PART I

Nasal Dorsum

1

CONUNDRUM 1

Combined Linear Closure and Burow's Graft for a Dorsal Nasal Defect

Daniel S. Behroozan[1] *& Leonard H. Goldberg*[2]
[1]DermSurgery Associates, Houston, Texas
[2]Department of Medicine (Dermatology), University of Texas, MD Anderson Cancer Center, Houston,Texas

An 80 year old man with a history of nonmelanoma skin cancers of the head and neck presented for treatment of a basal cell carcinoma of the nose. Physical examination revealed a poorly defined, exophytic, ulcerated nodule of the mid-dorsal nose. Given the size, location, and ill-defined margins of the tumor, Mohs micrographic surgical excision was indicated. The tumor was excised in three stages with microscopic control. The final defect was full thickness of the dermis, sparing the underlying muscle and measuring 3.2 × 2.4 cm on the mid-dorsal, supratip, and lateral aspects of the nose (Figure 1). How would you repair this defect?

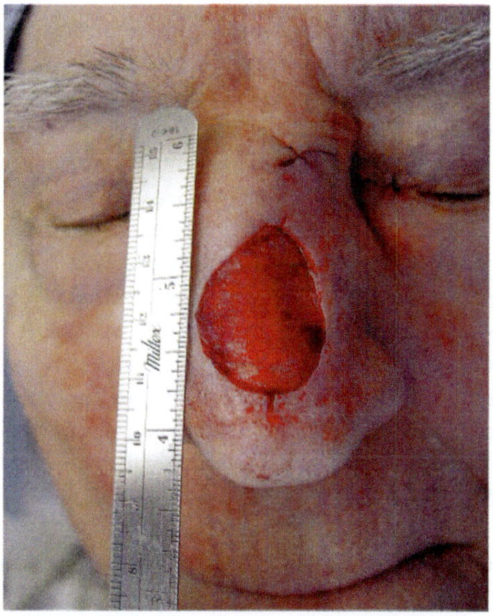

Figure 1 Anterior view of the nasal defect following Mohs micro-graphic surgery.

Resolution

This is an interesting case in that a large defect on the dorsal nose was created by tumor excision, resulting in a challenging reconstructive dilemma. Our patient was experienced with reconstructive options following Mohs micrographic surgery given his extensive history of facial skin cancers. His concern with the ultimate cosmetic outcome, coupled with his insistence on the ease of postoperative care and rapidity of healing, was the basis of the resolution of this reconstructive conundrum.

Perhaps the easiest option in this situation would be a full-thickness skin graft (FTSG). FTSGs are useful for larger skin defects, given their simplicity, good cosmetic outcome, and lack of distortion of adjacent structures. The disadvantages of full-thickness grafting include the need for a donor site offering enough similar quality of skin for coverage, the possibilities of poor graft take and

Reconstructive Conundrums in Dermatologic Surgery: The Nose, First Edition. Edited by Désirée Ratner, Joel L. Cohen and David G. Brodland.
© 2014 American Society for Dermatologic Surgery. Published 2014 by John Wiley & Sons, Ltd.

poor color and texture match at the recipient site, and the need for a bulky bolster dressing for at least a week. In addition, given the depth and size of the defect at hand, a FTSG from the pre- or postauricular region may have resulted in a large secondary defect, which may have been difficult to close.

Second-intention healing is a time-honored method of healing that is especially useful for older patients with loose skin. Granulation and epithelialization of defects are often expected in 6 to 12 weeks, and the cosmetic results are often excellent. The advantages of this technique lie in its simplicity and lack of need for further surgical procedures for reparative needs. The disadvantages include the length of time for complete healing and the need for prolonged daily wound care. In addition, the cosmetic outcome following contracture of tissue with large defects is difficult to predict. As such, wound healing on convex surfaces such as the nose may result in hypertrophic scarring in the vicinity of free tissue margins and suboptimal outcomes.

A forehead flap for repair of large defects of the dorsal nose is another option for postoperative reconstruction. Many different designs of this two-stage flap have been described, but the paramedian or midline flaps are most commonly used and often give the best overall results. The vascular supply to these flaps is excellent, with good flap viability. A second procedure 2 to 3 weeks later is necessary to divide the resulting pedicle, and additional procedures may be necessary to debulk the flap further. A secondary donor site on the forehead is created that may be closed primarily but usually results in a visible scar. Second-intention healing may be necessary for larger secondary forehead donor sites. The main advantage of this reconstructive option is the large amount of skin that the forehead provides and its good color and texture match for nasal skin. Precise and detailed explanation of postoperative wound care and large bandages that may be necessary to cover what the patient may perceive to be a disfiguring flap on the face must be understood prior to pedicle take-down by the patient and family.

Our experience with vertical linear closures for defects of the dorsal nose has been outstanding, and, as such, it has become our closure of choice for midline and paramedian dorsal nasal lesions. The long-term postoperative cosmetic results are so good that we have tried to incorporate this closure for larger defects in this anatomic location. Tension resulting from closing larger defects on the nasal dorsum may cause elevation of the nasal ala. Usually, this elevation is temporary, with improvement and resolution over the next few weeks. When there is a slight permanent residual raising of the ala, patients perceive an enhanced cosmetic look and an ease of breathing through the nostrils, which may help with snoring problems at night. Another result of the midline closure is thinning of the nasal tip, which results from the removal of the inferior dog-ear from this region. This has also been perceived by patients as a potential cosmetic benefit.

When repairing defects of the nasal dorsum, undermining of the lateral sides of the defect can be done at the subdermal level or above the cartilage and bone of the nasal sidewall. At this deep level, the undermining can be safely carried out onto the maxillary bone and cheek. This undermining provides a large amount of movement of skin medially. When using this wide undermining technique, even larger defects can be closed on the nasal dorsum. The vertical closure technique is thus more versatile for defects of larger sizes, which can be closed with excellent cosmetic results.

When a defect on the nasal dorsum is so large that an attempt to close primarily is unsuccessful, the superior or inferior dog-ear can be used as an FTSG to complete the closure. We initially tried to close this defect as a vertical linear closure but found that the superior dog-ear was needed as an FTSG to complete the closure. This technique is demonstrated in this case report.

In this case, the large defect following Mohs micrographic surgery could not be closed primarily despite wide lateral undermining (Figure 2). We chose to reconstruct this defect with a linear closure combined with a local Burow's (dog-ear) graft. A dog-ear was removed superiorly, and the resulting defect was closed in a linear side-to-side fashion using 5-0 subcutaneous buried poliglecaprone (Monocryl) sutures (Figure 3).

The Burow's (dog-ear) graft was then sutured centrally into the area of the defect that could not be closed primarily. To graft the dog-ear, 6-0 nylon (Ethilon) running sutures were used (Figure 4), and a bolster dressing was applied. The bolster dressing and sutures were removed after 1 week; the graft was pink, with 100% take (Figure 5).

Four-week follow-up results are shown in Figure 6. Elevation of the nasal ala is imperceptible, and the nasal passages are widely patent (Figure 7). The use of

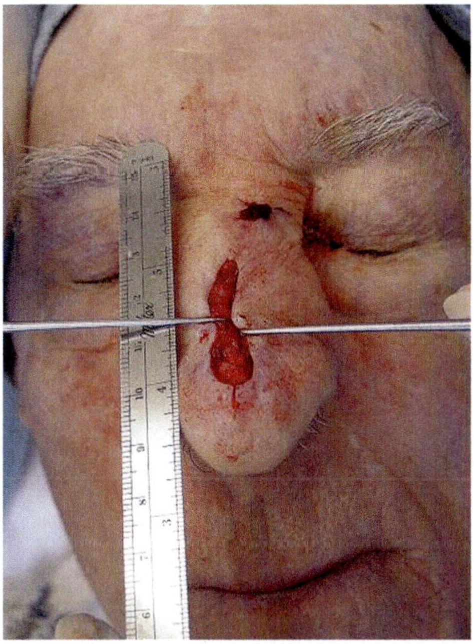

Figure 2 Anterior view showing inability to completely close the defect primarily.

local-tissue skin grafts from the nose allows for excellent cosmesis, with precise color and texture match. The patient was very pleased with the appearance of his nose and has not required further follow-up for scar revision.

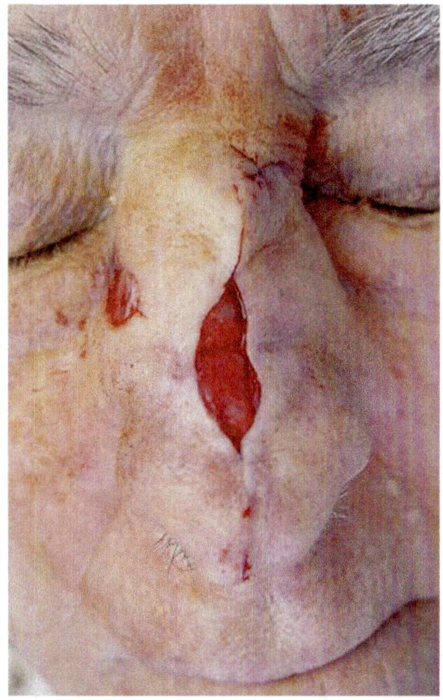

Figure 3 Removal of superior and inferior dog-ears prior to use as a full-thickness skin graft centrally.

Conundrum keys

- Large defects of the nose can be particularly challenging, but there are a vast number of reconstructive options for repair.

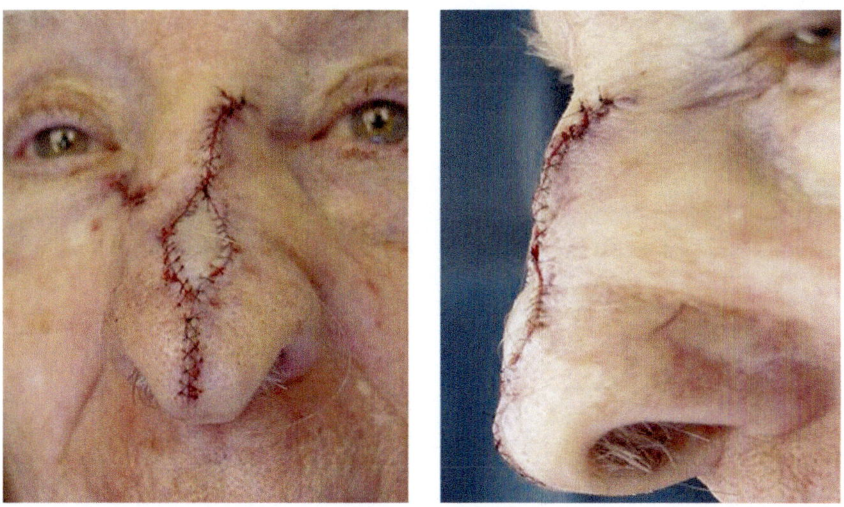

(a) (b)

Figure 4 Anterior (a) and lateral (b) views of combined linear closure with a Burow's graft centrally.

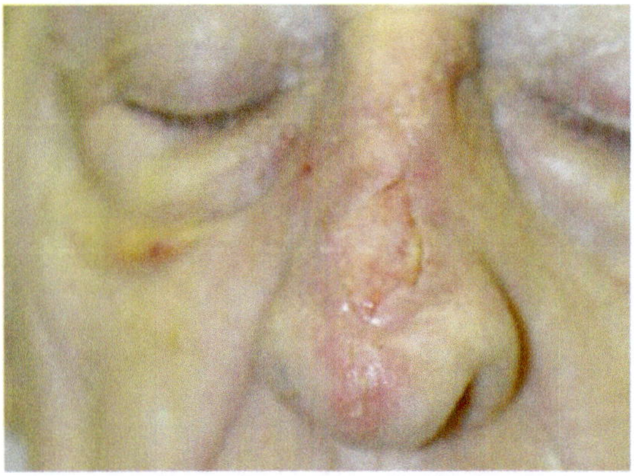

Figure 5 One-week follow-up.

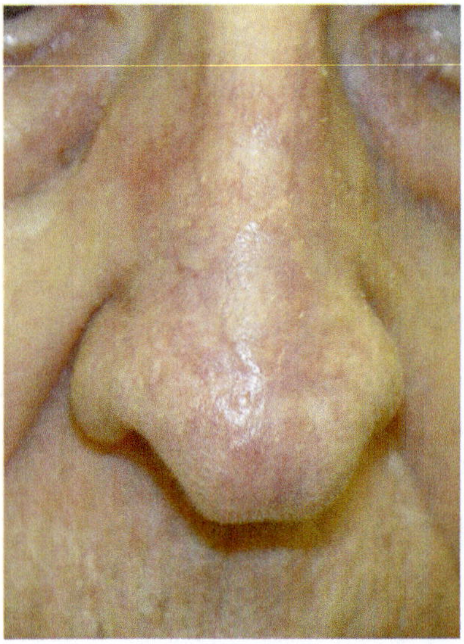

Figure 6 Four-week follow-up.

· When choosing a reconstructive option, both the patient and the surgeon must understand the pre- and

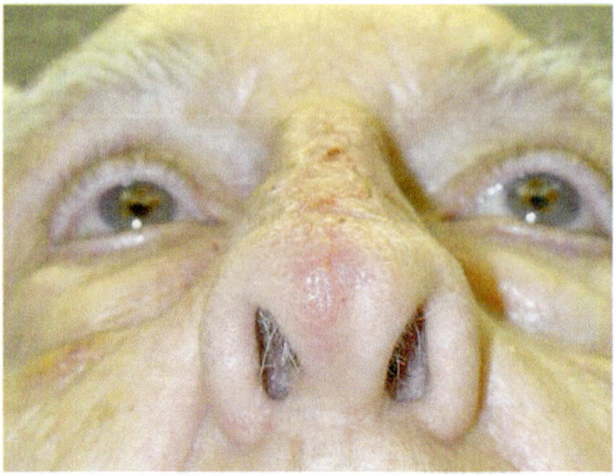

Figure 7 The nasal ala are widely patent, and elevation of the ala is imperceptible at 4 weeks.

postoperative implications, complications, and potential outcomes of a chosen reparative option.

· Linear closures, when feasible, are an outstanding option for dorsal nasal defects.

· For larger dorsal nasal defects that are not amenable to complete primary closure, local Burow's grafts provide superb color and texture match and facilitate an excellent cosmetic outcome.

Additional readings

Chester EC Jr. Closure of a surgical defect in a nose using island grafts from the nose. J Dermatol Surg Oncol 1982;8:790–1.

Chester EC Jr. The use of dog-ears as grafts. J Dermatol Surg Oncol 1981;7:956–9.

Cook J, Zitelli JA. Primary closure for mid-line defects of the nose: a simple approach for reconstruction. J Am Acad Dermatol 2000;43:508–10.

Kaufman AJ. Adjacent-tissue skin grafts for reconstruction. Dermatol Surg 2004;30:1350–3.

Zitelli JA. Burow's grafts. J Am Acad Dermatol 1987;17:271–9.

Commentary on conundrum 1

This case highlights several important principles in caring for patients with skin cancer. The first has to do with patients' involvement in choosing the reconstruction. As illustrated by the authors, there are a number of viable options for closure of this defect and early on, the authors imply that the patients were consulted regarding their goals and expectations for their repair. Every cutaneous surgeon has his or her own style. Some surgeons involve patients and allow them to play a significant part in determining which of several options they would prefer, while others make the decision independently. Neither extreme is ideal; soliciting the patient's participation is one facet of informed consent, and requires taking the time to assess patients' capacity to provide input and then clarifying their expectations. Some patients will gladly leave the entire decision process up to the surgeon, while others will give an opinion on how extensive a surgery they are willing to undergo and the level of cosmesis they require. This mutual participation process is invaluable in obtaining a reconstructive result that patients will find acceptable. However, it is surprising how often patients express a strong opinion on how involved a procedure they are willing to undergo, which may differ from the preconception of the surgeon. It would be advisable to have at least a preliminary conversation with patients regarding their goals and expectations.

The advantages and disadvantages of full-thickness skin graft closure are well known. The most common cause of a poor outcome with this method is the failure of continuous graft contact with the wound bed – which is usually avoidable – and if it occurs, will lead to an undesirable cosmetic result. It should be noted that in a case, such as this, in which the adjacent skin has been partially advanced, the depth of the wound base is often greater relative to the adjacent skin edges than it would have been otherwise. It is therefore even more important to assure graft contact with the wound base as there is a greater risk of unwanted lifting of these grafts from their recipient bed. Bolster dressings and basting sutures are effective ways to minimize this risk.

The second most common cause of partial graft failures is frictional trauma that avulses an area of the graft. Avulsion injury is most often seen when grafts are located on more prominent or projecting facial sites such as the nose and ears, but can occur in any location. This type of injury most frequently occurs within a month of the procedure. After the initial dressing has been removed, it is prudent to advise the patient to wear a protective, cushion-like bandage for about a month after the surgery to minimize the risk of this complication.

The authors' description of the advantages of linear closure on the nose, as described by Cook and Zitelli, is excellent. Critical to optimization of this technique is extensive undermining of the skin lateral to the defect. Deep-plane undermining just above the periosteum and cartilage is most effective on the nose. As described, undermining carried out beyond the nasal sidewall onto the cheek often affords a quantum increase in tissue movement. A previously unclosable wound can often achieve reapproximation merely by extending the plane of undermining onto the maxillary bone and cheek.

The authors also describe a "plan B" intraoperative decision. While it is always preferable to have a well-designed and workable plan preoperatively, the experienced surgeon realizes that having a backup plan, even one devised intraoperatively, can be invaluable.

As noted in Figure 3, the defect was reduced in size by 70%, which means that the majority of the wound was closed with perfectly matching adjacent skin. The concept of minimizing wound size when placement of a graft is contemplated is appropriate in most situations because minimizing graft size is generally desirable. However, when deciding upon the size of the graft to be harvested, the actual extent of the tissue loss, not the gaping wound, should be taken into consideration. The ideal scenario is to have the smallest possible graft filling the defect – with the graft stretched to its natural state of expansion. Assessing the true extent of tissue loss, which is usually less than the size of the defect due to the gaping phenomenon, is therefore critical because a correctly sized graft is esthetically superior to the one that is either oversized and redundant, or undersized and stretched to an unnatural degree.

In summary, on tight skin or in areas where tissue conservation needs to be at a premium, a Burow's graft combined with a partial closure can be an ideal solution. It is important to note, however, that Burow's grafting necessitates a high degree of confidence that tumor-free margins have been obtained. A wound resulting from Mohs surgery fosters the ideal scenario for use of such adjacent grafts. However, when a wound results from excisional removal with less meticulous tissue examination compared with the Mohs technique, the option of a Burow's graft should be considered much more cautiously, as unwittingly grafting tumor-containing skin into such a defect may result in a relatively rapid recurrence.

Commentary by Dr. Brodland

2

CONUNDRUM 2

Reconstruction of Two Nasal Defects Following Mohs Surgery

Alison O. Moon & Michael E. Lutz
Department of Dermatology, Mayo Clinic, Jacksonville, Florida

A 61-year-old woman had two defects involving the nose from Mohs micrographic surgery for basal cell carcinoma. The patient, an otherwise healthy non-smoker, was referred by her primary care physician for evaluation of a possible recurrent basal cell carcinoma of the nasal dorsum. On examination, a 5 mm × 7 mm area of hyperkeratotic erythema was observed. In addition, a 2 mm × 3 mm firm white papule was found on the right nasal ala, which the patient stated was new. Histologically both lesions were basal cell carcinoma.

After Mohs surgery the nasal dorsum defect was 1.0 cm in diameter and the nasal ala defect was 1.2 cm × 1.0 cm (Figure 1). How would you manage these wounds?

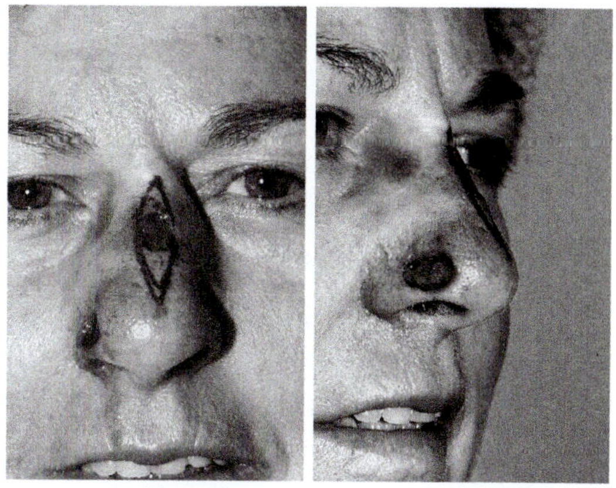

(a) (b)

Figure 1 a) Defect on the nasal dorsum after excision. b) Defect on the nasal ala after excision.

Resolution

There are several reconstructive options in this scenario. In our case, a primary closure of the midline defect of the nasal dorsum was designed with the additional intention to use the inferior Burow's triangle as a full-thickness skin graft for the alar defect. Although primary closure for nasal dorsum defects has not classically been considered an ideal option, this approach has been refined to yield predictable cosmetic results. In keeping with the technique advocated by Cook and Zitelli,[1] the standard 3:1 length/width ellipse design was extended to preserve the nasal profile. In our case, the inferior Burow's triangle was extended farther than the superior triangle to provide sufficient graft tissue. With meticulous trimming, defatting, and contouring to fit the graft bed dimensions, the donor skin reproduced the normal external contour of the ala. This tissue was an ideal donor site for the nasal ala for color, sebaceous texture, and thickness (Figure 2).

Because the patient was a nonsmoker and in good health, she was considered an acceptable candidate for a full-thickness graft. The long-term results were cosmetically pleasing, with minimal discordance between the graft and surrounding skin (Figure 3). There was no distortion of the nasal profile.

Reconstructive Conundrums in Dermatologic Surgery: The Nose, First Edition. Edited by Désirée Ratner, Joel L. Cohen and David G. Brodland.
© 2014 American Society for Dermatologic Surgery. Published 2014 by John Wiley & Sons, Ltd.

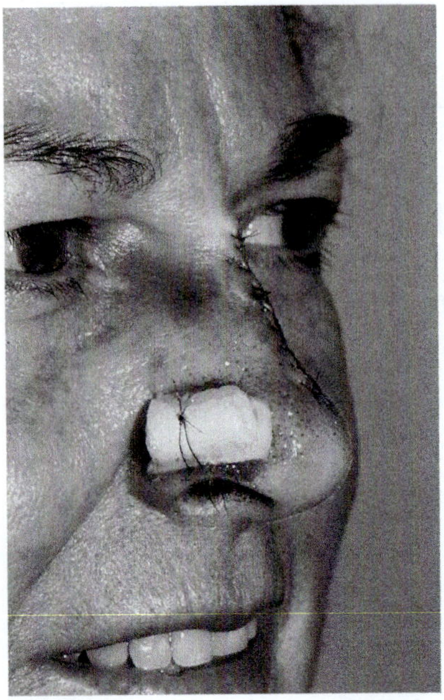

Figure 2 Immediately after reconstruction.

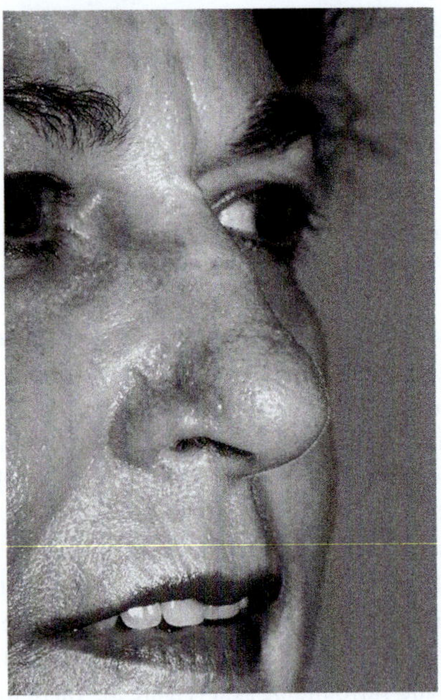

Figure 3 Two months after reconstruction.

Other options for reconstructing the nasal ala include a nasolabial transposition flap or a bilobed transposition flap; however, these often distort or ablate the alar groove. An alternative reconstructive approach is the nasolabial interpolation flap; however, this is a staged procedure and can be cumbersome for the patient postoperatively. In addition, more cosmetic units are involved with these methods. In repairing the nasal ala, allowing the wound to heal by second intention results in a poor texture match as well as wound contraction that may distort the free margin of the alar rim. Also, the resulting scar contracture may lead to nasal valve malfunction because of elevation of the alar margin. This causes the alar and lateral cartilages to move inward, thereby rendering the nasal valve immobile. This may also be a consideration for the other flap reconstruction options.

When evaluating various reconstruction options, alteration of sensation should be considered. Although the recovery of sensory innervation occurs earlier with flaps than with grafts, sensation of the nasal ala is less critical than for other facial sites.

Conundrum keys

- If there is more than one defect on the nose, including the nasal ala and dorsum, consider primary closure of the dorsal defect using a Burow's triangle as a full-thickness donor site. There is no better match for the ala than this nearby skin.
- Tailor the size of the Burow's triangle to accommodate the recipient site.
- Keep the number of involved cosmetic units to a minimum.

Reference

1 Cook JL, Zitelli JA. Primary closure for midline defects of the nose: a simple approach for reconstruction. J Am Acad Dermatol 2000; 43:508-10.

Commentary

Drs. Moon and Lutz present a technique of reconstruction for multiple defects that is virtuous in not only the excellent results it provides but also in its efficient use of tissue and hence tissue conservation. The side-to-side closure of the defect on the mid-line nasal dorsum is a simple, reliable, and reproducible reconstructive technique recently advocated by Cook and Zitelli. The use of a Burow's triangle as a graft for reconstruction of another defect has several important implications. First, the surgeons must be as certain as possible that the graft skin does not contain either residual tumor or additional primary skin cancers. The former is assured by microscopic margin control as accomplished by the authors with the use of the Mohs micrographic surgical technique. Careful inspection preoperatively of the prospective graft skin is the best way to ensure the absence of second primary tumors being transferred into the other defect. Studies performed 30–40 years ago on the transplantability of basal cell carcinoma indicate that it is not transplantable. I believe, based on anecdotal experience, that BCC can be transplanted within a full-thickness skin graft provided the tumor is a small percentage of the total graft. Squamous cell carcinoma is thought to be transplantable based on experimental models.

DAVID BRODLAND, MD *Clairton, Pennsylvania*

Commentary on conundrum 2

When approaching nasal reconstruction, it is important to remember that no two noses are exactly alike and that each patient's nasal skin must be evaluated individually. Some patients have thin, delicate skin over the upper two-thirds of the nose, with thicker, more sebaceous skin over the tip and ala, while other patients have a more uniformly sebaceous nose. There are times when linear closure can be an excellent option for closure of a dorsal nasal defect, and one or both of the Burow's triangles can be used for repair of a second nasal defect, as in this case. It is also possible that a Burow's triangle taken from the nasal dorsum would not be an optimal tissue match, in which case it becomes worthwhile to consider other options for repair of the alar defect, including transposition flaps from the adjacent cheek or nasal skin. Depending on the patient's dorsal nasal laxity, a linear closure like the one shown here could also affect sidewall laxity, such that a contemporaneous alar flap repair would need to be very carefully planned. Such a flap would likely be inferolaterally based so as to utilize the laxity of the lateral nasal sidewall and medial cheek, without requiring secondary movement from the nasal dorsum.

Although alar defects do not always require a cartilage graft for rim stabilization, if the defect is deep or if functional preservation of the nasal valve is a concern, a cartilage graft needs to be considered as well. In fact, the 2-month view shown here (Figure 3) reveals a slight retraction of the alar rim, suggesting that contraction had already begun to take place. A cartilage strut placed along the inferior alar margin would have bolstered the alar rim against these forces of contraction, thereby helping to prevent alar retraction. When evaluating alar defects, either individually or in the context of a second nearby defect, it is therefore essential to take this possibility into consideration as such a complication can often be avoided. When minimal retraction is present at 1–2 months, cosmesis can often be salvaged by an intensive 2–3 months of graft site massage. Aggressive massage by the patient for a suggested 30 seconds 10 times a day can help to reverse the retraction. Of course, intralesional steroids may be helpful as well, which may be injected as early as several weeks after the procedure and repeated at 2- to 4-week intervals, usually with rapid resolution of the unwanted scar tissue.

Commentary by Dr. Ratner

3

CONUNDRUM 3

Repair of Adjacent Nasal Defects with One Double-Rotation Flap Closure

Joseph P. Janik[1], *Joanna Lee Harp*[2], *& Ida Orengo*[1]

[1]Department of Dermatology, Baylor College of Medicine, Houston, Texas
[2]Medical Student, Baylor College of Medicine, Houston, Texas

A patient underwent Mohs micrographic surgery for the removal of adjacent nasal skin carcinomas. The patient was an 82-year-old male with a basal cell carcinoma removed from the right dorsum of his nose (Figure 1) and a second from the left nasal sidewall and ala (Figure 2). The surgery resulted in defects measuring 1.5 × 1.5 and 2.4 × 1.4 cm respectively, leaving cartilage exposed bilaterally. What is the most appropriate reconstructive technique for these surgical defects?

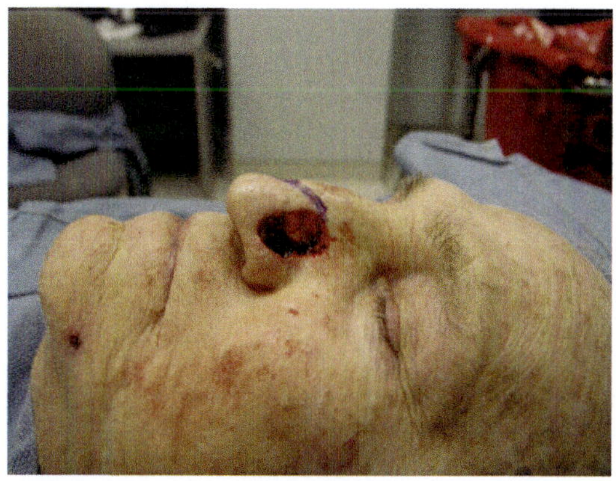

Figure 2 Defect on left nasal sidewall and ala.

Resolution

In this case, the size of the defects, their close proximity to one another, and their location on either side of the nose created a unique reconstructive challenge, especially considering the complex contour of the nose as well as its varying skin properties. Based on the size and location of the defects, and the risk of postoperative hemorrhage, infection, and deformity from scarring, we decided that closure of the adjacent defects was necessary. We chose the method of closure after considering these factors as well as the patient's wishes and general medical condition.

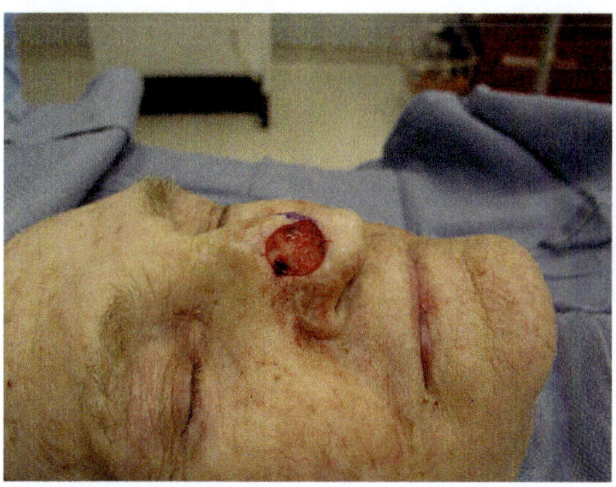

Figure 1 Defect on right dorsum of nose.

There is a step-by-step process that all cutaneous surgeons must go through to decide how best to close a defect. This process can be considered the art of reconstructive repair. A simple option for all repairs is to allow healing by secondary intention, which is best to use on concave surfaces. Unfortunately, this was not a feasible

Reconstructive Conundrums in Dermatologic Surgery: The Nose, First Edition. Edited by Désirée Ratner, Joel L. Cohen and David G. Brodland.
© 2014 American Society for Dermatologic Surgery. Published 2014 by John Wiley & Sons, Ltd.

option for our case given the convexity and sebaceous content of the nasal areas involved. Additionally, the proximity of the defects and the nature of the underlying structures made scar contracture with subsequent bilateral alar flare and collapse of the nasal passages a likely outcome in this case if left to heal secondarily.

Another option that cutaneous surgeons must always consider is primary closure with either vertical or horizontal side-to-side movement; however, this method was also not appropriate for our patient. In this case, there were two moderately sized defects in close proximity to one other, which significantly limited tissue availability in the area. Closure using this technique would have placed excessive tension on the wound and would have caused distortion of the nose leading to permanent deformity and probable dehiscence.

Full-thickness skin grafting was the first feasible reconstructive option that we considered. However, our optimism for its success was dismal given the size and depth of the defects; the exposed cartilage at the base of both lesions, which would not contribute to the revascularization process; and the patient's limited healing capacity due to multiple other medical problems. Despite these issues, the patient was still given the option of grafting. He and his family declined, stating that they did not want him to undergo additional procedures given his frail condition and other pending health issues. With his refusal for further surgery at a site away from the nose, this not only restricted grafting as an option, but also limited other aggressive closure techniques such as paramedian forehead flaps, bilateral cheek-to-nose transpositions, or interpolation flaps.

Limited by our patient's request for a simple local closure and taking into account his comorbidities, the conundrum began. How do you close two adjacent defects on the nose with limited tissue using a local flap? Flaps use adjacent tissue to fill in defects allowing optimal skin texture and color match. In a rotation flap, the skin adjacent to the defect is partially incised, undermined, and then rotated around a pivot point to fill in the defect. Rotation flaps are beneficial in areas where tissue is limited because they allow for the redistribution of tension along the entire flap to help decrease the risk of wound dehiscence and provide a better cosmetic result. In this case, the two defects on opposite sides of the nose required a double-rotation flap technique. An incision was made diagonally in the tissue connecting the two defects (Figure 3). Next, the appropriate tissue

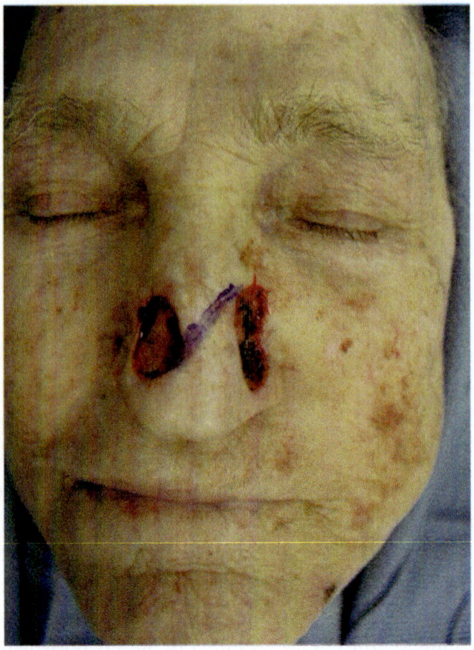

Figure 3 Both nasal defects shown. Blue line represents where the diagonal incision will be made connecting the two defects. Note the long length of the nose from the glabella to the distal tip and how the nasal tip droops down.

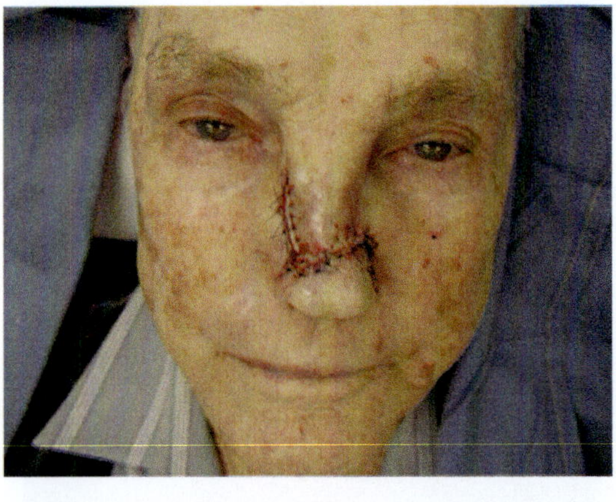

Figure 4 Final closure. The length of the nose from the glabella to the distal tip is shorter and the tip of the nose has been raised compared to Figure 3.

was undermined just superior to the cartilaginous plane, and the two curvilinear flaps were rotated in opposite directions to fill in the two defects as one closure with equal distribution of tension vectors and tissue (Figure 4). The defect was closed using interrupted 5-0 synthetic, absorbable poliglecaprone 25 sutures deep and vertical

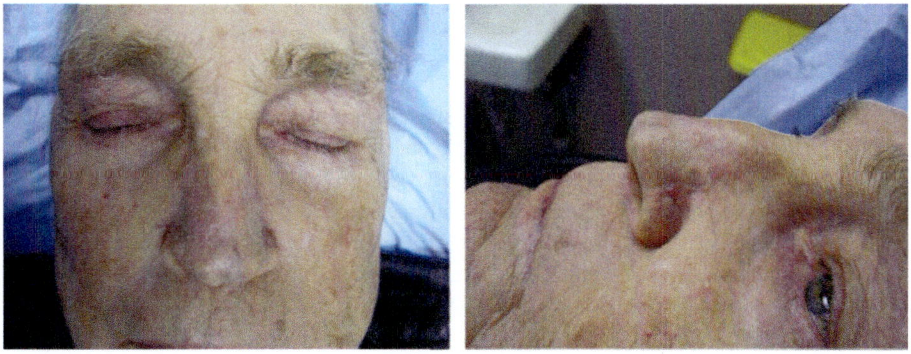

Figure 5 Two month follow-up. The overall size of the nose has been decreased, and the nasal tip has been elevated giving a more youthful appearance.

mattress 6-0 synthetic, nonabsorbable nylon sutures superficially for optimal eversion. Although the length of the nose was shortened when measuring from the glabella to the distal tip, the overall architecture of the nose was well preserved (Figure 5). In fact, over time, the nasal tip tends to droop in the elderly and raising it slightly can be of benefit. The use of a double-rotation flap in this case allowed the basal cell carcinomas to be removed and the defects closed with a single surgery and within one surgical area, minimizing operative and recovery time as well as postoperative management. The patient was extremely pleased with his cosmetic result and has had no complications.

Conundrum keys

Always take into account the comorbidities and wishes of your patients. These factors will limit closure options.

- When two defects are in close proximity to one another, connecting them can allow for a single closure and easier postoperative care for the patient.
- Making a diagonal incision that connects two similarly sized defects on opposite sides of the nose can create bilateral mirror-image rotation flaps, which allow for redistribution of shared tissue as well as tension vectors, thus leading to conservation of overall nasal architecture.

Commentary on conundrum 3

The conundrum in this case lies in the fact that there are two defects in close proximity to one another. This is a scenario that may be seen not only on the nose but also nearly anywhere on the head and neck. Each defect individually is challenging enough but when located within a centimeter or two of one another on the same anatomic structure, the real issue becomes the magnitude of each repair and the need to be as efficient as possible with the available skin. The beauty of this particular closure is that the surgeons astutely realized that each repair could be done synergistically with the other, thereby maximizing tissue efficiency and capitalizing on the adjacency of these two defects.

Although the title of this conundrum is "double-rotation flap closure," the reports in the literature with flaps of this name actually refer to two rotation flaps being performed on opposite sides of a large defect to close it. The surgical technique presented here is commonly used in my practice and is termed a "complimentary Burow's advancement flap." The semantic argument as to whether these are rotation flaps or advancement flaps has to do with whether the flaps are developed using a curvilinear line or a straight line. In Figure 3.1, it is evident that the tangent extending between the two defects is more of a straight-line. In fact, if one considers what a true rotation flap is, the creation of two arcs moving in opposite directions is, in practice, not possible. I therefore view these flaps mechanistically as the use of a single-tangential incision made from the inferior margin of one defect to the superior margin of the second defect. The descriptive name for a Burow's flap is "single-tangent advancement flap."

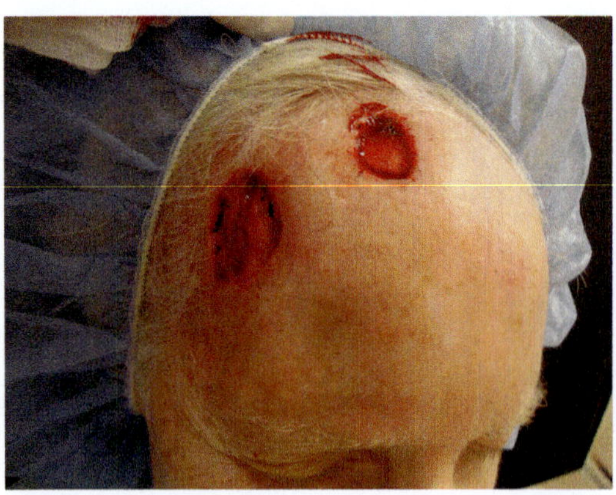

Figure 3.1 Mohs surgical defects of the right upper forehead and central upper forehead at hairline.

Complimentary single-tangent advancement flaps, or Burow's flaps, are synergistic and tissue conservative in that each flap uses the other flap's defect as the displaced Burow's triangle that would normally be removed to correct for skin edges of unequal length created by the advancement. In other words, the complimentary advancement flap "saves" two Burow's triangles, which would have been removed had each individual defect been closed independently. Although it is not well seen on the defect of the left nose, Burow's triangles have been removed at the rotation points of the flaps, as they would be when performing a Burow's flap anywhere else.

It appears that the Burow's triangle was minimized on the patient's left because it would have impinged upon the free margin of the left alar rim. Because these are large defects and the closure design does put the free margin at some risk for distortion, an interesting question arises. "Can this closure be performed on similar defects on any patient's nose?" The answer is absolutely not. The authors correctly describe the process of deciding how best to close a defect as the art of reconstructive repair. Truer words could never have been said. If reconstruction is considered an art, the reconstructive surgeon must realize that, in contrast to most other artists, we do not get to choose our canvas or our materials. We must instead work within the constraints of the canvas and achieve artistry while taking these constraints into consideration to maintain both function and form.

A quick calculation would suggest that in this case, over 20% of the entire nasal surface is missing after cancer removal. Obviously, the canvas in this case allowed for the redistribution of the nasal skin in an esthetic and functional manner. The tissue conservation of the flap was critical to its success. Its success was also undoubtedly due to mobilization of the majority of the nasal and medial cheek skin. The authors note that the length of the nose was shortened but that, because the patient had some preexisting nasal ptosis, this was an acceptable esthetic change. It is also fortunate that the patient's nose was not particularly petite. A smaller nose with a narrower tip and less laxity of the nasal dorsum could not have tolerated the tissue movement required by this closure.

The authors discuss other alternatives that they considered including second-intention healing because of the fact that the defects involved concave surfaces of the nose. As clarified by Zitelli, the best places to consider second-intention healing are on concave surfaces such as the medial canthus, the alar crease, and the concave region between the base of the ala and the melolabial fold.[1] The size and the depth of these defects are the most obvious mitigating factors in second-intention wound healing.

The authors also considered side-to-side closure of these defects and correctly point out that because of their close proximity to one another, excessive tension would have caused nasal distortion. Use of the complimentary advancement flaps, however, cleverly distributed exactly one half of the tension of each closure to each side of the nose, which accounts for the minimization of distortion.

Full-thickness skin grafting is always a consideration and obviates the problem of inadequate tissue mobility or tissue reservoirs to close a given defect. In essence, the surgeon imports skin from elsewhere to replace what was lost and avoids any tension-induced distortion of the surrounding tissues. The reasons given for not performing skin grafting in this case have to do with the fact that the patient and his family were not willing to undergo "additional procedures" because of his frail health condition. Presumably, the additional procedures refer to donor-site surgery, which is always one of the disadvantages of grafting as it creates another wound elsewhere. Similar reasons were given for not proceeding with other options including the paramedian forehead flap, cheek interpolation flap, and the nasolabial transposition flap. In the end, a single-stage procedure was best for this patient's situation.

It is appropriate to take a moment to emphasize the often overlooked factor that should be considered in most reconstructions. The opinion of the patient and his or her family, taken together with their current medical problems and social issues, can mean the difference between a successful surgery and happy patient. It is obvious that the surgeons discussed the options available to them with this patient and his family and allowed them to participate in the decision-making process.

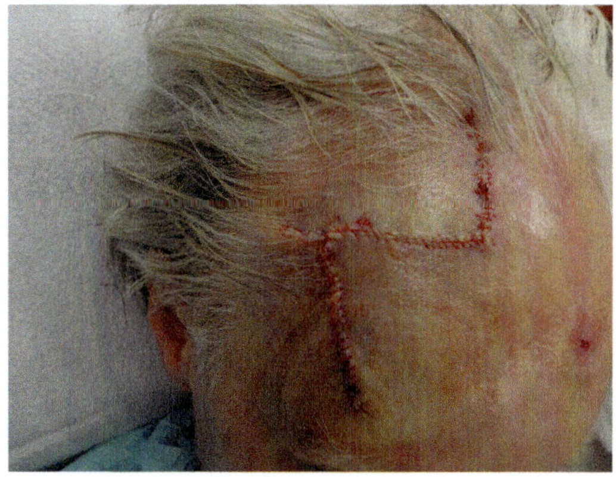

Figure 3.2 Complimentary Burow's advancement flaps sewn into place.

Shown here is another case of a complimentary Burow's advancement flap, or complimentary single-tangent advancement flap (Figures 3.1 and 3.2). Here again, there was synergy in performing a two-flap closure without doing much more surgery than if a single flap had been used for either defect. The synergy manifests itself in the saving of two Burow's triangles, and was advantageous to the patient in that this closure was less involved than it could have been, was under less tension, and therefore had a greater chance of success.

Commentary by Dr. Brodland

Reference

1 Zitelli JA. Wound healing by secondary intention: a cosmetic appraisal. J Am Acad Dermatol 1983;9(3):407–15.

4

CONUNDRUM 4

Contralateral Nasolabial Flap for a Large Nasal Defect

Pedro Ponte[1], *João Goulão*[2], *& José Rosa De Almeida*[3]
[1]Department of Dermatology, Centro Hospitalar de Lisboa Central, Lisbon, Portugal
[2]Department of Dermatology, Hospital Garcia de Orta, Lisbon, Portugal
[3]Department of Plastic Surgery, Instituto Português de Oncologia Francisco Gentil, Lisbon, Portugal

A 78-year-old woman was referred with a multicentric basal cell carcinoma (BCC) on the dorsum of the nose and a nodular BCC on the left nasolabial groove (Figure 1). The 5-mm-margin excision performed resulted in a defect that involved the whole nasal dorsum, nasal walls, tip, and left ala, with exposure of the cartilage and extended to the left nasolabial area (Figure 2). How would you manage this wound?

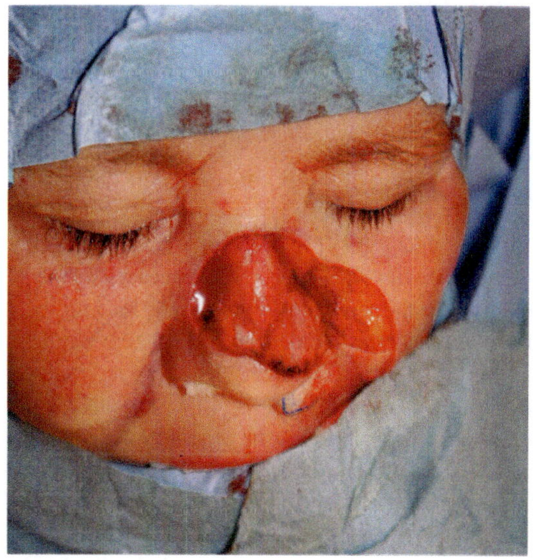

Figure 2 Surgical defect.

Resolution

Reconstruction of nasal defects presents a challenging problem for the surgeon, mainly because of the complexity of the nasal surface lines and the diversity of the color, texture, and appearance of its lining skin. The limited availability of mobile, adjacent skin increases the difficulty of the repair. Defects of nasal cover after cancer-ablative procedures have been treated with numerous reconstructive modalities, including free skin grafting and local flaps. Each technique differs according to the depth and size of the defect, the quality and availability of the donor site, and the skills of the surgeon.

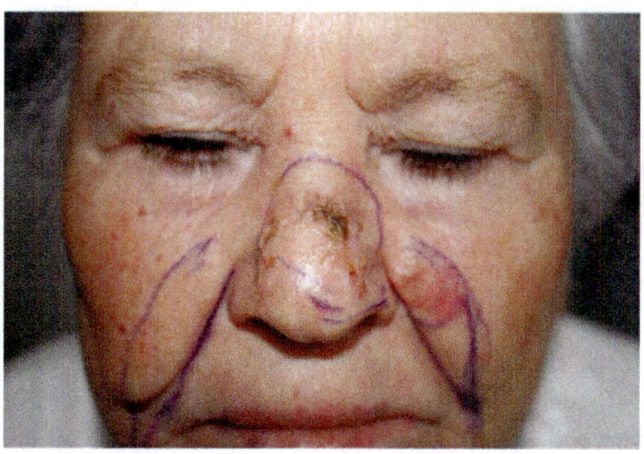

Figure 1 Basal cell carcinomas and surgical planning.

Reconstructive Conundrums in Dermatologic Surgery: The Nose, First Edition. Edited by Désirée Ratner, Joel L. Cohen and David G. Brodland.
© 2014 American Society for Dermatologic Surgery. Published 2014 by John Wiley & Sons, Ltd.

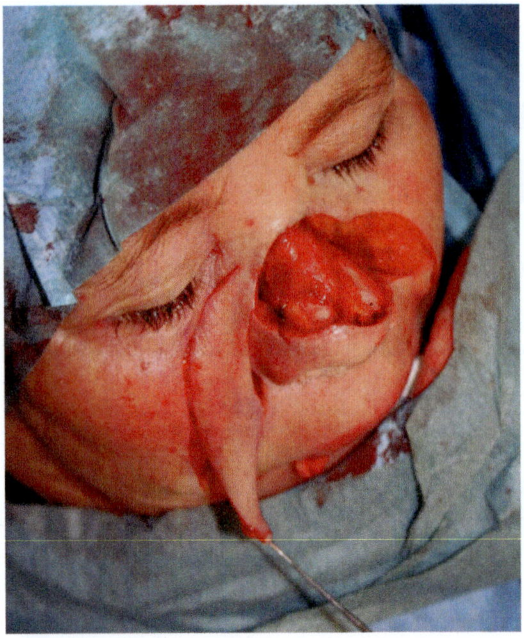

Figure 3 Isolation of the flap.

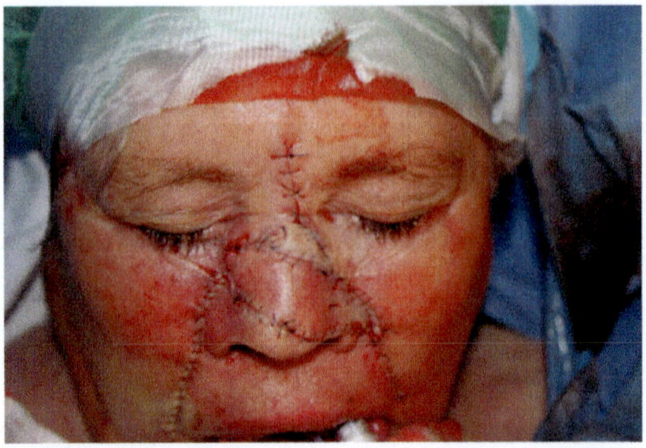

Figure 4 Closing of the defects.

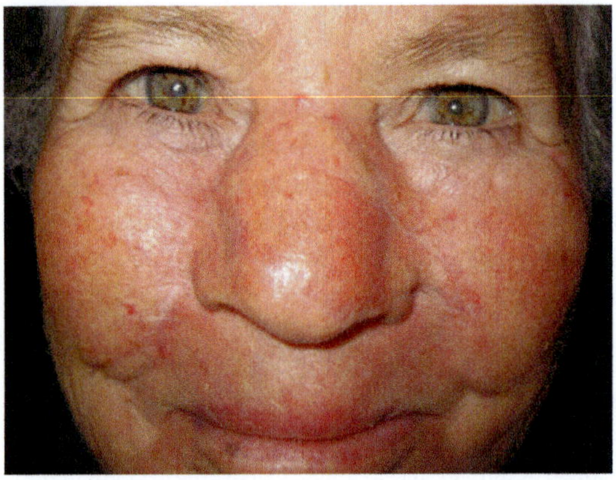

Figure 5 1-year follow-up.

The nasolabial flap (NLF) is one of the most versatile and robust flaps for facial defects.[1] It has been widely used for defects on the cheek, nose, lower eyelid, and lip.[2] In this case, because the traditional ipsilateral NLF was not available for reconstruction of the defect, we resorted to the contralateral region.

After adequate hemostasis, the superiorly based right NLF was created (Figure 3). The inferior border of the flap was the right nasolabial crease. The flap was shaped roughly like a banana, with a maximum width of 1.5 cm. The flap was incised through the skin, with the distal end elevated in the subcutaneous plane above the facial musculature. The pedicle was 0.5 cm wide and was located between the defect and the lower eyelid.

The adjacent tissues of the right cheek were undermined for closure of the donor site in the nasolabial fold. The flap was elevated, defatted, and transposed into the nasal defect over the remaining right alar skin. The lower border of the flap was then sutured to the lower border of the nose defect. The left nasolabial fold was closed primarily, which reduced the nasal defect dimensions. Because the skin flap was not wide enough to close the upper one-third of the nasal defect without the risk of causing left lower eyelid ectropion, a minor vertical glabellar flap was made to fill in the defect (Figure 4).

There were no postoperative complications. No scar or flap revision was needed. The final nasal contour, symmetry, and function were still good when the patient was seen 1 year after surgery, even though a certain degree of trapdoor effect was evident (Figure 5). No tumor recurrences were detected during follow-up.

The NLF is a choice flap for nasal defects because it provides local skin with an exact color, thickness, and contour match for the nasal skin. The unique features of vascularization in this area make the NLF a safe flap in facial reconstruction. It is mostly supplied by the facial artery, which, in the majority of cases (70.5%), ends up at the angular artery or at the nasal ala.[3] The angular artery itself usually has anastomoses to the external nasal, dorsal nasal, supratrochlear, or ophthalmic arteries. Because the pedicle of our flap was so close to this anastomosis bundle, it is safe to say it is based on these vessels.

However, one must not disregard that there is no single axial vessel in the skin of this area because the facial and angular arteries lie at a deeper level, passing through levator labii superioris.[4] Moreover, as has been previously demonstrated,[5] a rich pattern of vascularization from the facial and infraorbital arteries consisting of small, densely populated musculocutaneous perforating arteries supply the anterior face. This pattern allows the surgeon to safely make axial flaps along the vascular axis between the medial canthus and the submental area. One can thus obtain flaps with a length-to-width ratio greater than 5:1, clearly superior to the 2:1 or 3:1 length-to-width ratio of random-pattern skin flaps. Therefore, we consider this to be a variation of an axial flap. We believe, as Herbert has suggested before,[4] that the nasolabial flap can have its pedicle reduced to 0.5 cm without endangering the blood supply.

The advantages of using the NLF also include the simplicity and time saving that the procedure provides, in addition to minor donor site morbidity and the possibility of use in a wide variety of situations. Some of its limitations are the width of the flap and the somewhat limited arc of rotation.[6] Execution of the flap can render the loss of the nasal cheek junction and minor donor site morbidity (dog ear). Surgical revision of these effects is sometimes needed and can provide adequate aesthetic results, even though this flap is usually a single-stage procedure. As with any other flap, the number of procedures required to reach the final results, complications, donor site morbidity, and the contraction and degree of color match usually affect the cosmetic outcome of reconstruction.[7]

Conventionally pedicled NLF applications can range from intraoral reconstruction of the palate to small local repairs of the nasal wall.[8] The superiorly based NLF is best suited to lateral nasal reconstructions and occasionally to covering midline wounds of the nasal dorsum and supratip areas.[9] We believe that NLF surpasses these indications and that it can be used in an even wider range of applications.

Contralateral NLF has been previously reported for medial canthus reconstruction[10] and nostril defects,[11] in which additional complications of the trapdoor effect and possible collapse of the nasal ala may occur.

Our case provides some evidence that contralateral NLF can be used in medium to large nasal defects, even with a narrow-width pedicle. It illustrates that it is a safe, reliable, and cosmetically acceptable option to consider in repairing defects for large nasal lesions extending to the cheek, particularly ones that preclude the use of a flap from the ipsilateral nasolabial fold.

Conundrum keys

- Contralateral NLF can be used in the reconstruction of medium to large nasal defects when the use of the ipsilateral nasolabial fold is compromised.
- NLF can have its pedicle reduced to 0.5 cm without endangering the blood supply.

References

1 Zitelli JA. The nasolabial flap as a single-stage procedure. Arch Dermatol 1990;126:1445–8.
2 Schmidt BL, Dierks EJ. The nasolabial flap. Oral Maxillofac Surg Clin North Am 2003;15:487–95.
3 Brüe E, Bey E, Cariou JL. Facial artery. Embryological review, descriptive and functional anatomy based on a review of the literature. Ann Chir Plast Esthet 2000;45:461–84.
4 Herbert DC. A subcutaneous pedicled cheek flap for reconstruction of alar defects. Br J Plast Surg 1978;31:79–92.
5 Whetzel TP, Mathes SJ. Arterial anatomy of the face: an analysis of vascular territories and perforating cutaneous vessels. Plast Reconstr Surg 1992;89:591–603.
6 El-Marakby HH. The versatile naso-labial flaps in facial reconstruction. J Egypt Natl Canc Inst 2005;17:245–50.
7 Menick FJ. Defects of the nose, lip, and cheek: rebuilding the composite defect. Plast Reconstr Surg 2007;120:887–98.
8 Morgan RF, Chambers RG, Jaques DA, Hoopes JE. Nasolabial flap in intraoral reconstruction. Review of 55 cases. Am J Surg 1981;142:448–50.
9 Rohrich RJ, Conrad MH. The superiorly based nasolabial flap for simultaneous alar and cheek reconstruction. Plast Reconstr Surg 2001;108:1727–30.
10 Santos OA, Pappas JC. Repair of nostril defect with a contralateral nasolabial flap. Plast Reconstr Surg 1976;57:704–6.
11 Le-Quang C. Reversed vascular full-thickness nasolabial flap. Ann Chir Plast Esthet 1994;38:273–8.

Commentary on conundrum 4

This is a complex defect involving multiple nasal subunits as well as the left medial cheek. The novel repair described in this case provides a complex yet successful option for reconstruction. The author does not review alternative options to repair this type of defect, however, and there are certainly other options that could be considered.

A more conventional approach would entail treating the nasal and cheek defects separately. An inferiorly based sliding cheek advancement flap[1] with periosteal suspension sutures could repair the cheek component and at the same time recapitulate the alar groove. With the cheek advancement flap, placement of these suspension sutures at the level of the periosteum is key to avoid blunting the lateral alar groove (which is seen in Figure 5 along with the trapdoor effect that they describe) as well as to avoid visible "pulling" on the flap. Placement of long-lasting absorbable anchoring sutures to the inferior bony orbital rim would also be advisable to prevent lower eyelid ectropion.

After closure of the cheek defect, either a paramedian forehead flap or even a full-thickness skin graft could be employed to close the large nasal defect. A graft would most likely need to be harvested from the supraclavicular fossa or upper inner arm skin to ensure a sufficient amount of skin for defect coverage. Although a graft would provide a simple, straightforward solution to close this defect, it would likely fail to restore the volume lost after tumor resection. Delaying the graft until a few weeks later to fill in some of the depth of the defect might have made more sense. Depending on the patient's comorbidities and the ability to tolerate a two-staged procedure, a paramedian forehead flap could provide coverage of the entire nasal defect and importantly restore this lost volume.[2] Removal of the remainder of the distal nasal skin at the right nasal tip would help to camouflage the surgical scars within cosmetic subunit boundaries. Had this defect consisted solely of the nasal component shown in this example, bilateral superiorly based one-stage nasolabial flaps sewn together could have been employed to provide sufficient volume replacement for the depth of the defect while resurfacing it in its entirety.[3]

Commentary by Dr. Cohen

References

1 Hussain W, Tan E, Salmon P. Inferiorly based crescentic "sliding" cheek flaps for the reconstruction of paranasal surgical defects. Dermatol Surg 2012;38:249–55.

2 Baker S. Chapter 18: Reconstruction of the nose. In: Local flaps in reconstruction, 2nd Edition. St Louis: Mosby, 2007: p. 468–9.

3 Baker S, Swanson N. Chapter 12: Melolabial flaps. In: Local flaps in facial reconstruction, 1st Edition. St Louis: Mosby, 1995: p. 188.

PART II
Nasal Sidewall

5

CONUNDRUM 5

Dual Nasal Sidewall and Lip Defects Combined into a Single Arcuate Advancement Flap

David J. Kouba[1], Ronald L. Moy[2], & Edgar F. Fincher[2]

[1]Department of Dermatology, Henry Ford Health System, Detroit, MI

[2]David Geffen School of Medicine, University of California, Los Angeles, CA

A 67-year-old Caucasian male presented with a 6-month history of enlarging, pearly plaques of the distal nasal sidewall and upper medial lip. Past medical history was significant for transient ischemic attacks and numerous nonmelanoma skin cancers. Medications included warfarin, but not aspirin. Biopsy had confirmed the diagnosis of basal cell carcinoma at both locations. The tumors were removed under local anesthesia using the Mohs micrographic technique in two (nose) and three (lip) stages, yielding the two defects shown in Figure 1. The nasal sidewall defect was 0.9 cm and the upper lip defect was semicircular with greatest diameter of 1.3 cm. How would you repair these two defects?

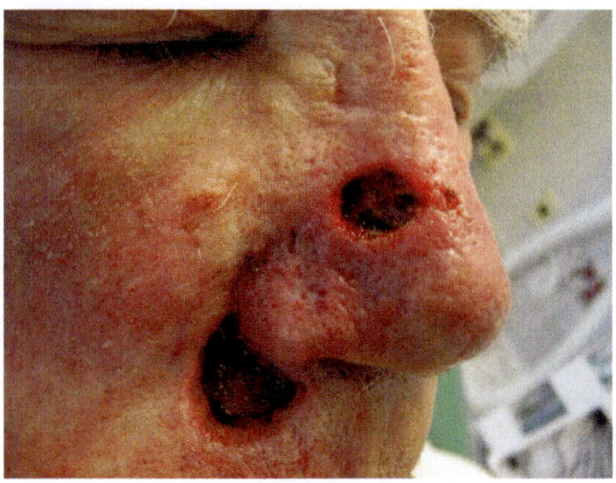

Figure 1 The nose and lip tumors were cleared by Mohs micrographic surgery in two and three stages respectively, resulting in two separate defects.

Nature of the conundrum

The absence of tissue laxity and the nonbony platform of the distal nose often precludes primary closure of distal nasal sidewall defects. To do so can result in pulling and elevation of the alar rim. Therefore, these defects often require adjacent tissue transfer for closure. Traditional approaches used to repair these defects frequently involve transposition flaps such as the bilobed transposition flap as described by Zitelli.[1] Alternatively, a laterally based rhombic transposition with the standing cone taken superiorly, pointing toward the glabella can be used. Other options for closure of these defects include tissue rotation, such as the dorsal–nasal (Rieger) flap.[2] For defects less than 1 cm, an angled advancement flap would suffice. Here, one cone of the advancement is angled up toward the glabella and one cone perpendicular to the first, angled toward the right cheek.[3] Both secondary intention healing and full-thickness skin grafting were both inferior options for this closure. Secondary intention healing on a defect of this depth would leave a highly visible atrophic scar and grafting often results in either color or texture mismatch, which can also be quite noticeable cosmetically.

Reconstructive Conundrums in Dermatologic Surgery: The Nose, First Edition. Edited by Désirée Ratner, Joel L. Cohen and David G. Brodland.
© 2014 American Society for Dermatologic Surgery. Published 2014 by John Wiley & Sons, Ltd.

The lip defect posed a more challenging reconstructive dilemma, because the defect had become somewhat semicircular and immediately adjacent to the alar rim after tumor extirpation. Likely the best reconstructive options for this closure would be either an island pedicle advancement or a rotation flap. With the island pedicle flap, incision lines could be partially camouflaged into the melolabial fold. In a rotation flap, a vertical, inferiorly placed Burow's triangle would act as the pivot, and the arc of the rotation would create an incision line along the melolabial fold. Again, other less desirable options would include skin grafting and secondary intention healing because of the depth of the wound and the frequently inferior tissue match of a full-thickness skin graft.

Individually, these two defects are relatively straightforward cases for closure. Unfortunately, the real conundrum for the surgeon is the underlying problem that all of these repairs are unrelated. If one chose any number of the aforementioned combinations of closures, the result would be multiple incision lines both on the nose, cheek, and lip. Therefore, we sought to find a way to combine these two defects into one closure. In that way, we could minimize the area of the reconstruction and simultaneously reduce visible incision lines.

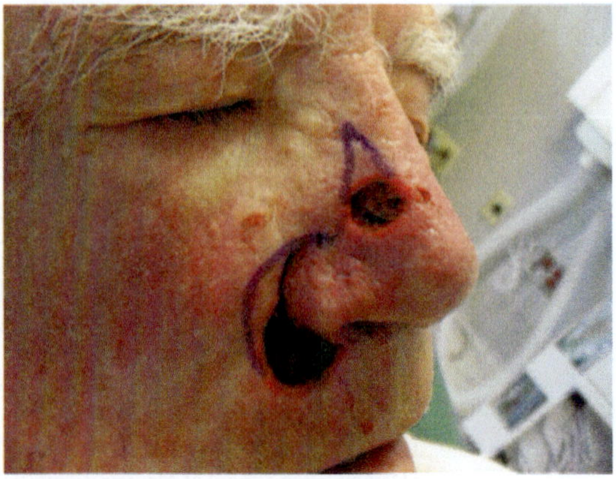

Figure 2 The proposed incision lines are marked.

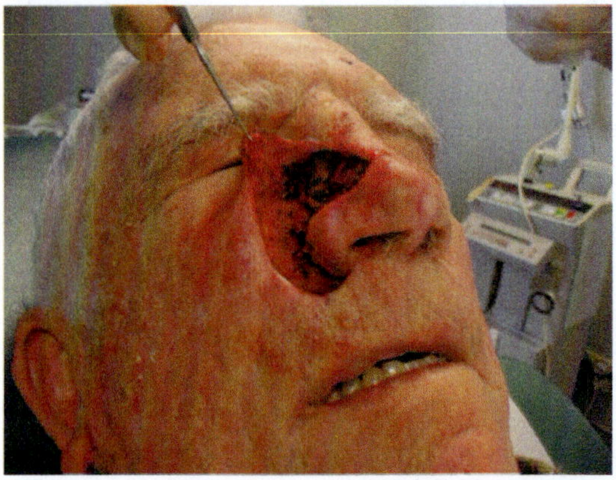

Figure 3 The secondary defects are incised; the flap is undermined and is shown reflected.

Resolution

The two defects were combined into one closure by creating a single, arcuate advancement flap that concealed the majority of incision lines into the alar groove. This flap shares some similarities with the crescentic advancement flap described by Mellette and Harrington.[4] After prepping the surgical site with chlorhexidine, a sterile gentian violet marking pen was used to plan the proposed flap (Figure 2). We then anesthetized the area with 1% lidocaine and 1:100,000 epinephrine and a No. 15 blade was used to extend the lip primary defect into a lazy arc around the upper alar crease, where it met the inferior border of the nasal primary defect. The secondary defect was excised and the cheek tissue immediately lateral to the alar rim and nasal sidewall was undermined and reflected (Figure 3). Hemostasis was achieved and we began our deep plane closure.

The most challenging aspects of this reconstruction were first, rotating the curved, inferior Burows triangle into the alar crease, and second, ensuring that there was no cheek elevation which would effectively blunt the nose/cheek junction. To perform these maneuvers, we took advantage of the inherent malleability of the upper lip tissue. We first used a buried, simple suture of 4-0 polyglactin (Vicryl, Johnson & Johnson, New Brunswick, NJ) to elevate the flap toward the nose/cheek junction and pexed the mid-portion of the flap into the base of the nasal bone periosteum. This suture both helped to relieve tension on the lip and nose defects and, more importantly, helped pull the flap downward, into the melonasal junction.

We then used buried, simple 4-0 polyglactin sutures to slide the inferior, lip portion of the flap into the alar sulcus. Because the lip defect was so large relative to the ala, there was excess lip tissue lateral to the alar rim. Once we secured the midportion of this lower part of the flap, we placed additional simple, buried sutures according to the principle of the "rule of halves."[5] Simple buried sutures were again used to secure the upper or nasal portion of the flap. Subsequently, a running suture of 5-0 fast-absorbing gut was used to evert the wound edges. At the inferior portion, there was some excess bunching of tissue lateral to the alar rim. This excess tissue was leveled by using a running suture that pleated the side of excess together and downward, into the alar sulcus.[6] The patient was swollen in the immediate postoperative period (Figure 4a) but there was no distortion of the alar rim or upper lip (Figure 4b).

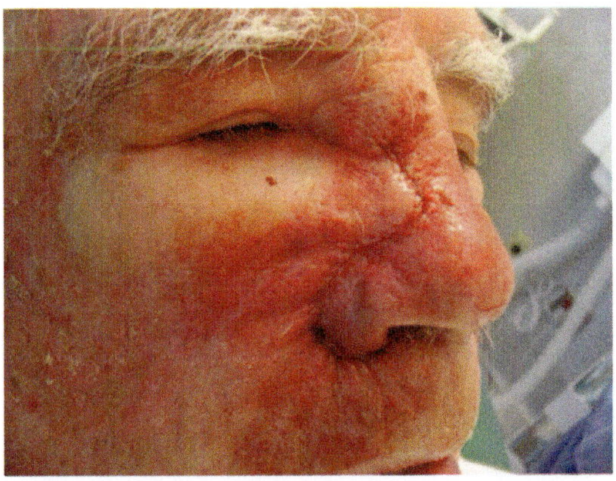

(a)

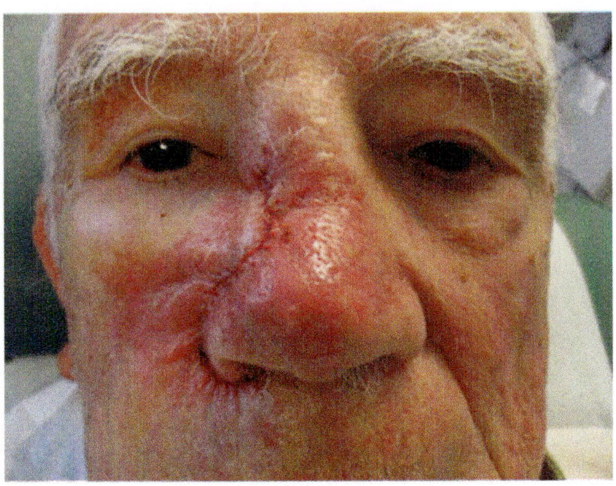

(b)

Figure 4 Immediate postoperative result is shown from (a) the lateral view, and from (b) the frontal view, showing edema, but no distortion of the lip or alar rim.

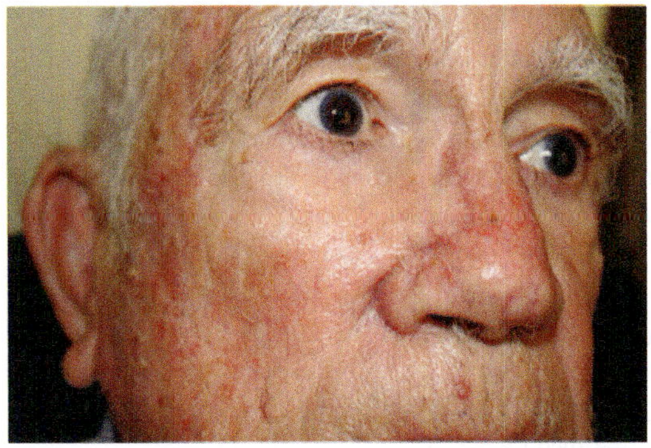

(a)

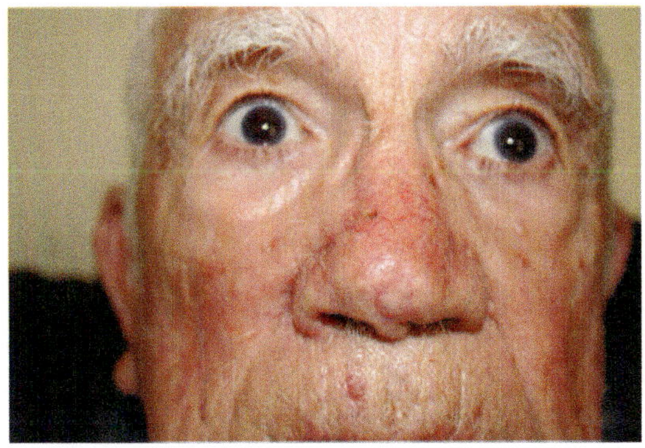

(b)

Figure 5 Three-month postoperative result shown from (a) the oblique view and from (b) the frontal view which both show no lip distortion.

At 3 months postoperation, the patient had healed well, with most of his incision line concealed in the alar groove and nasal sidewall (Figure 5a) and without distortion of either the lip or alar rim (Figure 5b). There was some slight blunting of the nose/cheek junction and a modest pincushioning of the nasal portion of the flap. While the traditional approach to avoiding pincushioning deformities is extensive undermining,[7] we were less aggressive in this patient because of his anticoagulant use. Some have also proposed that squaring off edges of a semicircular flap can help avoid this complication.[8]

Conundrum keys

- Wide undermining of the upper lip and cheek was required to allow elevation and advancement of the flap without causing distortion of the lip and alar rim.

· Pexing sutures from cheek secondary defect should be secured to the nasal bone periosteum to prevent tenting over the cheek/nose cosmetic boundary.

· Excess tissue on the lateral lip/cheek was distributed into the alar sulcus according to the principle of halving sutures.

References

1 Zitelli JA. The bilobed flap for nasal reconstruction. Arch Dermatol 1989;125:957–9.

2 Johnson TM, Swanson NA, Baker SR, et al. The Rieger flap for nasal reconstruction. Arch Otolaryngol Head Neck Surg 1995;121:634–7.

3 Zeikus PS, Maloney ME, Jellinek NJ. Advancement flap for the reconstruction of nasal ala and lateral nasal tip defects. J Am Acad Dermatol 2006;55:1032–5.

4 Mellette JR Jr, Harrington AC. Applications of the crescentic advancement flap. J Dermatol Surg Oncol 1991;17:447–54.

5 Bennett R. Basic excisional surgery. In: Roenigk RK and Roenigk, editors. Fundamentals of cutaneous surgery, Vol. 1. St Louis: Mosby, 1988:p. 355–443.

6 Kouba DJ, Miller SJ. "Running pleated" suture technique opposes wound edges of unequal lengths. Dermatol Surg 2006;32:411–4.

7 Koranda FC, Webster RC. Trapdoor effect in nasolabial flaps. Causes and corrections. Arch Otolaryngol 1985;111:421–4.

8 Field LM. Peripheral tissue undermining is not the final answer to prevent trapdooring in transposition flaps. J Dermatol Surg Oncol 1993;19:1131–2.

Commentary on conundrum 5

It is not uncommon for patients with skin cancer to have metachronous malignancies, sometimes in close proximity to one another. Because Mohs surgeons can be confident that their patients' defects are free of cancer, they can plan closures that recruit available adjacent tissue in a complimentary fashion to allow the repair of more than one defect at a time. With this unique reconstructive perspective, a well-trained Mohs surgeon can creatively develop a flap that closes more than one defect in a tissue efficient, esthetically elegant, and cost-effective manner, resulting in lower morbidity for the patient. In this case, a single flap was utilized to close two defects in close proximity to one another but in different cosmetic subunits. Ultimately, all incision lines were designed to fall within cosmetic subunit junctions or relaxed skin tension lines.

It is also important to note that this patient was on anticoagulants as a preventative measure. Although no mention is made of the International Normalised Ratio (INR), in this instance, it goes almost without saying that patients on anticoagulants with therapeutic INR levels have an increased risk of postoperative bleeding. However, as clarified by Kovich and Otley, the danger of discontinuing the anticoagulant far outweighs the slight risk of bleeding.[1] The question is "how slight is the risk?" A study by Merritt et al. of a cohort of 1550 patients found that patients taking anticoagulants did have an increased rate of postoperative bleeding, although that rate did not reach statistical significance when compared with the nonanticoagulated group ($p = 0.08$).[2] Therefore, while it is prudent to keep this risk factor in mind, it probably should not substantially change most surgeons' standard approach to reconstruction. The author points out that while extensive undermining may help to avoid a pincushion deformity, undermining was not performed in this case because the patient was on warfarin. The implication is that pincushioning might have been avoided by more extensive undermining. Given the low risk of complications associated with therapeutic anticoagulation, adherence to usual surgical technique, including extensive undermining, would have been justifiable in this case.

There are other considerations with respect to the phenomenon of pincushioning. First, if it occurs early after an extensive flap procedure, it may improve and even completely resolve over time. An underappreciated and underutilized technique to reduce pincushioning is aggressive daily massage of the incision lines and flap. It is believed that the mechanical effect of massage induces a softening and remodeling of the contracted portion of the scar. Counseling the patient to massage the entire area with fingertips at least 10 times daily for 15–30 seconds, for a minimum of 2–3 months, beginning 1 month after surgery, can sometimes generate significant clinical improvement. Alternatively, or in addition, the surgeon can consider intralesional corticosteroid injections beginning 2–6 months postoperatively. The last resort is to reoperate and debulk the undersurface of the flap. Although occasionally necessary, surgical reintervention is often avoidable if these more conservative approaches have been instituted early.

Another important principle illustrated by this case involves the use of periosteal tacking sutures. In Figure 3, the medial aspect of the malar fat pad is shown in its normal anatomic position. However, upon advancement of the overlying skin, it is likely that despite adequate undermining, the fat pad will be displaced medially out of its normal position onto the nasal sidewall. Furthermore, the tension created by redraping the lateral nasal sidewall and cheek skin into the nasal defect leads to a tendency for the nasofacial sulcus to "tent." This tenting along with the medial migration of the malar fat pad leads to blunting of the normal contour of the nasofacial sulcus. The periosteal tackdown suture is the ideal solution to this problem. A carefully placed tackdown suture not only counteracts the tendency toward tissue tenting but also provides a physical barrier to medial migration of the malar fat pad. Correct placement of these sutures to recreate the contour of the nasofacial sulcus entails a vertically oriented suture "bite," usually at the most lateral aspect of the nasal bone. The flap is then pulled into position using a skin hook, and the corresponding location on its undersurface is identified by envisioning where the new "sulcus" should be once it is sutured into place. The suture needle is passed with a small bite perpendicular to the direction of arterial blood flow so as to avoid inadvertent suture constriction of vital vessels. The suture is then tied. Normally, there is a very subtle dimple on the flap at the site of the suture. This technique can and should be used any time that maintenance of skin and soft tissue contour over bone is desirable. It can also be used to protect free margins from distortion due to countertension created by flap movement.

Careful review of the surgical technique in this case indicates that the author correctly used buried absorbable sutures as the foundation for flap movement. In contrast to superficial skin sutures, these sutures represent a longer lasting, stabilizing force for several months after surgery while the wound edges undergo the later stages of healing. Because the normal tensile strength of a freshly made wound at 1 month is less than 10% of its original strength, and because the superficial sutures are removed long before then, it makes sense to have longer lasting supportive sutures in place to maintain the correct skin position and allow the remodeling process to occur in a relatively tension-free environment. Furthermore, when dermal sutures are placed using the subcutaneous vertical mattress technique, tissue eversion is maintained for a greater period of time, thereby counteracting the contraction that naturally occurs perpendicular to the skin surface at all suture lines.[3] More prolonged support of the skin in the everted position may ultimately diminish the degree of inversion created by the transdermal, perpendicular scar contraction. When the wound edges are well everted with dermal sutures, the superficial suture layer serves to refine and precisely level the epidermal edges.

In Figure 5, an excellent restitution of the natural contour at the junction between the ala, upper lip, and nasolabial fold is seen. In essence, the tissue movement that resulted in the closure of this defect took advantage of the same principle that makes an island pedicle flap a reasonable consideration here – which is based on the fact that there is a significant pool of donor tissue inferiorly and laterally on the upper lip parallel to the nasolabial fold. Smaller defects in this area can sometimes be closed by direct advancement of this tissue obliquely toward the base of the ala, resulting in tissue redundancy that can be "sewn out" by the rule of halves or addressed by removing a more conventional but diminutive Burow's triangle medially and laterally. If the running pleated suture technique cannot entirely obviate the problem of wound edges of unequal lengths, it can certainly diminish the size of Burow's triangles, which must be removed on either end of the closure. For any wound smaller than the one presented here, direct closure utilizing this donor pool inferior and lateral to the alar base should be considered.

Commentary by Dr. Brodland

References

1 Kovich O, Otley CC. Thrombotic complications related to discontinuation of warfarin and aspirin therapy perioperatively for cutaneous operation. J Am Acad Dermatol 2003;48(2):233–7.

2 Merritt BG, Lee NY, Brodland DG, Zitelli JA, Cook J. The safety of Mohs surgery: a prospective multicenter cohort study. J Am Acad Dermatol 2012;67(6):1302–9.

3 Zitelli JA, Moy RL. The buried vertical mattress suture. J Dermatol Surg Oncol 1989;15:17–9.

6

CONUNDRUM 6

Advancement Flap in the Reconstruction of a Lateral Nasal Sidewall Defect

Pedro Redondo
Department of Dermatology, University Clinic of Navarra, Pamplona, Spain

A 61-year-old woman presented with a defect of the lateral nasal sidewall after Mohs surgery for a basal cell carcinoma, which had already been treated by normal excision. The final defect was geometric, and measured 2 × 3 cm in size at the greatest diameter (Figure 1).

A common site for the development of skin cancers is the junction between the nose and cheek along the nasofacial sulcus. Several goals must be considered in the reconstructive surgery of the anterior cheek and lateral nasal sidewall: the maintenance of the natural grooves, lines and cosmetic units, and optimal scar camouflage by placement of scars adjacent to the mesolabial crease and inferior orbital rim, whenever possible. How would you reconstruct this defect? (Figure 2).

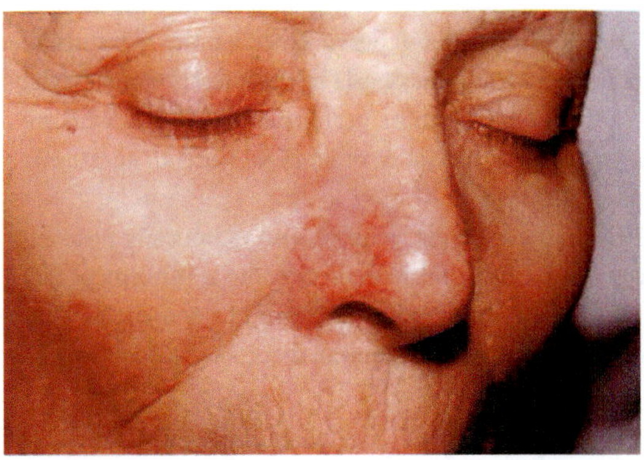

Figure 1 Preoperative photo of cheek – lateral nasal sidewall basal cell carcinoma.

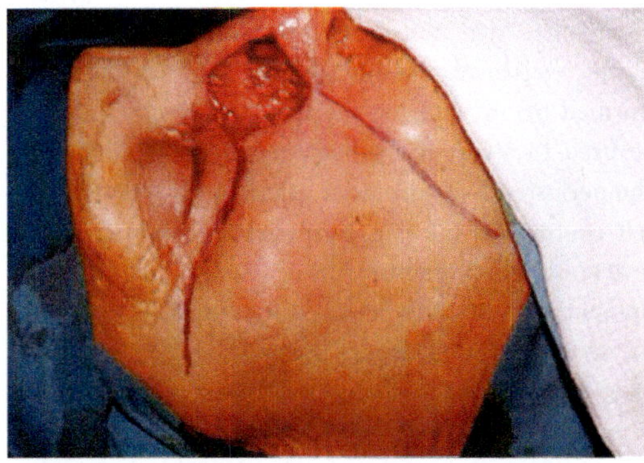

Figure 2 Defect after Mohs excision. Advancement flap is designed with borders of flap coinciding with the border of facial esthetic units (eyelid and cheek). Incisions are performed parallel to melolabial sulcus and infraorbital rim.

Resolution

Reconstructive techniques of the anterior cheek and lateral nasal sidewall include simple closure along relaxed skin tension lines, full-thickness skin grafting, secondary intention healing, or tissue rearrangement. Local and regional flaps are the first choice. Transposition flaps can

Reconstructive Conundrums in Dermatologic Surgery: The Nose, First Edition. Edited by Désirée Ratner, Joel L. Cohen and David G. Brodland.
© 2014 American Society for Dermatologic Surgery. Published 2014 by John Wiley & Sons, Ltd.

be used on the cheek and lateral nasal sidewall. These flaps (rhombic or bilobe flaps) often require incisions that may not fit into the natural lines of the face, and the esthetic result can be disappointing with a trapdoor deformity.[1,2]

After tumor removal, the mobility of the surrounding tissue was determined. The defect was segmented and closure lines were planned to place in the junctions of cosmetic units without crossing the junctions. The advancement flap had two lateral curvilinear incisions tangential to the defect superiorly along the lower eyelid cheek junction and inferiorly along the nasolabial fold. The flap was undermined at the upper level of the subcutaneous fat, mobilized and advanced medially, and gently pulled into place with a hook. The flap was appropriately thinned in the region of the lower eyelid for a better tissue match. Meticulous hemostasis using atraumatic pinpoint electrocoagulation of bleeding vessels was performed before suturing the flap. Suspension sutures were used to attach the subcutaneous-advanced tissue to the periosteum of nasofacial sulcus, and to sculpt the rolled contour on the flap. Suspension sutures help to relieve tension on the suture line of the distal flap, and to maintain the nasofacial sulcus. These sutures advance the tissue to the preferred closure line at the junction of the cosmetic units.[3] An absorbable suture such as 3-0 and 4-0 Dexon suture was used, avoiding vascular compromise of the flap. Burow's triangles of redundant skin in temple and nasolabial fold, caused by tissue advancement placed into appropriate relaxed skin tension lines, were excised. At the nasal cheek junctions, suspension sutures can adequately reconstitute the nasofacial sulcus obliterated by the movement of the tissue. The "puckering" of the surface of the flap is avoided with a good design. Skin edges were approximated with 6-0 silk sutures (Figure 3).

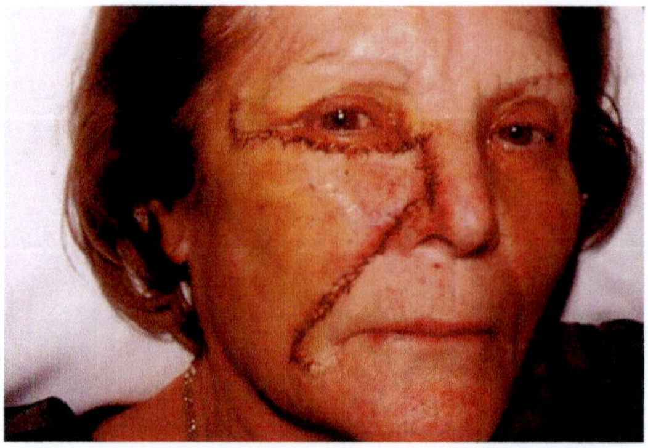

Figure 3 Excision of Burow's triangles and suspension suture attaching the dermis of the flap to the periosteum of the naso-facial sulcus.

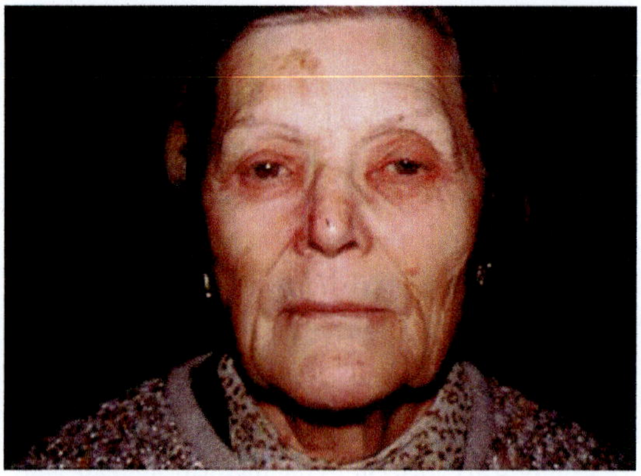

Figure 4 Appearance 8 years postoperatively.

Advancement flap of the cheek maintains the borders of cosmetic units, avoids distortion of anatomic structures, and allows closure lines to be placed discretely along the lower eyelid cheek junction and nasolabial fold. The cheek is an excellent reservoir of skin, with a rich vascular network that allows a large superficial area to be lifted with a very low risk of necrosis. This flap permits the advancement of the cheek upward and toward the medial aspect of the face until it covers the defect. The only pitfall can be the superficial temporal branch of the facial nerve that crosses near our upper incision at the zygomatic arch, approximately following a line drawn from 0.5 cm below the tragus to a point 1.5 to 2 cm above the lateral eyebrow. With a good nerve block of the infraorbital foramen and local anesthesia of the lateral branches, the present procedure can be performed in patients who are not excessively anxious; otherwise, general anesthesia can be used (Figure 4).

This flap is a simple, reliable, and esthetically pleasing reconstruction option. We consider the advancement flap to be the gold standard for the repair of extensive anterior cheek and lateral nasal sidewall defects.

Conundrum keys

- Segmental facial reconstruction places incisions at the junction of cosmetic units and uses an advancement flap of the cheek to replace resected tissue with similar tissue, thereby restoring facial contours without distorting surrounding functional and esthetic structures.

· Suspension sutures are used to attach the advanced tissue to deeper structures, such as deep subcutaneous, or muscle insertions on the bone, and to sculpt the rolled contour on the nasofacial sulcus. These sutures advance the tissue to the preferred closure line at the junction of the cosmetic units.

· Judicious placement of Burow's triangles or half moons of redundant skin along natural esthetic borders can enhance the final result of the reconstruction.

Additional readings

1 Robinson JK. Segmental reconstruction of the face. Dermatol Surg 2004;30:67–74.
2 Dzubow LM, Zack L. The principles of cosmetic junctions as applied to reconstruction of defects following Mohs surgery. J Dermatol Surg Oncol 1990;16:353–5.
3 Salasche SJ, Jarchow R, Feldman BD, et al. The suspension suture. J Dermatol Surg Oncol 1987;13:973–8.

Commentary on conundrum 6

Recreation of the nasofacial sulcus is essential when repairing defects straddling the medial cheek and lateral nasal sidewall. In this reconstructive conundrum, suspension sutures attaching the subcutaneous tissue of the flap to the underlying periosteum were effective in recreating the nasofacial sulcus and preserving facial symmetry. There are some instances, however, in which defects like this one are best reconstructed as two separate units, a medial cheek portion and a nasal portion; for example, in patients with a deep or prominent crease within the nasofacial sulcus. This type of repair is usually performed by first advancing the cheek skin medially to close the lateral portion of the defect, with standing cones taken superiorly and inferiorly so that the suture line is placed within the nasofacial sulcus, extending downward into the nasolabial fold. The remaining nasal defect can then be repaired with a Burow's full-thickness skin graft taken from whichever standing cone constitutes a better tissue match for the nasal skin.

In the accompanying case, a large lateral nasal sidewall defect is present, which also extends onto the medial cheek (Figure 6.1). In this instance, there was sufficient cheek laxity such that a Burow's triangle could be removed inferiorly, and the cheek skin advanced medially, thereby placing the suture line within the nasolabial fold. The Burow's triangle was sufficiently large that it could be used as a full-thickness skin graft for the remaining nasal defect (Figure 6.2). Because adjacent skin tends to have a similar color, thickness, and texture, it tends to provide a cosmetically superior match compared with grafts harvested from more distant locations. At times, however, particularly in elderly patients, grafts can become hypopigmented, resulting in a flat white scar (Figure 6.3).

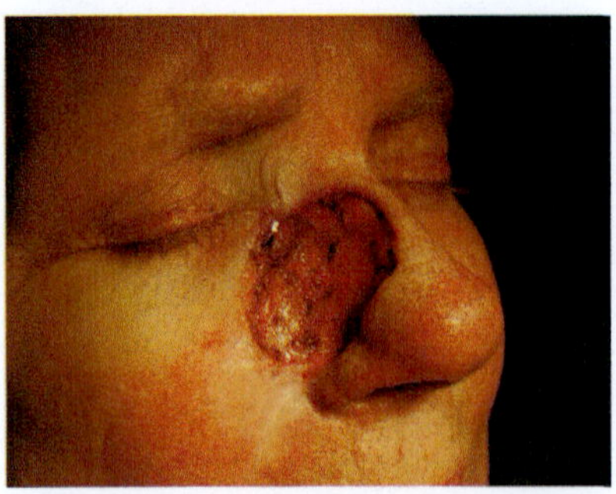

Figure 6.1 Lateral nasal sidewall defect after Mohs excision.

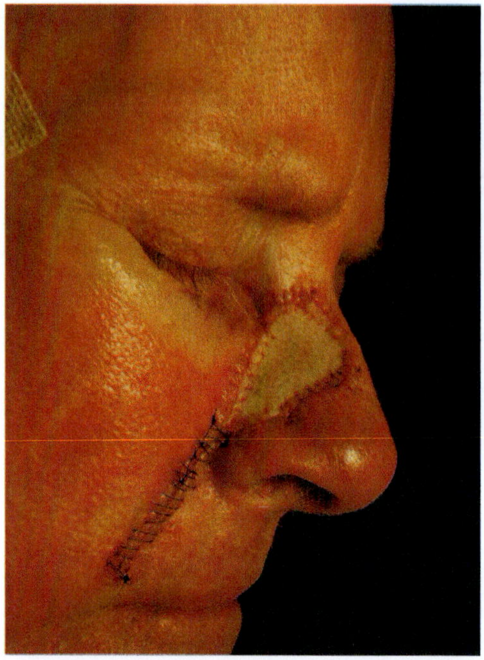

Figure 6.2 Excision of lower Burow's triangle with closure of medial cheek defect along the nasolabial fold and Burow's full-thickness skin graft placed within the remaining nasal sidewall defect.

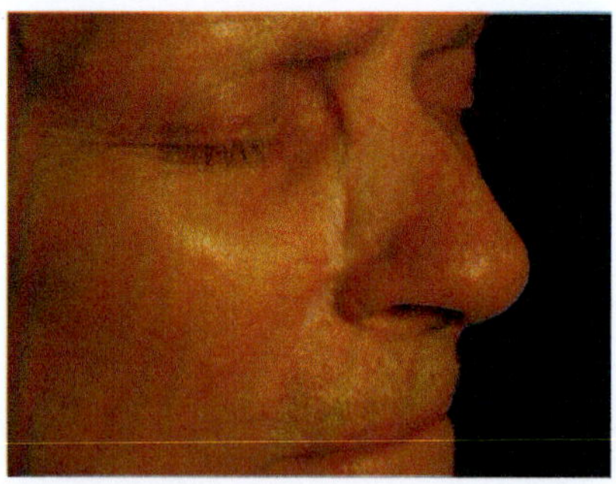

Figure 6.3 Follow-up view at 6 months. Hypopigmentation of graft and suture lines can sometimes occur, but scars are nearly imperceptible if patient applies make-up.

Both of these cases highlight the desirability of placing incisions in cosmetic unit junction lines. They also illustrate the advantages of using adjacent cheek skin to repair extensive lateral nasal sidewall defects, thereby restoring facial contours without distortion and optimizing the ultimate esthetic result.

Commentary by Dr. Ratner

7

CONUNDRUM 7

Repair of the Left Nasal Sidewall, Nasofacial Sulcus, and Medial Cheek

Steven Bernstein
Hôtel-Dieu de Montreal, Montreal, Quebec, Canada

This 42-year-old man was referred to our department for the treatment of a recurrent infiltrating basal cell carcinoma clinically involving the left nasal sidewall (Figure 1). Mohs micrographic surgery was considered the procedure of choice. Tumor extirpation resulted in a defect of the left nasal sidewall as well as the nasofacial sulcus and medial cheek. The postoperative defect measured 2.6 cm × 1.8 cm and extended through the subcutaneous tissue of the lateral nose to the nasalis muscle and to the subcutaneous tissue on the cheek. Nasal cartilage was not involved.

Areas of concern with respect to reconstruction involve a desire to avoid displacement of the nasal ala and to replace missing tissue with tissue possessing a similar texture, color, sebaceousness, thickness, and photodamage. An additional concern is that this defect involves more than one facial cosmetic unit.

How would you manage this wound?

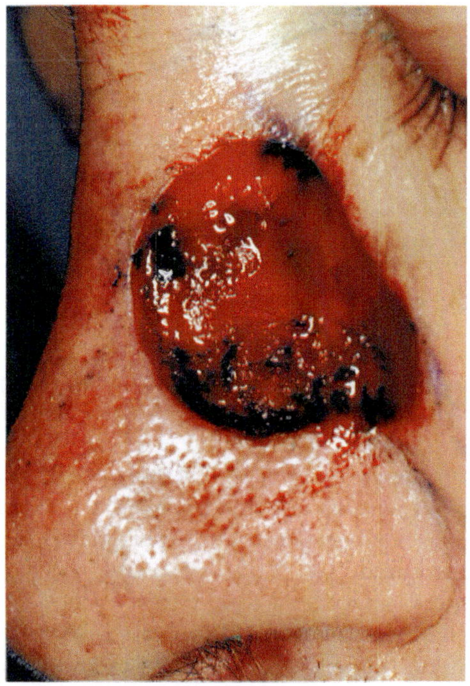

Figure 1 Postoperative defect.

Resolution

The challenge and pleasure of reconstruction stems from the fact that no two lesions are identical. Even if a defect possesses similar characteristics as to size and anatomic location, the tissue properties from patient to patient are often variable. Aesthetic reconstruction never relies on a cookbook approach. Reconstruction of the relatively large nasal defect is often limited by the lack of availability of nasal skin. Most often we are forced to look to the more lax and mobile cheek skin for repair of the larger nasal defect. This implies either a transposition flap which is inferolaterally based, or a large advancement/rotation-type flap of the cheek. The former comes with the inherent risks of creating a bridge between the cheek and nose or a trapdoor deformity. The latter demands a large

Reconstructive Conundrums in Dermatologic Surgery: The Nose, First Edition. Edited by Désirée Ratner, Joel L. Cohen and David G. Brodland.
© 2014 American Society for Dermatologic Surgery. Published 2014 by John Wiley & Sons, Ltd.

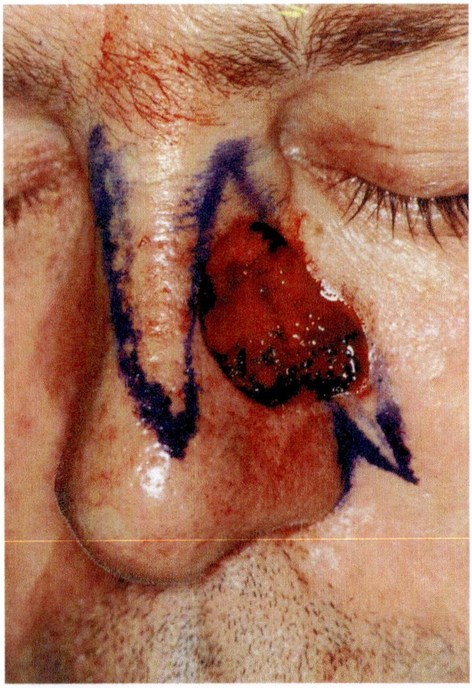

Figure 2 Defect divided into cosmetic units.

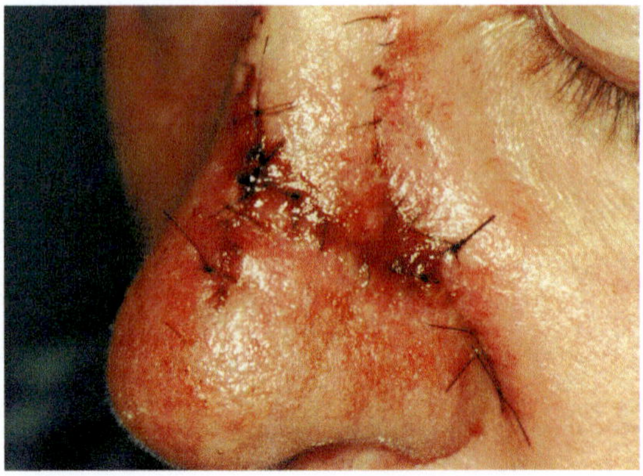

Figure 3 Post-reconstruction.

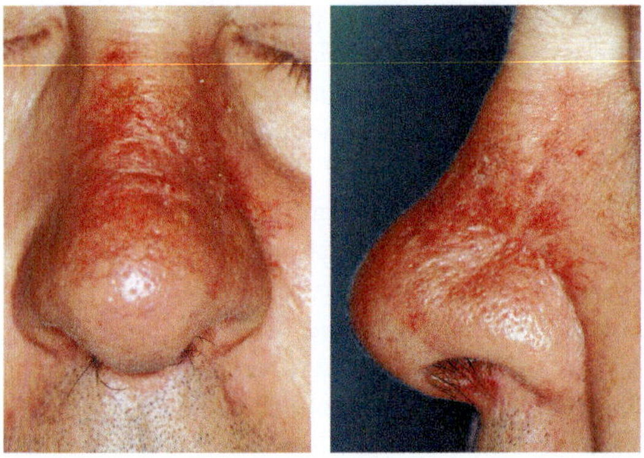

Figure 4 2 months post-reconstruction.

incision and extensive undermining, and would greatly risk blunting the naso-facial sulcus and creating facial asymmetry.

Finally, an appropriately chosen full-thickness skin graft can often give satisfactory results, but implies a second surgical site for donor skin, risk of necrosis, and less than ideal tissue match.

I decided to simplify the repair by dividing the defect into cosmetic units (Figure 2). The medial cheek defect was first repaired by removing a small Burrow's triangle at the ala/cheek junction and then advancing the cheek skin medially to the nasofacial sulcus. Consequently I was able to confine the tissue replacement part of the repair to the cosmetic unit of the nasal sidewall.

Of interest, this young patient had a good tissue reservoir medial to the surgical defect over the bridge of the nose and inferior glabellar area. A transposition flap was thus designed superiomedially to take advantage of this relatively lax area to reconstruct the entire remaining defect (Figure 3). Of importance, the flap was designed very exactingly, with enough length and width to avoid nasal retraction or distortion, but not too wide as to encourage pin cushioning.

The result of reconstruction 2-months postoperatively is seen in Figure 4. The shape of the nose as well as the nasofacial sulcus have been preserved, as the skin match is excellent. Incision lines are well concealed in cosmetic unit junction lines and will fade considerably with time.

Conundrum keys

- Identify tissue donor site(s). In this case, the nasal dorsum and medial cheek.
- View the defect as smaller parts of a whole (the medial cheek portion plus the nasal sidewall portion).
- Reconstruct within cosmetic units.

Commentary

Dr. Bernstein utilizes several fundamental reconstructive principles in the repair of the large defect on the side of this young patient's nose. He recognizes the donor pools of this location which include the medial cheek, the nasal root/glabella, and a less traditional donor site, the nasal dorsum. The cheek is almost always an ample source for donor skin. A recent article by Cook and Zitelli underscores the often-overlooked utility of midline nasal laxity.[1] Not all noses have a great deal of midline laxity, however, in appropriately selected cases, 1 cm or more of flap skin may be available. I note on Figure 3 what appears to be a small area of necrosis visible at the confluence of the alar crease and nasofacial junction. I believe that this is most likely due to the length of the incision made on the medial-most portion of the transposition flap. I would submit that this incision need only extend superiorly to the level of the tissue island over which the flap will be transposed. Indeed, it appears in Figure 3 that the superior half of this incision has been simply resutured and therefore has not materially contributed to the wound closure. In fact, I believe that the superior extent of this incision may have actually severed valuable random blood supply from the right angular artery and limited the vascular supply to that which could be derived from the glabella. In my experience, superiorly based nasal dorsum flaps which transect the vascular contributions from both the right and left angular arteries are at increased risk for partial flap necrosis. Nonetheless, despite this potential design flaw, the consequences are minimal as demonstrated in Figures 4 and 5. The end result is, as pointed out by Dr. Bernstein, without structural, functional, or anatomic distortion and with a skin match that would be difficult to improve upon with the use of a graft.

David Brodland
Clairton, Pennsylvania

Reference

1 Cook JL, Zitelli JA. Primary closure for midline defects of the nose: a simple approach for reconstruction. J Am Acad Dermatol 2000; 43:508-10.

Commentary on conundrum 7

Combined defects of the lateral upper nasal sidewall and medial cheek can be challenging to repair, particularly in younger patients, whose tissue laxity can sometimes be limited. While the author of this conundrum successfully utilized adjacent nasal skin in a transposition flap to execute an elegant repair, the more lax and mobile cheek skin is more often used to repair similarly large nasal defects. Regardless of the repair selected, it is essential to preserve the cosmetic junction lines of the face and to re-create the preexisting facial symmetry to the greatest extent possible.

The defect shown here (Figure 7.1) is similar to Figure 1 in that it also involves both the nasal sidewall and medial cheek but differs in that it is broader than it is tall. Furthermore, this patient is young with a fairly delicate and thin-skinned nose. In this instance, there was insufficient nasal laxity even to consider performing a transposition flap from adjacent nasal skin to close that portion of the defect. It became evident that a large advancement flap, extending down the nasofacial sulcus into the nasolabial fold, would likely provide the best coverage for this repair. As shown in Figure 7.2, when the flap was advanced medially, the most lateral portion of the defect was displaced medially into the medial canthus and could not be closed with the existing flap laxity. The decision was therefore made to use the standing cone removed from the superior

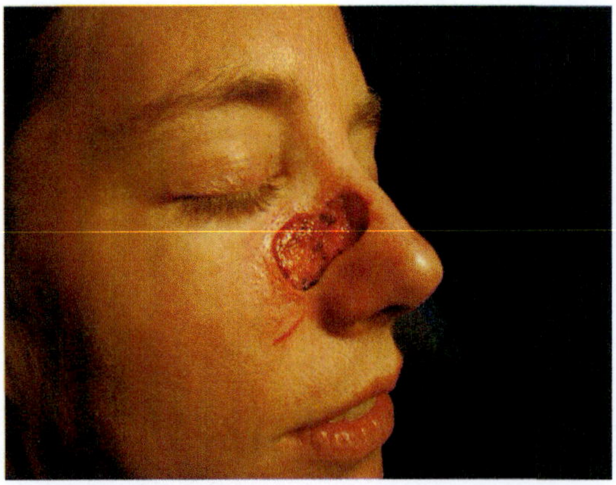

Figure 7.1 Defect of the right upper nasal sidewall extending onto the medial cheek.

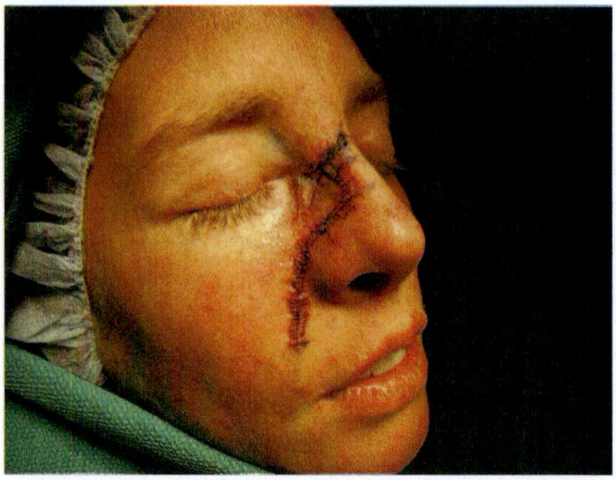

Figure 7.2 Cheek advancement flap with Burow's full-thickness skin graft to close the residual medial canthal defect.

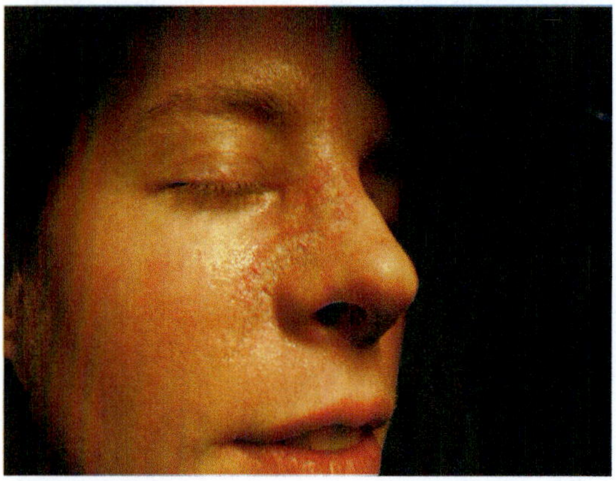

Figure 7.3 Suture removal at 2 weeks.

aspect of the flap as a Burow's full-thickness skin graft for the remaining portion of the defect. To avoid distortion of the canthus and to provide more effective scar camouflage, the standing cone was angled medially along the superior border of the nasal dorsum, thereby allowing the suture line to be concealed within the upper nasal crease. At the time of suture removal 2 weeks later (Figure 7.3), the flap lines had already blended into the natural facial contours, and the graft was barely recognizable as a distinct portion of the repair.

In both of these cases, available tissue donor sites were identified, and each defect was divided into its component parts – a medial cheek portion and a nasal portion. The tissue laxity dictated the nature of the repair to be selected – a transposition flap from the nasal skin in one instance and a cheek advancement flap in the other. In both cases, the larger defects were conceptualized as smaller parts of a whole, and the incision lines were placed along the cosmetic unit junction lines so as to optimize the final esthetic results for each patient to the greatest extent possible.

Commentary by Dr. Ratner

PART III

Nasal Tip

8

CONUNDRUM 8

The Dorsal Nasal Flap for Reconstruction of Large Nasal Tip Defects

Marc S. Zimbler
Department of Otolaryngology-Head & Neck Surgery, Beth Israel Medical Center, New York, NY

A 49-year-old male was referred for nasal reconstruction following Mohs micrographic re-section of a basal cell carcinoma. The patient had undergone three stages of Mohs surgery, and physical examination revealed a 2.0 × 2.0-cm defect of the nasal tip and supratip centered off to the patient's right side. The defect involved the full thickness of the nasal skin but underlying nasal perichondrium and tip cartilages were not disturbed (Figure 1). How would you manage the defect?

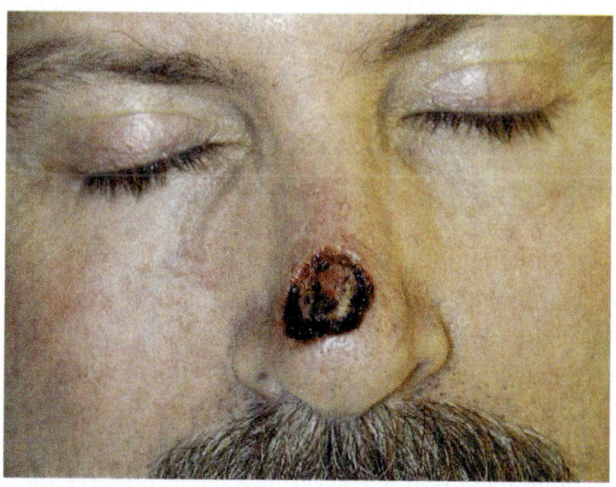

Figure 1 Mohs nasal tip defect measuring 2.0 × 2.0 cm in greatest diameter.

Resolution

Reconstructing large surgical defects of the nasal tip and lower third of the nose presents a unique challenge for the surgeon because of its cosmetically prominent location. Treatment options include second-intention healing, full-thickness skin grafts, various local flaps, and the paramedian forehead flap. Owing to the unique texture and color of nasal skin, it is always preferable that like-tissue be replaced by like-tissue. Scars are best placed at the junction of aesthetic facial units, while reconstruction should adhere to nasal "subunit" principles.

Before contemplating various reconstructive options, however, there are certain patient-dependent physical characteristics that are worth mentioning that can affect one's decision when choosing a reconstructive technique. First, what is the texture of the nasal skin? Thick sebaceous nasal skin often results in a poor texture and contour match when utilizing skin grafts for reconstruction. However, a thin-skinned patient with a fair complexion (Fitzpatrick I or II) will often do quite nicely with skin grafting. The depth and size of the defect will also determine the location of the skin graft donor site. Other variables include patient's age, comorbidities, and cosmetic expectations. Some patients may be very

Reconstructive Conundrums in Dermatologic Surgery: The Nose, First Edition. Edited by Désirée Ratner, Joel L. Cohen and David G. Brodland.
© 2014 American Society for Dermatologic Surgery. Published 2014 by John Wiley & Sons, Ltd.

willing to undergo a two- or three-staged distal flap reconstruction, while for other more elderly patients this may not be a viable option. Finally, I consider the actual size of the nose along with skin laxity. Mobilizing large flaps in a younger patient with a petite nose is often difficult and can cause nasal distortion and asymmetry. However, in an elderly patient with a larger nose many considerable defects can be closed with local tissue rearrangement. Moreover, correction of tip ptosis can be obtained in the senile nose, which to the patient may not only be cosmetically appealing but could also improve the nasal airway.

Because of the size of the defect and the high cosmetic expectations of this patient, second-intention healing was not considered. A full-thickness skin graft is a very reasonable option and highly considered. For female patients who can utilize makeup for camouflage, a skin graft is often a very good option. However, in the male patient, if the graft healed with pigmentation differences or skin texture differences, the outcome would be less than ideal. Local flaps are always my primary choice on the nose; however, size often dictates whether they can be utilized. Once defects approach the 2-cm mark, it becomes difficult to rotate local tissue. My primary flap choice in nasal reconstruction is the modified Zitelli bilobed flap,[1] which works particularly well with more laterally based nasal defects. However, when defects are located centrally over the tip, one often gets some nasal asymmetry or alar distortion when trying to rotate larger flaps. A paramedian forehead flap is an excellent choice for this patient; however, my personal philosophy is that I am hard-pressed to perform a forehead flap for a skin-only defect. For defects that are through and through, or involve the alar rim requiring cartilage reconstruction, I am quite comfortable performing forehead flaps. However, for skin-only defects I am not convinced that the combination of donor site morbidity plus a two-to three-staged procedure is a reasonable trade for the cosmetic outcome.

The dorsal nasal flap is a local flap that utilizes nasal skin for a single-stage reconstruction. It involves rotation advancement of dorsal nasal skin from the upper two-thirds of the nose and glabella to the lower nose. The dorsal nasal flap is used for defects of the distal third of the nose that are at least 5 mm away from the alar rim. I use a broad random pedicle that is typically based ipsilateral to the lesion to improve flap rotation. Incisions are marked before infiltration with local anesthetic. Flap design starts above the inner canthus and extends into glabellar frown lines, but should avoid extending well above the medial brow if possible (Figure 2A). The skin of the dorsum, through the defect, is undermined in a submuscular plane with Kaye scissors before flap incision. Using a No. 15 blade, the skin-muscle flap is incised; however, in the glabellar region only skin is elevated with the flap. Meticulous hemostasis is achieved with bipolar cautery, making sure not to injure the undersurface of the flap. If more advancement or rotation is required, the skin incision can be lengthened to the level of the medial canthal ligament. The lateral incision should be placed at the nasofacial junction, making sure not to violate the nasal sidewall subunit. A small amount of lateral undermining in the cheek region is performed to decrease flap tension by advancing cheek skin. Excision of the standing cone deformity is performed in an oblique direction to the defect on the ipsilateral side of the flap pedicle. Flap contour and inset is optimized by sculpting the undersurface of the flap and thinning the soft tissue of the recipient bed. The glabellar donor site is closed in a V-Y fashion. All incisions are closed in two layers, with 5-0 monocryl subcuticular and 6-0 nylon for skin (Figure 2b). Particular attention with meticulous skin eversion is performed at the tip level and lateral naso-facial junction, making sure to allow for discrepancies in skin thickness. Tension is minimized at the distal aspect of the flap to prevent alar retraction or asymmetries secondary to flap tension (Figure 3). I routinely evaluate for incisional interface dermabrasion at 6 weeks postoperatively; however, this was not required in this particular case.

The dorsal nasal flap was originally described by Gillies[2] as a bishop's miter flap. However, it was Rieger[3] who in 1967 published his design that popularized the flap for its use in defects of the nasal tip. I prefer the nasal dorsal flap for larger distal nasal defects because it is a one-stage reconstruction that replaces like-tissue with skin of similar kind.[4] Reconstruction of nasal skin defects should use remaining nasal skin whenever possible to preserve the unique color and texture of the nose.

Conundrum keys

- Placing donor site incisions in glabellar frown lines while minimizing cephalad extension to the level of the medial brow.

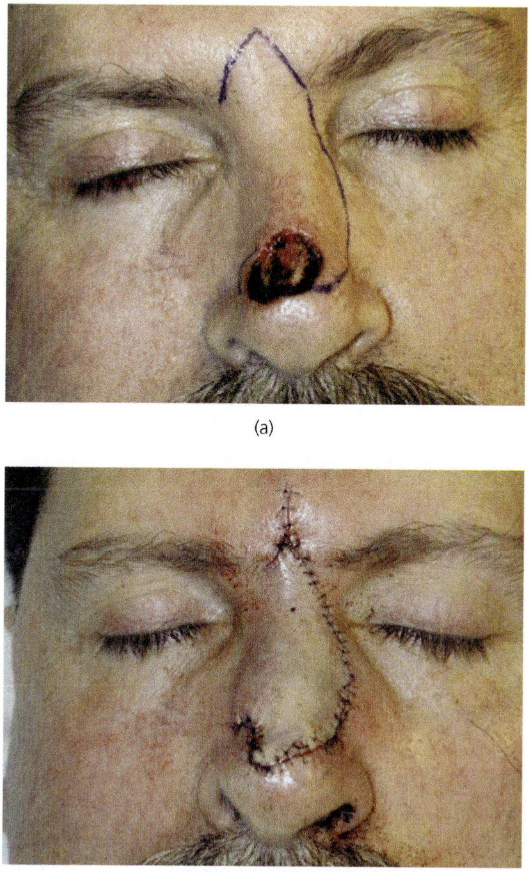

(a) (b)

Figure 2 (a) Flap design: donor incision within glabellar frown lines with limited cranial extension. Lateral incision at nasofacial junction. Obliquely marked standing cone deformity excision ipsilateral to flap pedicle. (b) After closure of defect.

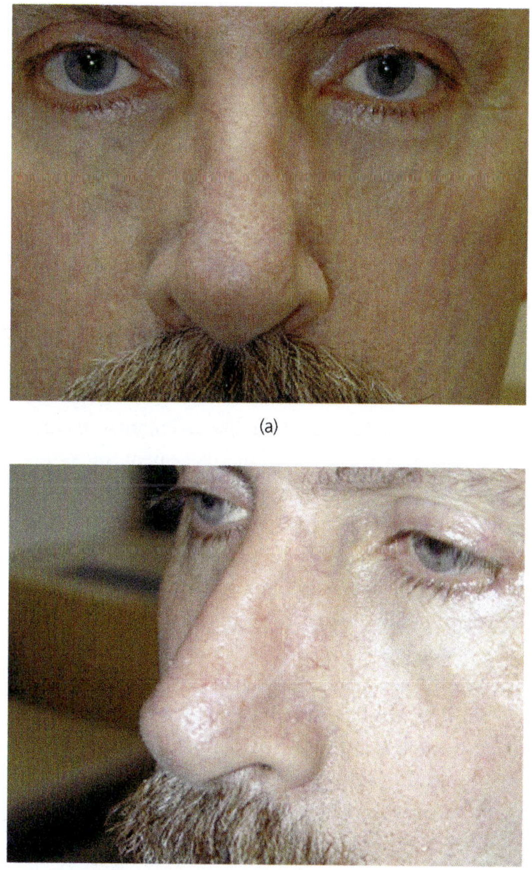

(a) (b)

Figure 3 (a) Six-month follow-up. (b) Oblique view with sidewall scar.

· Lateral incisions at the nasofacial junction, making sure not to violate the nasal sidewall subunit.

· Obliquely marked standing cone deformity excision ipsilateral to flap pedicle.

· Contouring the undersurface of the flap and soft tissue recipient bed before flap inset.

· Meticulous flap closure with 5-0 monocryl for deep tissue and 6-0 nylon for skin, making sure to allow for discrepancies in skin thickness.

· Consider postoperative dermabrasion at 6 weeks for mild contour correction.

References

1 Zitelli JA. The bilobed flap for nasal reconstruction. Arch Dermatol 1989;125:957–9.

2 Gillies HD. Plastic surgery of the face. London: Oxford Medical Publishers, 1920.

3 Rieger RA. A local flap for repair of the nasal tip. Plast Recon Surg 1967;40:147.

4 Zimbler MS, Thomas RJ. The dorsal nasal flap revisited: aesthetic refinements in nasal reconstruction. Arch Facial Plast Surg 2000;2:285–6.

Commentary on conundrum 8

This defect is one that dermatologic surgeons encounter fairly frequently. As with any defect, there are several possible repair strategies, including local flaps and grafts. In choosing among them, the surgeon should attempt to select an option that provides optimal color and texture match while minimizing visible scar lines. The skin surrounding the defect pictured in this case, located on the distal one-third of the nose, is sebaceous, so skin from a similarly textured area should be chosen. The dorsal nasal flap can be an excellent choice for defects in the range of 2 cm in this location. Its advantages include repair with adjacent nasal skin, placement of suture lines principally along the nasofacial sulcus and glabellar crease, and avoidance of extranasal suture lines. When using this flap, care must be taken to compensate for rotational shortening by designing it with a wide leading edge lateral arc. Failure to do so can result in disruption of alar symmetry.

The choice of a dorsal nasal flap in this case was an excellent one. The fact that this flap is large (something that can be quite scary for patients initially) and continues across the entire dorsum of the nose, however, translates to a good deal of suturing and the possibility of prominent lines along the proximal two-thirds of the nose. Nevertheless, these flaps tend to produce excellent results because the suture lines are generally hidden in the lateral "shadow" of the nasofacial sulcus. In Figure 3, these hypopigmented scars are, in fact, visible and could likely be improved or minimized with postsurgical ablative options including dermabrasion, traditional laser resurfacing, or even newer fractional laser modalities, whether ablative or nonablative. Figures 8.1a and b show the utility of two treatments of fractional ablative laser resurfacing to improve scar texture and color.[1] As the superior V to Y portion of the flap in this example directly overlies the corrugator muscles, perisurgical botulinum toxin injections could also be helpful in decreasing underlying muscle contraction, thereby decreasing tension on the overlying scar.[2]

The bilobed flap is another workhorse for reconstructing distal nasal defects, although the diameter of 2 × 2 cm for this particular defect is at the upper limit of what can be successfully repaired without disruption of alar symmetry. These flaps are generally employed for defects 1.5 cm or less on the nose, and the secondary lobule should be designed perpendicular to the alar rim to avoid contralateral alar elevation.[3] A laterally based bilobed flap would be a good choice for this defect, although secondary defect closure can at times produce unwanted tension on the medial canthus. If more than 90 degrees of rotational movement was required or if the flap was medially based, a trilobed flap could also

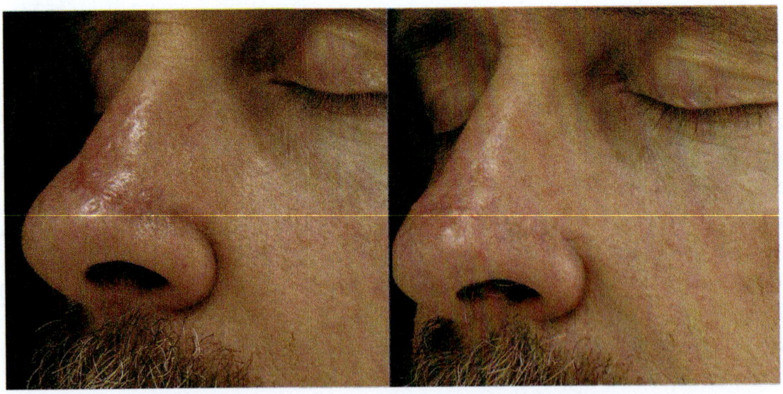

Figure 8.1 Five months after advancement flap repair of Mohs surgical defect of distal nasal sidewall and 6 weeks after second fractional ablative erbium laser resurfacing of scar. At this point, pulsed dye laser could be used to minimize persistent neovascular blush.

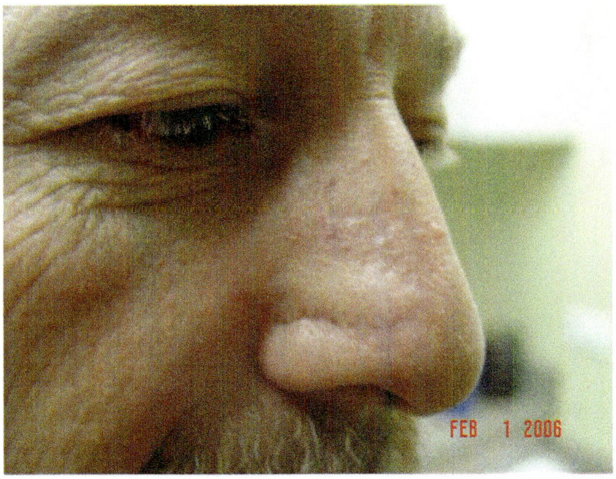

Figure 8.2 Pincushioned appearance of distal lobe of bilobed flap 5 months after Mohs surgical repair.

be considered.[4] "Pincushioning" of both types of flaps (Figure 8.2) may be minimized with careful suturing technique, aggressive undermining, and postoperative intralesional steroids. Occasionally, there is sufficient mobility of the nasal tissue to permit a simple linear closure of a rather larger defect (Figure 8.3). At times, an east–west advancement flap can also be considered, especially if the defect is considerably smaller than 2 cm (Figure 8.4).

Given the shallow nature of this particular defect, a full-thickness skin graft would also have been a good option, although a sebaceous donor site (such as the conchal bowl or glabella) would be essential for a male patient with prominent pores on his perilesional skin. Although nasolabial donor sites have been described, they are frequently unacceptable in men since the graft may transfer hair-bearing skin to the nose.[5] While a preauricular graft avoids the donor site morbidity of a granulating conchal bowl donor site and allows the scar to be hidden in the preauricular crease, this skin does not always match the sebaceous quality and texture of the distal nose. A Burow's full-thickness skin graft from

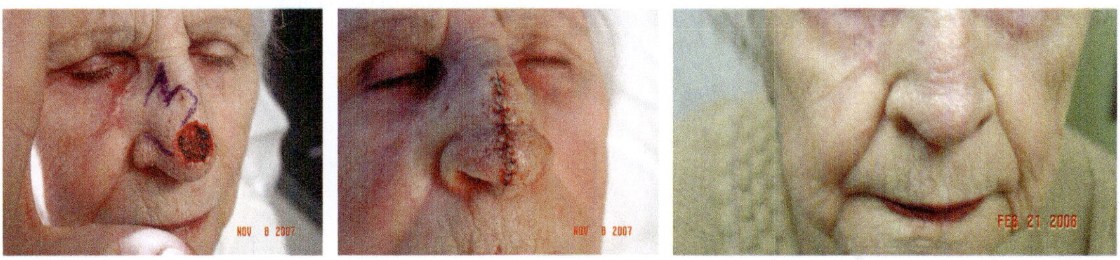

(a) (b) (c)

Figure 8.3 (a) A bilobed flap was planned for repair of this 1.4-cm Mohs defect. (b) With wide undermining, there was enough mobility to repair the defect in a linear fashion. (c) Follow-up at 3 months.

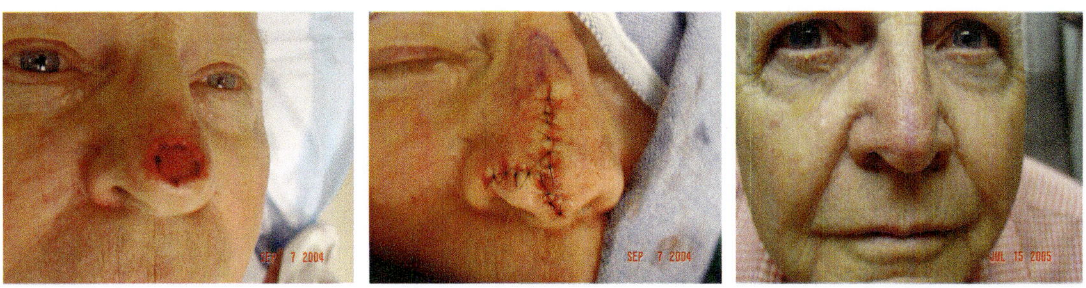

(a) (b) (c)

Figure 8.4 (a) Distal nasal defect; (b) repair with east-west advancement flap; (c) follow-up at 10 months.

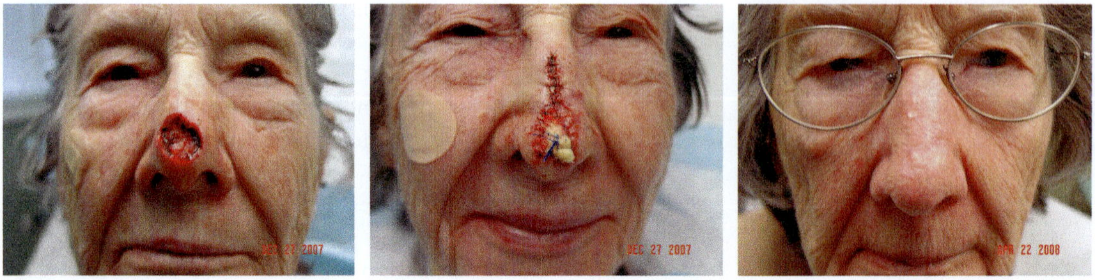

(a) (b) (c)

Figure 8.5 (a) Distal nasal defect; (b) repair with Burow's full-thickness skin graft from superiorly located triangle; (c) follow-up at 4 months.

closely matching superiorly located skin could therefore be considered in this location as well (Figure 8.5).

Commentary by Dr. Cohen

References

1 Vasily D, Cerina M, Ziselman E, Tannous Z. Non-ablative fractional resurfacing of surgical and post-traumatic scars. J Drugs Dermatol 2009;8(11):998–1005.

2 Flynn T. Use of intraoperative botulinum toxin in facial reconstruction. Dermatol Surg 2009;35(2):182–8.

3 Braun M, Cook J. The island pedicle flap. Dermatol Surg 2005;31(8 pt 2):995–1005.

4 Albertini J, Hansen J. Trilobed flap reconstruction for distal nasal skin defects. Dermatol Surg 2010;36(11):1726–35.

5 Hussain W, Hafiji J, Salmon P. The nasofacial sulcus as a primary donor site for full-thickness skin grafts of the nasal alar and distal nose. Dermatol Surg 2012;38(6):926–8.

9

CONUNDRUM 9

Adjunctive Use of Primary Nasal Tip Closure to Facilitate Local Flap Closure of Challenging Nasal Defects

Laura Gilman[1] & Galen Fisher[2]

[1]School of Medicine, Virginia Commonwealth University, Richmond, Virginia
[2]Laser and Skin Surgery Center of Richmond, Richmond, Virginia

Closure of large nasal tip and dorsum defects after Mohs micrographic surgery (MMS) is a challenge that Mohs reconstructive surgeons encounter frequently. When designing these closures, attention must be paid to functional preservation and esthetic restoration. Options for nasal reconstructions include healing by second intention, primary closure, skin grafting, local nasal flap repair, and staged interpolation flap reconstruction.

A 78-year-old Caucasian woman presented to our clinic for Mohs micrographic surgical extirpation of a persistent basal cell carcinoma of the nasal tip, which had been previously frozen. Following four stages of Mohs surgery, the site was deemed free of tumor and the resultant defect was ready for reconstruction.

Initially, all reconstructive options were considered for this case. Secondary intention was not felt to be a viable option for this defect. The defect was deemed too large for closure with a local flap such as a dorsal nasal rotation flap or a bilobed transposition flap. We next contemplated a full-thickness skin graft (FTSG), but because skin grafts on the nose often fail to match the local tissue in color and texture, we felt that our patient's cosmetic expectations would not be met with the use of a graft. Given the size of the lesion, we next discussed the use of an interpolated paramedian forehead flap. Pedicled forehead flaps are an excellent choice for optimal functional and esthetic restoration of large nasal defects. These flaps are highly vascular and versatile and have the advantage of resembling nasal tissue in contour, texture, and color. Despite the numerous advantages regarding final cosmesis and function of an interpolated paramedian forehead flap, morbidity associated with the procedure can preclude its use in patients who are not willing to undergo the staged procedure or who do not have a viable donor site. In our case, the forehead was deemed to be an excellent donor site, but the patient was not open to the use of an interpolation flap. Given the aforementioned parameters of patient expectations and closure options, we sought to modify the defect to allow for local flap closure in a single-stage procedure.

To achieve this goal, we devised a reconstructive approach that combined partial primary closure with a bilobed transposition flap. The use of partial primary closure of the nasal tip transformed her large nasal defect into a medium size nasal defect that was then suitable for closure with a traditional bilobed transposition flap. The patient had clinically appreciable nasal ptosis and a wide columella that allowed us to take advantage of

Reconstructive Conundrums in Dermatologic Surgery: The Nose, First Edition. Edited by Désirée Ratner, Joel L. Cohen and David G. Brodland.
© 2014 American Society for Dermatologic Surgery. Published 2014 by John Wiley & Sons, Ltd.

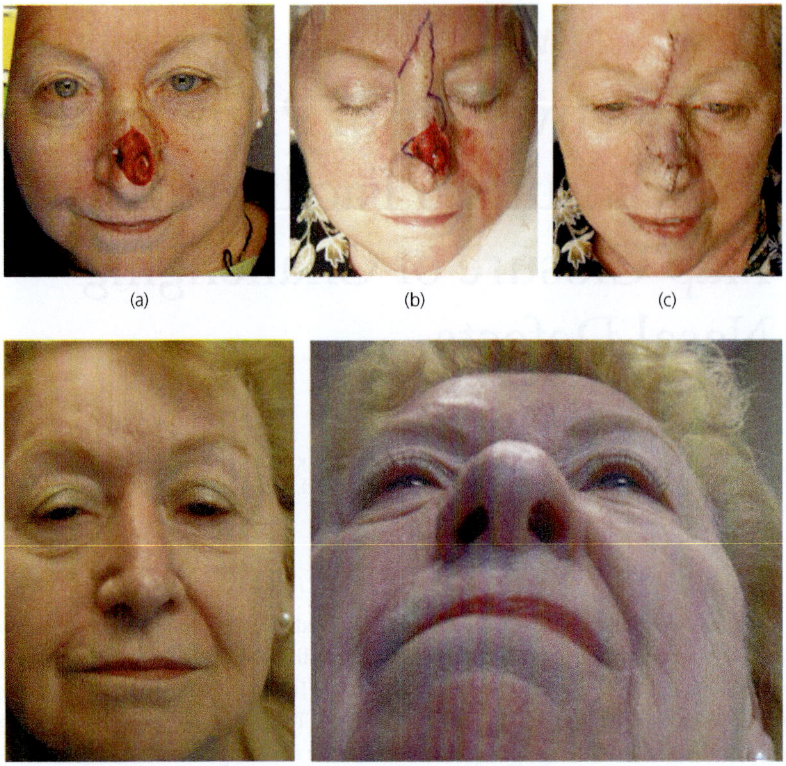

(a) (b) (c) (d) (e)

Figure 1 (a) Post-Mohs surgical defect of the nasal dorsum and tip. (b) Primary linear closure of the nasal tip complete and bilobed flap outlined. (c) Bilobed flap closure following primary partial closure of nasal tip. (d) Frontal and (e) caudal nasal views 11 months after surgery.

primary nasal tip closure to decrease wound size before bilobed flap reconstruction. The first step of her reconstruction was to excise a standard Burow's triangle from the caudal apex of the primary defect, which extended half the distance down the columella. After closure of this nasal tip Burow's triangle, a standard bilobed flap was designed and executed in standard fashion, taking care to undermine widely in the subnasalis plane. The primary lobe of the flap was cut to reflect the shape of the defect, although it was approximately 10% to 15% smaller in the vertical direction and was appropriately longer horizontally to account for rotational shortening of the flap. The small Y-shaped deformity at the cephalic margin of the primary closure was addressed using two subcuticular mattress sutures that were placed in the dermis and acted to mold the shape of this junction to the flap (Figure 1).

The mechanism by which this technique works is that the primary closure of the distal portion of the wound reduces the circumference of the wound; because tensions are shared relatively evenly around the perimeter of the wound, this results in smaller dimensions of the defect in the medial–lateral (horizontal) and the cephalad–caudad (vertical) directions. Although we have used this technique only with the bilobed flap, we believe that it is possible to apply it to other local flap closures such as the dorsal nasal flap. The technique could also theoretically be used intraoperatively, in the event that unanticipated nasal distortion or excessive flap tension arose with the originally designed flap; again, we have not had the opportunity to apply primary tip closure under this scenario but suspect that it could prove useful in a subset of patients (Figure 2).

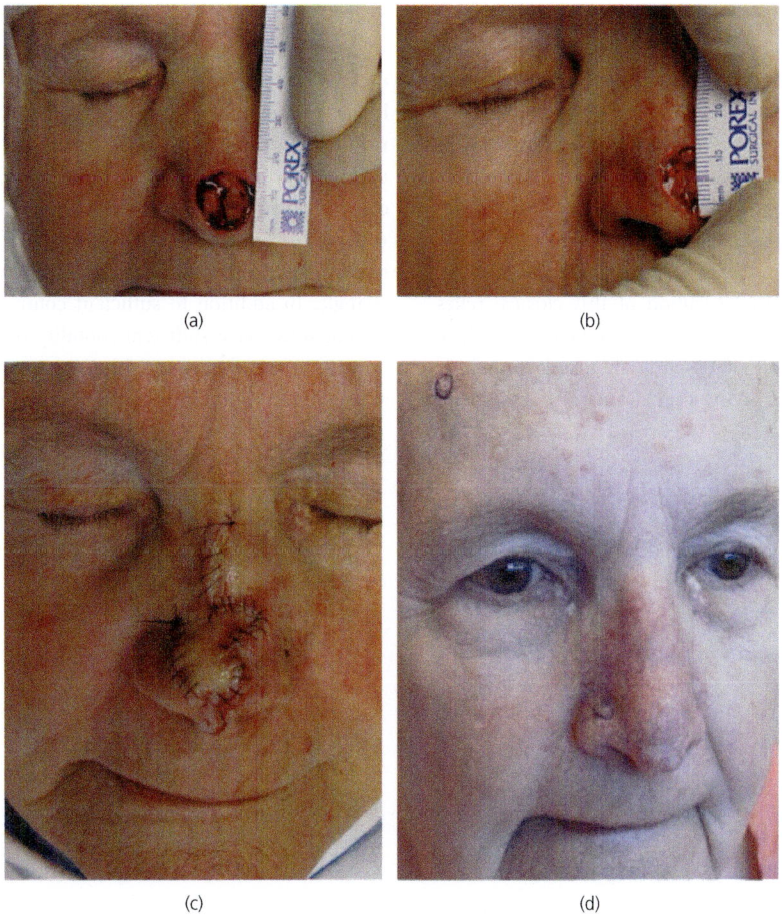

Figure 2 In this different surgical case, an 85-year-old woman underwent Mohs micrographic surgery for a basal cell carcinoma on the nose. (a) After Mohs surgical extirpation, wound measuring 1.7 cm in diameter. (b) The distal portion of the surgical defect was approximated with primary closure, leaving a defect measuring 1.3 cm in diameter. (c) Frontal view of bilobed flap repair after primary closure. (d) Frontal view of repair 12 months after surgery.

Notes regarding candidate selection and technical considerations

Patients with medium to large nasal defects that are limited to the tip and distal nasal dorsum may be good candidates for this type of closure. In our experience, defects that are 1.5 cm or smaller, on a typically dimensioned nose, can be successfully closed using local flaps, such as a dorsal nasal rotation flap or a bilobed transposition flap. Traditional local flaps involve simpler incision lines than the above-mentioned procedure, with surgical invasion into fewer anatomic subunits of the nose, but in cases in which the defect is larger than 1.5 cm in diameter, use of local flaps can cause significant distortion, and surgeons have traditionally used paramedian forehead flaps and FTSGs for closure. The use of primary nasal closure in combination with local flap closure transforms defects that are too large for traditional flap repair into defects that are of appropriate size for traditional repair while avoiding more morbid techniques such as pedicle forehead flap or less cosmetically rewarding approaches such as a FTSG.

After partial primary tip closure, the resultant defect could have been closed using a dorsal nasal or a bilobed flap. Although the lines of a bilobed flap are more complex than those of a dorsal nasal flap, it is the authors' experience that the bilobed flap is more predictable with regard to its mobility and final result, and for that reason we chose to use a bilobed transposition flap for closure once the tip had been reduced.

Care must be taken to assess each patient individually, because the successful execution of this closure relies on precise tissue rearrangement. In candidates who lack a significant reservoir of tissue in the caudal nasal tip and columellar area or the cephalic nasal dorsum and glabellar area, the final outcome may be less optimal. The success of this repair depends on partial primary closure decreasing the vertical dimension of the defect, and this hinges on adjacent tissue laxity and mobility in the tip region. Care should be taken to remove no more than 60% to 70% of the width of the columella. The nascent columellar width limits the effect of the flap. Patients with wider columellar width are inherently better candidates because they can tolerate excision of a wider Burow's triangle. In addition to sufficient columellar width, the patient must have sufficient mobility of the nasal skin, because a partial closure without enough mobility may affect only the horizontal width of the defect.

Commentary on conundrum 9

The primary message and the most important learning point in this case is the value of "strategic subclosures" to facilitate wound closure with local flaps. There are situations in which combining simple side-to-side closure of portions of a defect will facilitate closures that would otherwise be difficult to accomplish. This case illustrates that some wounds in which multistaged forehead flaps may be the first consideration can actually be repaired with a single-stage closure.

The surgeon must assess all aspects of the wound and its surrounding donor tissue and identify ways of reconfiguring the defect in a fashion that would be amenable to a local flap. Two conditions must be present. First, a portion of the defect must be amenable to some form of closure independent of the principal anticipated reconstruction. The second condition is that there needs to be ample laxity or donor skin in the area of "subclosure." With these conditions met, the creative reconstructive surgeon can often accomplish a single-stage closure that would not have ordinarily been possible.

The process of identifying potential areas for "strategic subclosures" involves assessing the laxity at the wound perimeter and identifying portions of the wound that may be enlarged due to areas of gaping. The surgeon must remember that upon excision of a tumor, the final defect size is usually considerably larger than the actual size of the tissue removed. Often, this can be a consideration in planning a primary flap closure and can also be used to identify loose skin amenable to side-to-side closure to decrease the overall size of the wound. Another case with a defect located on the zygoma shows how a partial closure of the superomedial portion of the defect makes possible a single-stage closure with a substantially smaller flap than would have been necessary otherwise (Figures 9.1–9.3).

Another instructive concept illustrated in this case is the level of undermining required for a bilobed flap. Inclusion of the nasalis muscle within the flap optimizes its vascularity, making the bilobed flap extremely robust and resistant to distal necrosis. Furthermore, undermining widely toward the nasofacial sulcus can optimize mobility and increase flap reach to the most distal portions of the defect. The risk of postoperative bleeding is minimized compared to when undermining is performed in the subcutaneous plane. It must be remembered that while suturing the primary lobe into the defect, the dermal sutures must be placed such that the slightly retracted muscularis layer is included in the suture bite on the flap side. This ensures that the thickness of the flap is uniform and promotes optimal contour postoperatively.

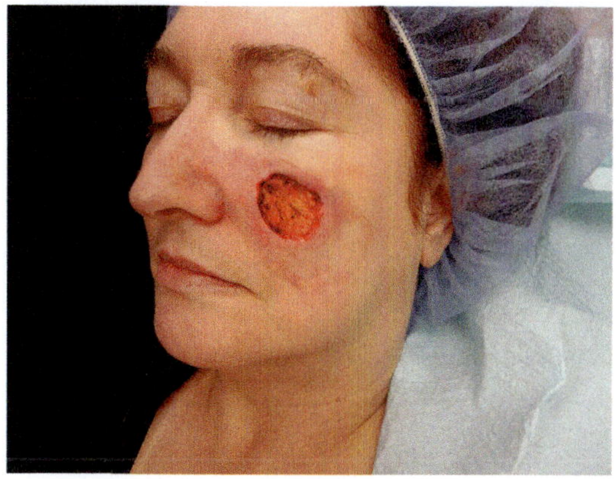

Figure 9.1 Large defect on the midcheek.

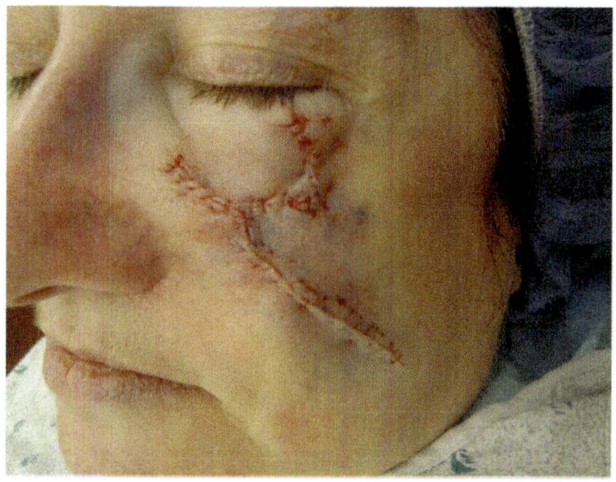

Figure 9.2 The partial closure of the medial portion of the wound, represented by the medial diagonal sutured line, enables closure of the remainder of the wound with a small rhombic flap.

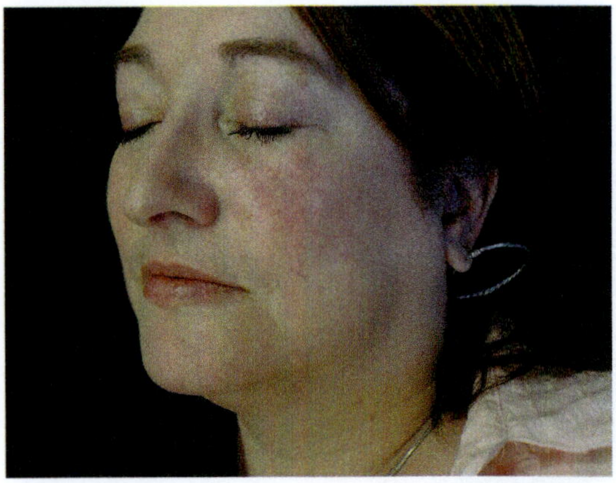

Figure 9.3 Three-month follow-up view with resolving suture lines and no eyelid distortion.

The second case depicted in Figure 2, in my estimation, may have not been as optimal an instance in which to consider primary closure of the nasal tip. In the long-term follow-up view, there seems to be a persistent flare of the alae and an undesirable downward protrusion of the nasal infratip resulting in unnatural tip angulation. The specifics of this case are unknown and the result may well have been worth it if a two-stage closure was avoided, and the patient could not have tolerated a forehead flap or cheek interpolation flap. However, this case clearly shows the potential for distortion of the lower third of the nose with relatively minor tissue movement.

Commentary by Dr. Brodland

10

CONUNDRUM 10

Repair of a Large, Exposed-Cartilage Nasal Tip Defect Using Nasalis-Based Subcutaneous Pedicle Flaps and Full-Thickness Skin Grafting

Diego E. Marra, Edgar F. Fincher, Julie Iwasaki, & Ronald L. Moy
David Geffen School of Medicine at UCLA and West Los Angeles VA Medical Center, Los Angeles, California

Large full-thickness nasal tip defects after Mohs surgery present a challenge to the reconstructive surgeon. The interpolated paramedian forehead flap is the standard modality to repair such defects, especially when exposed cartilage is present.[1] Despite providing an excellent cosmetic outcome, some patients are reluctant to undergo this procedure due to the associated temporary deformity, the permanent forehead scar, and the need for at least two stages to achieve a successful outcome.

A 62-year-old Caucasian man was referred for Mohs micrographic surgery for an infiltrative basal cell carcinoma on the nasal tip. Complete excision of the tumor required five surgical stages, resulting in a 2.3 × 2-cm defect through which exposed alar cartilages and upper lateral cartilages could be seen (Figure 1). How would you reconstruct this defect?

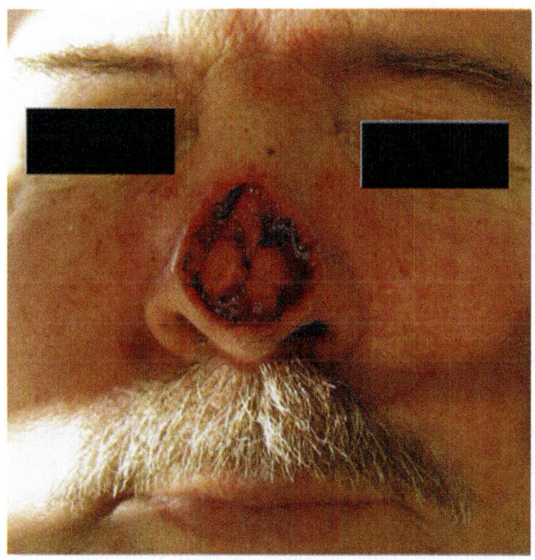

Figure 1 Surgical defect after Mohs micrographic surgery, measuring 2.3 × 2 cm. Exposed alar cartilages and upper lateral cartilages can be seen.

Resolution

The patient was an ideal candidate for the interpolated paramedian forehead flap, but refused to undergo the procedure. Given the depth of the defect and presence of exposed nasal cartilage, a full-thickness skin graft alone would have been unlikely to provide adequate coverage. We therefore designed nasalis-based subcutaneous

Reconstructive Conundrums in Dermatologic Surgery: The Nose, First Edition. Edited by Désirée Ratner, Joel L. Cohen and David G. Brodland.
© 2014 American Society for Dermatologic Surgery. Published 2014 by John Wiley & Sons, Ltd.

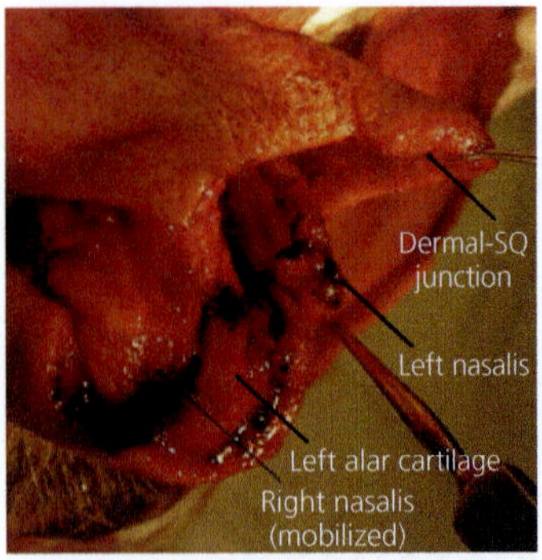

(a)

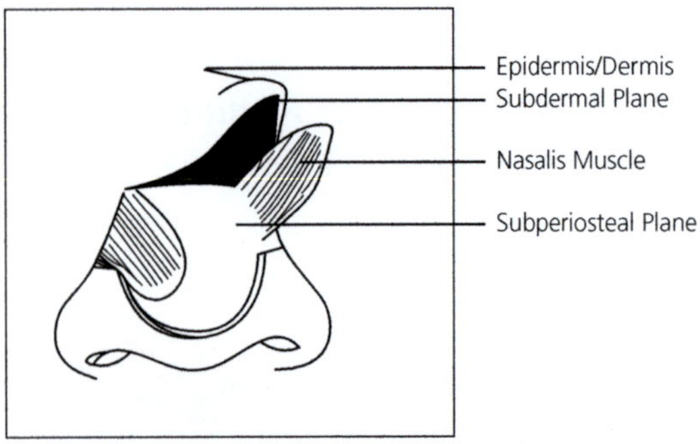

(b)

Figure 2 Intraoperative photograph (a) and schematic (b) showing elevation of nasalis-based subcutaneous pedicle flaps, created by dissecting first along the subdermal plane, followed by dissection along the subperiosteal plane. The nasalis muscle on the patient's right side has already been dissected and rotated into position. The lower skin hook on the photograph points to the left nasalis muscle, which is being elevated.

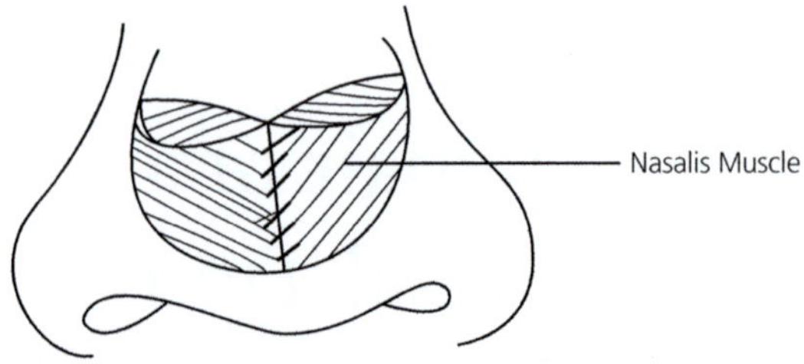

Figure 3 The right and left subcutaneous flaps are rotated and advanced inferomedially to the defect margin and secured to the underlying cartilage. The medial aspects of each subcutaneous flap are then sutured together in a corsetlike fashion to completely line all previously exposed nasal cartilage.

pedicle flaps to restore the nasal contour and provide a vascular bed suitable for grafting.

An incision was made along both alar grooves extending to the nasofacial sulcus to facilitate exposure and superolateral dissection. Nasalis-based subcutaneous pedicle flaps were elevated by dissecting first along the subdermal plane, followed by dissection along the subperiosteal plane (Figure 2). The midline aponeurosis connecting the two elevated nasalis muscles was then divided, and careful dissection and judicious back-cutting of each pedicle along its superolateral margin were performed to maximize tissue movement. The right and left subcutaneous flaps thus created were rotated and advanced inferomedially to the defect margin and secured to the underlying cartilage with 4-0 polyglactin absorbable sutures. The medial aspects of each subcutaneous flap were then sutured together in a corset fashion to completely line all previously exposed nasal cartilage (Figure 3). The overlying cutaneous flap was then advanced inferiorly to the tip-supratip aesthetic subunit junction and secured. Finally, a full-thickness skin graft was harvested from the supraclavicular area and used to line the tip.

At the time of suture removal 1 week later, complete survival of the graft was noted. Superiorly directed force vectors resulted in approximately 5 mm of nasal tip elevation immediately postprocedure; however, this had diminished significantly after 1 week and had nearly completely resolved after 2 months. Six months after the procedure and 6 weeks after manual dermabrasion, the area showed a smooth contour without indentation or irregularities (Figure 4).

Discussion

Combined full-thickness nasal tip and supratip defects represent a challenge to the reconstructive surgeon. The usual treatment of choice remains the paramedian forehead flap. Limitations for the use of this procedure, however, occasionally require alternative methods to reconstruct such defects.

The anatomy of the nasalis muscle and its application to flap design have been described in outstanding detail by Papadopoulos and Trinei.[2] The main (transverse) body of the nasalis muscle arises from the maxilla and inserts with the muscle of the opposite side into the midline aponeurosis as it crosses the dorsum of the nose.[3]

This aponeurosis joins and forms a broader fusion with the aponeurosis of the procerus muscle.[2] The muscle also

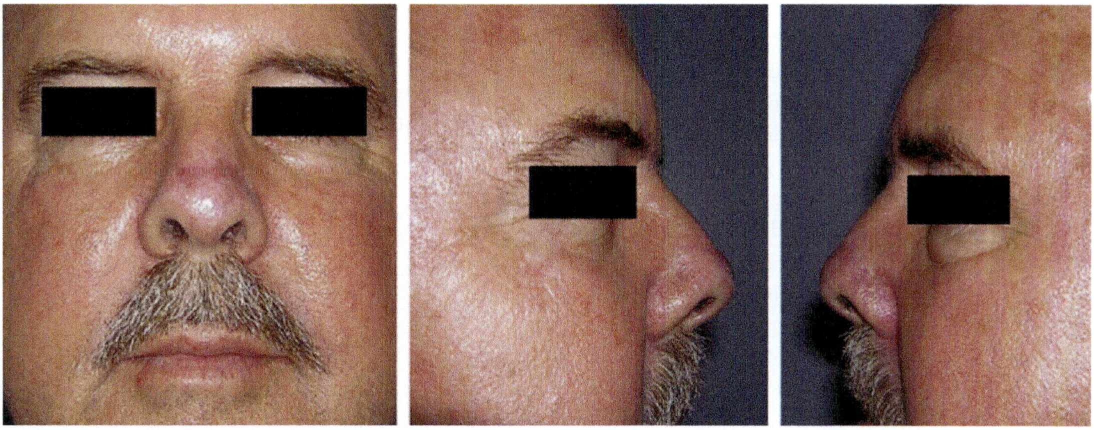

Figure 4 Appearance 6 months after the procedure. The patient underwent manual dermabrasion 6 weeks before this photograph.

inserts to some degree into the skin of the nasolabial sulcus.[3] The nasalis muscle has a rich blood supply based on the nasal artery.

These anatomic considerations, and the concept that skin can be sustained by its underlying muscle through perforating cutaneous vessels, was exploited by Papadopoulos and Trinei[2] to design a superiorly based myocutaneous island pedicle flap with bilevel undermining for reconstruction of nasal tip and supratip defects. Their technique relies on undermining that is carried out in two planes, a subcutaneous one (between the subcutaneous fat and nasalis muscle lateral to the flap) and a submuscular one (beneath the nasalis muscle and beneath the flap). This allows the surgeon to suspend the island of skin on two distinct muscular slings, which provides mobility and ensures proper arterial supply to the cutaneous component of the flap.[2] While extremely useful in the proper clinical setting, however, use of this flap is limited in large defects (especially those whose craniocaudal dimension exceeds 2 cm), in defects placed far distally on the nasal tip, and in patients with insufficient amounts of recruitable superior laxity. The patient presented here fit all of these criteria and was not considered a candidate for this repair option.

Building on these concepts and the principles of Papadopoulos and Trinei, we relied on the rich vascular supply of the nasalis muscle and the ability to create a vascularized sling following bilevel undermining to create purely subcutaneous flaps. These were then rotated and advanced inferomedially to provide both bulk to the deep defect, as well as a vascular bed suitable for grafting, which would not have been possible over exposed nasal cartilage. The technique has been described in the plastic surgery literature[4] and, more recently, in an excellent case series in the dermatologic surgical literature.[5] Our technique incorporates incisions along both alar grooves to facilitate exposure and superolateral dissection, which may be difficult to otherwise carry out safely when the defect is placed far distally on the nasal tip, as in this case.

Bilevel dermal undermining in conjunction with full-thickness skin grafting has been used to reconstruct defects of the nasal dorsum, with good results.[6] More recently, Salmon and Stanway[5] have published their experience with the nasalis flap and graft repair for denuded defects of the nose, utilizing either the nasalis anomalous or the nasalis transversus as the basis for the subcutaneous pedicle flap. Their series underscores the safety and reliability of the procedure. Of 26 patients undergoing reconstruction with the technique, 2 patients developed partial superficial graft necrosis involving less than one-third of the graft. In both cases, this resolved to leave a satisfactory contour and a small area of hypopigmentation. One patient developed postoperative infection, which resolved with oral antibiotics and without significant graft necrosis. In all patients, a natural contour was achieved following reconstruction.[5]

Several important technical aspects should be noted. It is important to carry the bilevel undermining sufficiently superolaterally to achieve maximum mobility without excessive back-cutting of the pedicle, which would compromise the flap's viability. Lateral dissection in the subcutaneous plane is likely to disrupt significant perforator vessels, and careful attention to hemostasis is required. This is partly the reason for extending incisions along the alar groove, as the necessary exposure for proper undermining and hemostasis would otherwise be difficult to achieve. In our experience, these incisions, which are closed without tension, generally heal with imperceptible scars. Patients must also be warned that the superior tension vector created by advancing the subcutaneous pedicle flap to the distal edge of the defect may result in significant nasal tip elevation. Although it is likely for this deformity to self-correct to a significant extent, that may not always be the case.

In conclusion, we have described the use of nasalis-based subcutaneous pedicle flaps for reconstruction of a large full-thickness nasal tip defect after Mohs surgery. This technique effectively restores nasal contour and provides a vascular bed for successful full-thickness skin grafting, even in the setting of exposed nasal cartilage. Given its well-defined anatomic basis, ease of execution, and ability to be performed in a single stage, this technique may be a valuable repair option in patients who are not candidates for, or do not wish to undergo, multistage interpolated reconstructive procedures. Furthermore, nasalis myofascial flaps combined with full-thickness skin grafts may be a valuable alternative to provide lining or bulk for smaller nasal defects when local skin flaps are not indicated.

References

1 Baker SR, Naficy S. Principles of nasal reconstruction. St. Louis: Mosby; 2002.
2 Papadopoulos DJ, Trinei FA. Superiorly based nasalis myocutaneous island pedicle flap with bilevel undermining for nasal tip and supratip reconstruction. Dermatol Surg 1999;25:530–6.
3 Salasche SJ, Bernstein G, Senkarik M. Surgical anatomy of the skin. East Norwalk (CT): Appleton & Lange; 1988.
4 Letourneau A, Daniel RK. The superficial musculoaponeurotic system of the nose. Plast Reconstr Surg 1988;82:48–57.
5 Salmon P, Stanway A. Nasalis flap and graft repair provides reliable closure for denuded defects of the nose. Dermatol Surg 2005;31:692–6.
6 Menaker GM, Moy RL, Lamb P. Surgical pearl: dermal advancement flaps for filling deep dorsal nasal defects under grafts. J Am Acad Dermatol 1998;39:478–80.

Commentary

The nose is the most common location for basal cell carcinomas, and dermasurgeons have become experts in the reconstruction of defects on the nose. There are numerous reconstructive options for defects on the nose. The goal of the surgeon is to pick the option that predictably yields the best functional and cosmetic outcome. The authors describe the use of bilateral "nasalis-based subcutaneous pedicle flaps" in reconstruction of a large, deep defect on the nose. This is essentially a double muscular hinge flap.[1] The nasalis muscles from each side are mobilized to replace a soft tissue defect and provide a vascular bed for a full-thickness skin graft. This is a viable alternative to a forehead flap. One can expect the graft to hypopigment over time, however. This is one of the drawbacks of a full-thickness skin graft that is typically not seen with a forehead flap.

Ali Hendi, MD
Jacksonville, FL

Reference

1 Fader DJ, Wang TS, Johnson TM. Nasal reconstruction utilizing a muscle hinge flap with overlying full-thickness skin graft. J Am Acad Dermatol 2000;43:837–40.

Commentary on conundrum 10

This nasalis-based subcutaneous pedicle flap followed by a full-thickness skin graft provided a wonderful cosmetic result for this nasal tip defect, although using periauricular rather than supraclavicular donor skin might have produced an even better tissue match and cosmetic result. As the authors point out, a paramedian forehead flap is often one of the best options for defects of this size and extent with exposed cartilage. Although this flap can almost "mimic" the exact tip subunit, it is a big procedure that necessitates a large forehead scar that can sometimes be prominent (Figure 10.1), and may require revision, making single-stage flap or graft procedures a more attractive option in selected cases. Given the depth and diameter of this defect, a paramedian forehead flap would offer a consistent, esthetically elegant result. Furthermore, the thickness of tissue provided by a paramedian forehead flap would be more likely to recreate the anterior projection of the distal nose, which has been lost in this case.

Another option not discussed in this review is the superiorly based one-stage nasolabial flap, which would be of sufficient size and bulk to cover this deep defect. In designing this type of flap, the leading edge cut would be placed at about the 3-o'clock aspect of the defect and would continue down the cheek parallel to the left nasolabial fold. Excision of a standing cone at the inferior aspect of the donor site would be required as well as excision of a standing cone at the superior aspect of the defect once the flap is inset. A periosteal tacking suture may help to preserve the concavity of the superior alar groove and avoid a blunted or flattened groove (Figure 10.2). Even so, this type of flap would still have a chance of requiring postoperative revision, either to diminish the thickness of any "trapdooring," or to blend the demarcation points of the suture lines using an ablative procedure. A one- or a two-stage nasolabial flap may also produce slight lower facial asymmetry due to blunting of the superior nasolabial fold (Figure 10.3). Large defects of the nasal tip can also be left to heal to allow a "delayed" full-thickness skin graft to be performed a few weeks after tumor extirpation.[1]

All in all, as illustrated by this case, hinge flaps can be quite useful for the repair of deep defects, particularly those with exposed cartilage, because they provide structural as well as vascular support over which these grafts

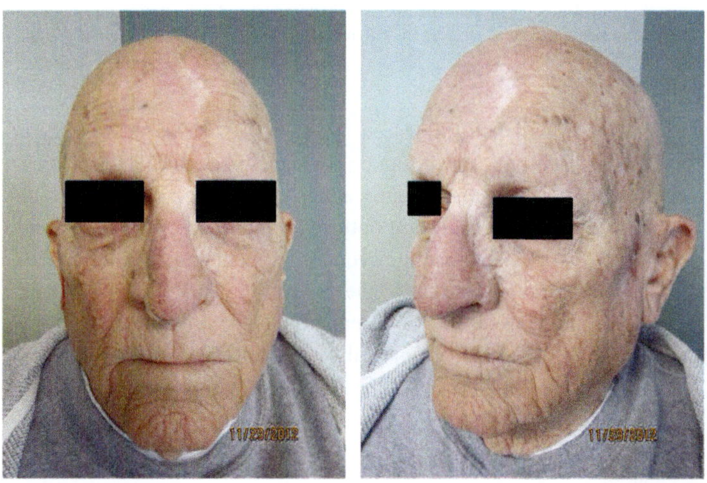

(a) (b)

Figure 10.1 (a) Anterior view showing forehead scar after paramedian forehead flap. (b) Side view of the forehead scar and final result of nasal repair.

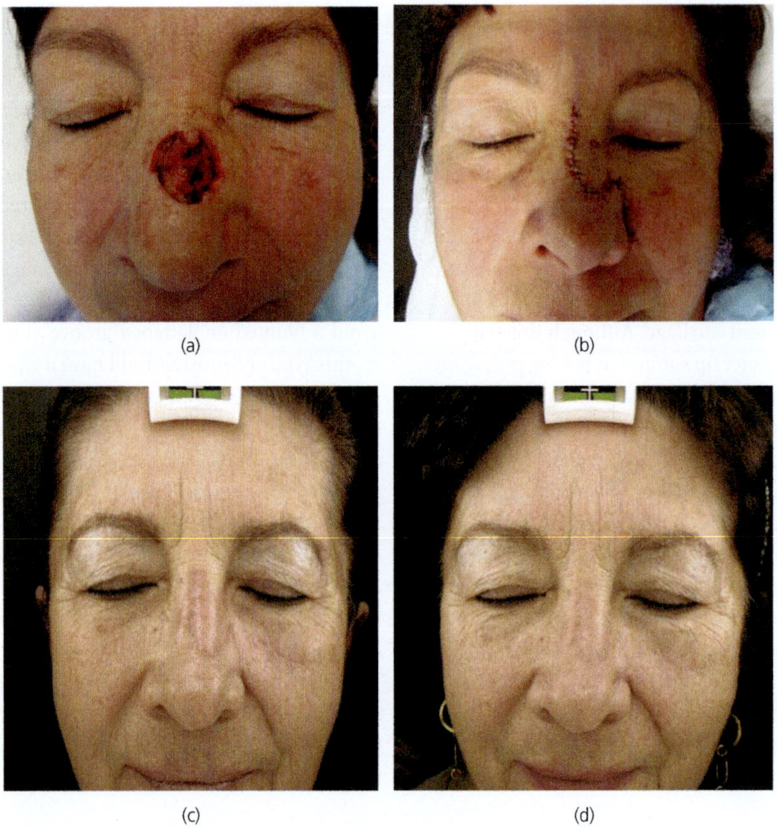

Figure 10.2 (a) Defect of the nasal dorsum after Mohs surgery. (b) Immediately post-repair with one-stage nasolabial flap. A periosteal tacking suture can preserve concavity of the superior alar groove. (c) Scar line prominence 4 months after repair. (d) Two months after second ablative fractional erbium resurfacing along the scar.

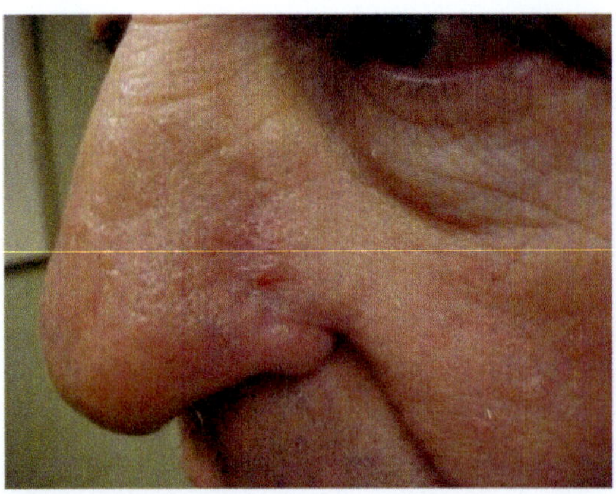

Figure 10.3 Blunted alar groove after one-stage nasolabial transposition flap.

can then be placed (Figure 10.4). However, regardless of the repair option ultimately selected, a discussion with patients using either drawings or photographs of potential closure options is important. Should postsurgical revision be required, patients are typically more understanding if the possibilities are discussed either at a consultation appointment before surgery or in a thorough fashion at the time of repair.

Commentary by Dr. Cohen

Reference

1 Robinson J, DIllig G. The advantages of delayed nasal full-thickness grafting after Mohs micrographic surgery. Dermatol Surg 2002;28(9):845–51.

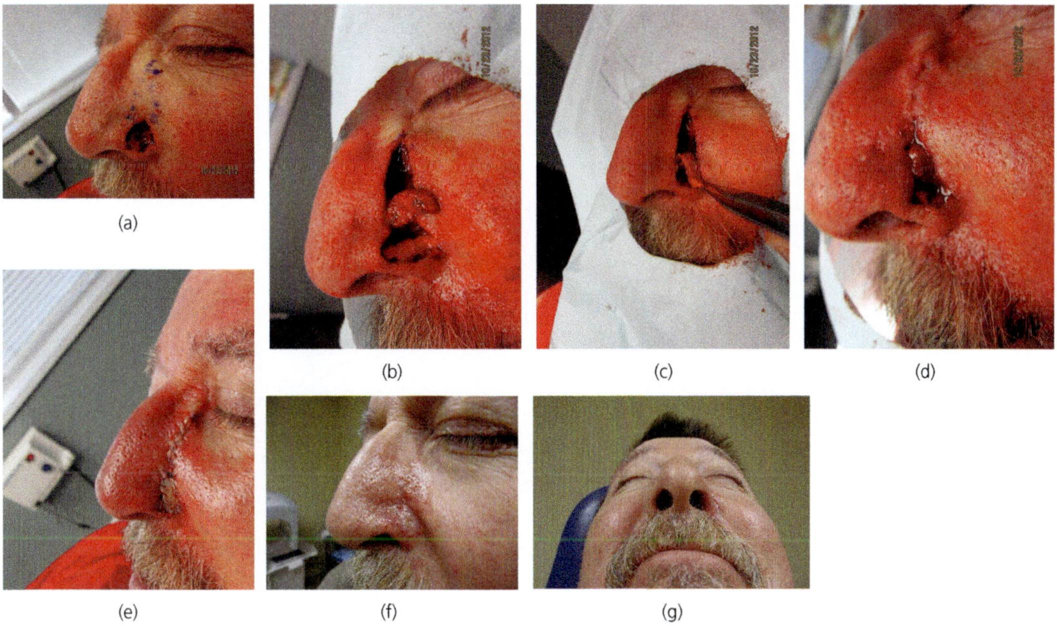

Figure 10.4 (a) Mohs surgical defect of the left nasal ala. (b) Cartilage strut in place, with hinge flap prepared from deep tissue of superior Burow's triangle. (c) Hinge flap transposed over the cartilage strut. (d) Linear closure of superior dog ear and tacking down of the hinge flap. (e) Burow's full-thickness skin graft sewn into place. (f) Lateral view 8 weeks post-repair. (g) Swimmer's view demonstrating alar symmetry after 8 weeks.

11

CONUNDRUM 11

Nasal Tip Wound Repair Using a Rhombic Transposition Flap with a Double Z-Plasty at Its Base

Adam M. Rotunda[1] *& Richard G. Bennett*[2]

[1]Department of Dermatology, University of Southern California School of Medicine, Los Angeles, CA
[2]Department of Medicine (Dermatology), University of California at Los Angeles School of Medicine, Los Angeles, CA

A 65-year-old Caucasian woman with a primary basal cell carcinoma on the nasal tip was referred for Mohs micro-graphic surgery. The patient had a history of breast cancer and mild hypertension and was a non-smoker. The tumor appeared as a red, smooth macule that measured 0.5 × 0.5 cm. The basal cell carcinoma was completely removed with two stages of Mohs micro-graphic surgery. The final surgical defect measured 0.9 × 0.8 cm on the midnasal tip and extended in depth to the midsubcutaneous tissue (Figure 1). How would you manage this wound?

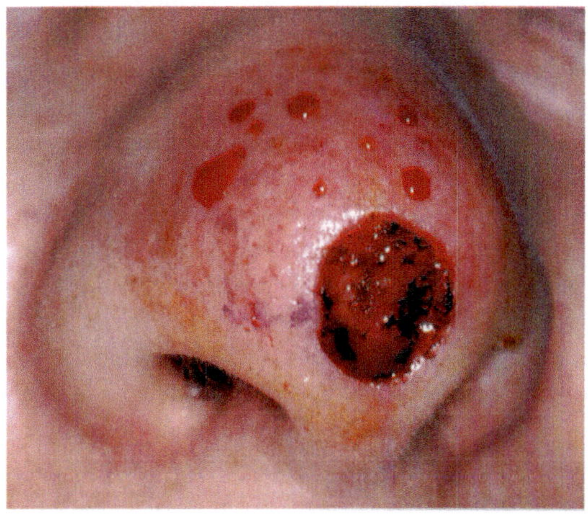

Figure 1 Postoperative Mohs defect on the nasal tip measuring 0.9 × 0.8 cm and extending to midsubcutaneous tissue. Note that the long axis of the elliptic defect is vertical and the short axis is horizontal. Also, the small angles for closure are superior and inferior.

Resolution

Small (<1-cm) nasal tip defects can be repaired in several ways. Our patient had a surgical defect that extended to the midsubcutaneous tissue and did not involve perichondrium or cartilage. Her nasal skin was smooth and not particularly porous. In addition, the skin surrounding the defect donor skin was not particularly mobile. The wound could granulate and close by second intention. This type of healing, however, takes approximately 6 weeks, and the cosmetic outcome is unpredictable. Sometimes, the resultant scar is depressed and quite noticeable, especially when the wound is relatively deep as in this case. A skin graft in a nasal tip defect can be considered. If the patient has porous nasal skin, however, the skin graft is generally a poor texture match. Some authors advocate grafting adjacent skin[1] or conchal bowl skin[2] to minimize the mismatched skin texture problem. Despite use of these donor sites, however, there may still be color and texture mismatch or a noticeable, round wound edge. Skin grafts, nevertheless, may be desirable

Reconstructive Conundrums in Dermatologic Surgery: The Nose, First Edition. Edited by Désirée Ratner, Joel L. Cohen and David G. Brodland.

© 2014 American Society for Dermatologic Surgery. Published 2014 by John Wiley & Sons, Ltd.

particularly for superficial, larger defects on the nose tip. It has been our experience that small skin grafts on the nasal tip are more noticeable than large skin grafts on the same area. This relative imperceptibility of a large skin graft is due to the fact that a complete or almost a complete nasal aesthetic unit is replaced.

A skin flap is the optimal method to repair a small, deep nasal tip defect. Because the surrounding skin is relatively immobile, however, options for local flaps are limited. Possible local flaps that may be considered in this area include a bilateral rotation flap (the "Peng" flap),[3] myocutaneous island pedicle flap,[4] or a bilobed transposition flap.[5] The bilateral rotation flap would result in nasal tip elevation and curvilinear lines along the sides of the nose. The myocutaneous island pedicle flap would also result in nasal tip elevation and, in our hands, is technically difficult. The bilobed flap is another possibility. In our present case, however, the 45° bilobed flap would tend to raise the ala and the 90° bilobed flap would shorten the tissue along the nasal bridge. In either case, in noses of certain size and shape, a saddle nose deformity may result. This latter contour issue is rarely pointed out in bilobed flap descriptions.[5]

We chose to repair the defect with a rhombic transposition flap with a double Z-plasty at its base. The wound as shown in Figure 1 is roughly an ellipse with the long axis vertically oriented and the short axis horizontally oriented. The angle of closure for a transposition flap is the small angle, which is superior and inferior in this case. Because of a lack of columella skin inferiorly, a rhombic flap design could only be done with a lateral and superior incision as shown in Figure 2. To enhance the flap movement and to preclude alar rim elevation, a second flap was necessary. We chose to add two small rhombic flaps (which we have formerly referred to as double Z-plasties[6]) instead of one additional rhombic flap, which would have created a birhombic flap. Using the smaller rhombic flaps (which are actually Z-plasties), we avoided alar rim elevation and, more importantly, dorsal nasal depression (saddle nose deformity).

The mobility of a rhombic transposition flap can be enhanced by the addition of a double Z-plasty.[6] The first Z-plasty triangle is created with a 90° to 105° angle to the rhombic flap and with one 60° angle in the Z-plasty tip, while the second Z-plasty triangle is created at a 90° angle to the first Z-plasty and a 60° angle in the second Z-plasty tip (Figure 2). Although the angle between the first and second Z-plasty was originally described as 60°, we have observed that a 90° angle works better.[7] The bilobed transposition flap uses a similar design concept. The bilobed flap, however, uses two large rounded donor flaps, rather than one rhombic flap and two smaller Z-plasty flaps. After healing, the rounded closure lines of the bilobed flap are more likely to be visible and cause trapdooring than the angulated closure lines of the rhombic flap with two Z-plasties. In addition, the bilobed flap can cause significant dorsal nasal depression and alar elevation.

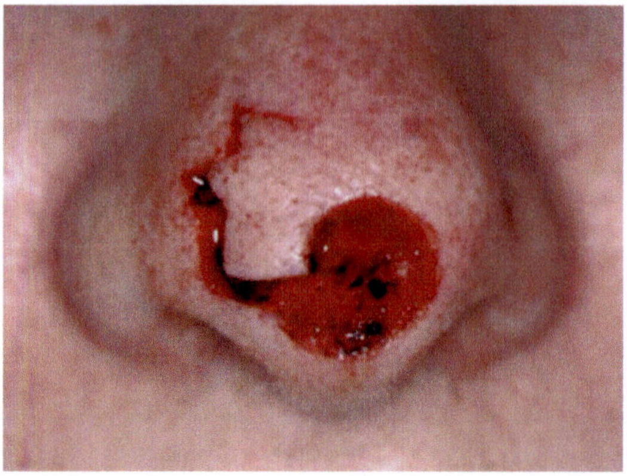

Figure 2 Rhombic flap with two Z-plasties, cut and undermined.

In our case, the 105° angle of the first Z-plasty allowed an additional medial and inferior movement to the rhombic flap (Figures 2 and 3). The second Z-plasty triangle at 90° to the first Z-plasty triangle further enhanced the same movement. The first Z-plasty triangle helped to close the rhombic flap donor defect. Thus, movement of

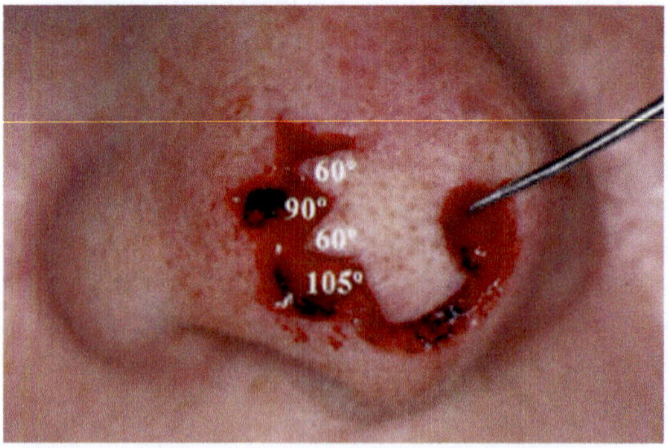

Figure 3 Flap mobilized. Note that the first Z-plasty will help close the rhombic flap donor site and thus will prevent alar rim deviation.

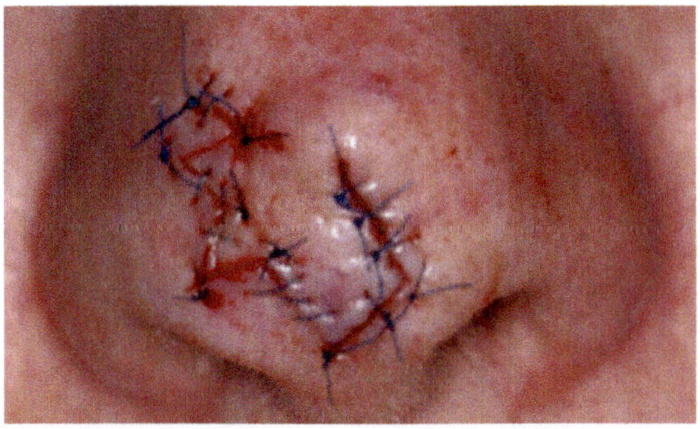

Figure 4 Flap sutured into place. Note that the recipient wound edges have been squared off to coapt the right angles of the rhombic flap.

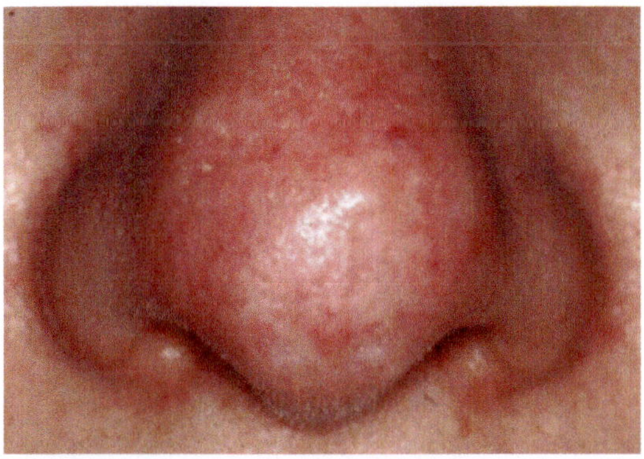

Figure 5 Healed nasal tip 2 years postoperatively. Note absence of alar rim distortion and the inconspicuous closure lines.

the flap into the donor site created minimal nasal distortion at the time of repair (Figure 4). A slight standing cone (dog ear) was created at the rhombic flap base. Since the rhombic flap base was narrowed by the two Z-plasties and to avoid cutting the blood supply to the flap, we chose not to remove the standing cone at the time of surgery. On physical examination 2 years after surgery, the patient had an excellent cosmetic result with an inconspicuous surgical scar and no structural nasal distortion (Figure 5). Although the standing cone is still slightly present 2 years after surgery, it is barely noticeable. On a relatively firm surface such as the nasal tip, the standing cone usually will improve slowly over about 6 to 12 months after surgery. We always leave the decision to correct the standing cone to the patient. Options for correction are injection with triamcinolone (Kenalog-10), pressure massage for 1 minute several times daily, or excision.

Conundrum keys

- Use of the Z-plasty at the base of a transposition flap, such as the rhombic flap, can enhance flap mobility.
- Properly constructed nasal flaps can prevent nasal tip and alar rim distortion.
- Local nasal tissue provides the best color and texture match for missing tissue.

References

1 Zitelli JA. Burow's grafts. J Am Acad Dermatol 1987;17:271–9.
2 Rohrer TE, Dzubow LM. Conchal bowl skin grafting in nasal tip reconstruction: clinical and histologic evaluation. J Am Acad Dermatol 1995;33:476–81.
3 Peng VT, Sturm RL, Marsh TW. "Pinch modification" of the linear advancement flap. J Dermatol Surg Oncol 1987;13: 251–3.
4 Papadopoulos DJ, Trinei FA. Superiorly based nasalis myocutaneous island pedicle flap with bilevel undermining for nasal tip supratip reconstruction. Dermatol Surg 1999;25:530–6.
5 Cook JL. Reconstructive utility of the bilobed flap: lessons from flap successes and failures. Dermatol Surg 2005;31: 1024–33.
6 Johnson SC, Bennett RG. Double Z-plasty to enhance rhombic flap mobility. J Dermatol Surg Oncol 1994;20:128–32.
7 Herman AR, Bennett RG. Reconstruction of a large surgical defect on the lower eyelid and infraorbital cheek. Dermatol Surg 2005;31:689–91.

Commentary on conundrum 11

Repair of small nasal tip defects can be deceptively straightforward at times, and at other times exceedingly tricky or complex, depending on the laxity, tissue quality, and position of the defect with respect to the free margins of the ala. The flap repair shown here, while clearly described and beautifully executed, is exceedingly complex. The two Z-plasties at the base of the flap had to be precisely designed so as not to cause alar rim elevation or dorsal nasal depression. The authors also recognized the fact that the standing cone at the flap base, if not removed, could require surgical correction later if it did not flatten completely.

A close look at this flap reveals that it is a variation on a trilobed flap, which is a modification of the bilobed flap.[1] Both bilobed and trilobed flaps work because of intrinsic Z-plasties that serve to shift skin in the direction of their middle arms. The main difference between this flap and the standard bilobed flap is that the secondary lobes are very small. As long as there is no distortion resulting from filling a larger defect with a smaller flap, this option efficiently repairs the wound with a flap limited to the cosmetic unit of the nasal tip. It is evident that this nose is relatively elastic as it nicely accommodates the flap. The decision to employ this particular repair option must be made based on the mobility of the adjacent skin.

Small nasal tip defects can sometimes be simply repaired with a layered closure, which may be vertically oriented or angled diagonally, depending on the relaxed skin tension lines, and can provide esthetically pleasing results without distortion of the nasal tip or ala. Advancement flaps of the type described by Goldberg and Alam, as well as Lambert and Dzubow, may be a better alternative when the laxity of the nasal tip skin is insufficient to perform a primary closure.[2,3] The advantage of these flaps is their ability to recruit adjacent tissue movement to close small- to medium-sized midline nasal tip defects without distorting the nasal architecture. Their disadvantage lies in the fact that their incision lines do not always match the relaxed skin tension lines of the nose and can therefore be difficult to camouflage. However, a similar design principle utilizing the available laxity of the lateral nasal tip and columella can be used to design and execute a modified primary closure for small nasal tip defects, as shown in the accompanying series of photos.

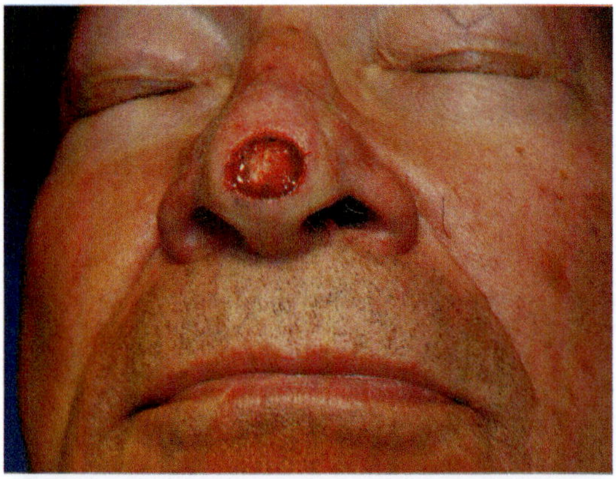

Figure 11.1 Nasal tip defect after Mohs surgery.

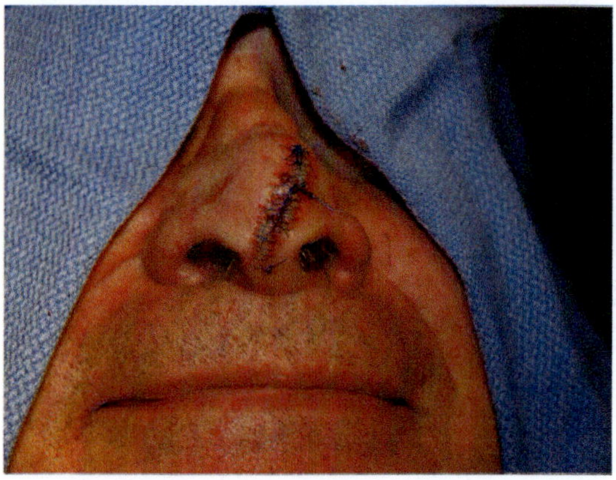

Figure 11.2 Final repair. Burow's triangles have been removed superior and inferior to the defect and displaced medially and laterally to take advantage of skin laxity in these areas.

A defect of the nasal tip is shown in Figure 11.1, which extends to the level of the perichondrium. Standing cones were designed with a slight curvature superiorly and inferiorly to take advantage of the available tissue laxity – in this case, on the left nasal tip skin superiorly and the columella inferiorly (Figure 11.2). The incision lines

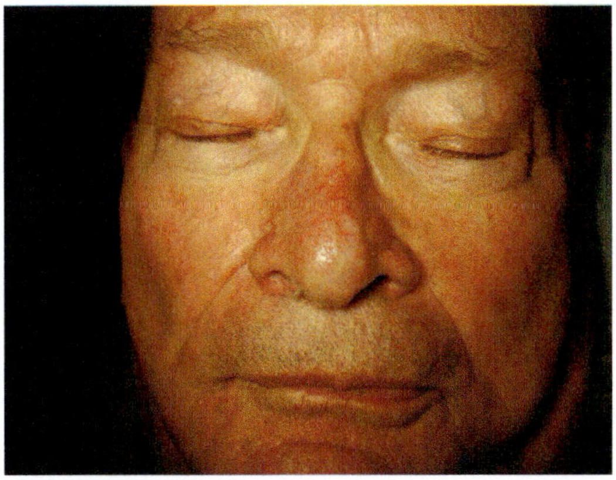

Figure 11.3 Follow-up at 6 months.

ultimately sit inconspicuously within the contour lines of the nose without distortion of the alar rim on either side or resultant dorsal nasal depression (Figure 11.3).

As the authors state, properly constructed nasal flaps can prevent nasal tip and alar rim distortion, with local tissue providing the best color and texture match for missing tissue. There is no doubt that use of the Z-plasty at the base of this nasal tip transposition flap enhanced its mobility, but it is important to recognize that, in some instances, a properly designed curvilinear closure may be an equally viable reconstructive option.

Commentary by Dr. Ratner

References

1 Albertini JG, Hansen JP. Trilobed flap reconstruction for distal nasal skin defects. Dermatol Surg 2010;36(11): 1726–35.
2 Goldberg LH, Alam M. Horizontal advancement flap for symmetric reconstruction of small to medium-sized cutaneous defects of the lateral nasal supratip. J Am Acad Dermatol 2003;49(4):685–9.
3 Lambert RW, Dzubow LM. A dorsal nasal advancement flap for off-midline defects. J Am Acad Dermatol 2004;50(3):380–3.

IV

PART IV
Nasal Ala

12 CONUNDRUM 12

Spiral Subcutaneous Island Pedicle Advancement Flap for Repair of Alar Defects

John G. Stoner[1] *& John G. Stoner*[2]
[1]York, PA
[2]Philadelphia, PA

The patient is a 55-year-old female who presented with a 6-month history of a bleeding patch on the left side of her nose. Physical examination revealed a 0.7 cm translucent red plaque just lateral to the alar groove (Figure 1). Biopsy revealed a basal cell carcinoma with an infiltrative growth pattern. The tumor was subsequently excised by the Mohs technique. Clear surgical margins were obtained after two Mohs stages. The patient was left with a 1.0 × 1.3 cm defect (Figure 2). How would you repair this defect?

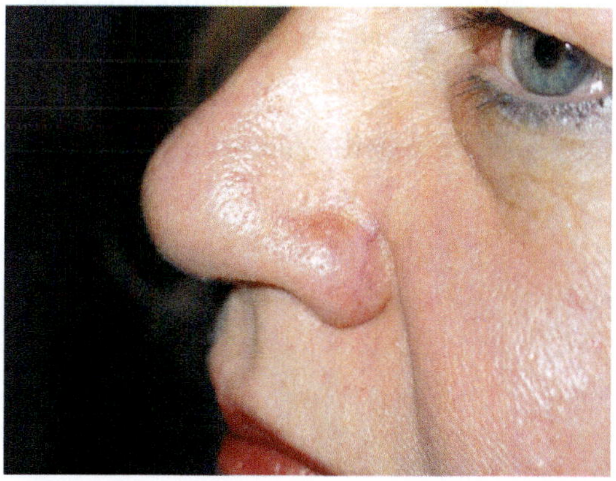

Figure 1 Patient 55 years old, pre-Mohs surgery.

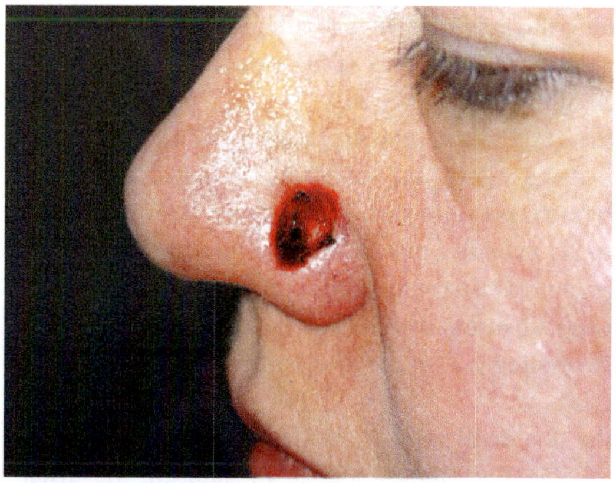

Figure 2 Defect 1.0 × 1.3 cm following Mohs surgery.

Resolution

Repair of alar defects is often challenging. Consideration of nasal valve deformity on inspiration, deformity of the alar rim, and contour deformity of the alar groove all need to be evaluated when planning a reconstruction.

Options for reconstruction include grafting and melolabial transposition flap. The latter flap frequently develops a "trapdoor effect," often distorting the normal

Reconstructive Conundrums in Dermatologic Surgery: The Nose, First Edition. Edited by Désirée Ratner, Joel L. Cohen and David G. Brodland.
© 2014 American Society for Dermatologic Surgery. Published 2014 by John Wiley & Sons, Ltd.

alar groove. An alternative solution for small- to medium-sized defects is the spiral subcutaneous island pedicle advancement flap. This flap is ideal for defects located over or just lateral to the alar groove. This flap is almost entirely confined to the nasal side wall; it almost never develops a "trapdoor effect" and actually recreates the alar groove instead of obliterating it. The flap is designed to spiral onto itself, moving tissue down from the upper nasal dorsum and medially from the nasal sidewall. When designed properly, there is little movement of the alar free margin. The flap is well vascularized on a myocutaneous pedicle, and viability has not been a problem.

The flap is designed as follows. The initial incision parallels the alar rim, extending superiorly and medially, approximately the width of the defect. The incision then extends in an arc-like fashion around the defect, maintaining the previously measured width. The flap is then incised down to the apex of the melolabial fold, where a back cut is made (Figure 3).

The distal third of the flap is dissected away from the underlying muscle and subcutaneous tissue. The flap is freed at the proximal portion by the apex of the melolabial fold. An extensive myocutaneous pedicle is maintained over approximately two-thirds of the proximal portion of the flap, ensuring an excellent blood supply. Superficial undermining is also carried out around the perimeter of the flap.

The free distal third of the flap is then spiraled onto itself. The key suture is placed by suturing the distal third of the flap onto the middle third (Figure 4). The free margin along the left nasal dorsum is then sutured to the arc-like portion of the flap. This up-and-down suturing anchors the flap in place and prevents distortion of the alar free margin. The alar margin is then sutured, followed by the side wall and subsequently the apex of the melolabial fold (Figure 5).

Slight dehiscence may occur where the flap has been spiraled onto itself but readily granulates. The contour of the alar groove is maintained and, in fact, is recreated by the design of the flap. One year following surgery, the scar is well healed, and no revisions have been necessary (Figure 6).

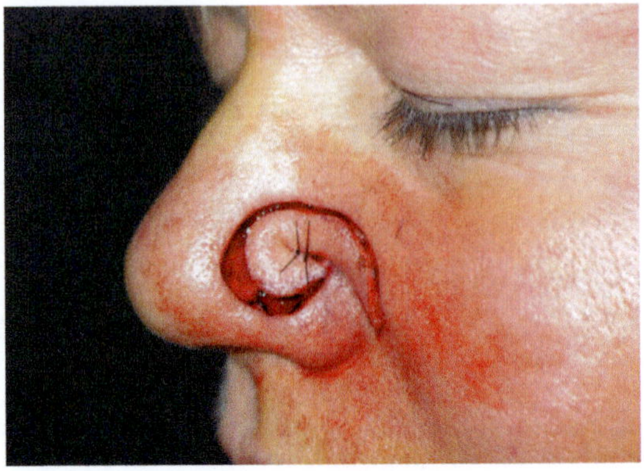

Figure 4 Flap incised, undermined, and spiraled unto itself. Key sutures placed connecting distal third to middle third of flap.

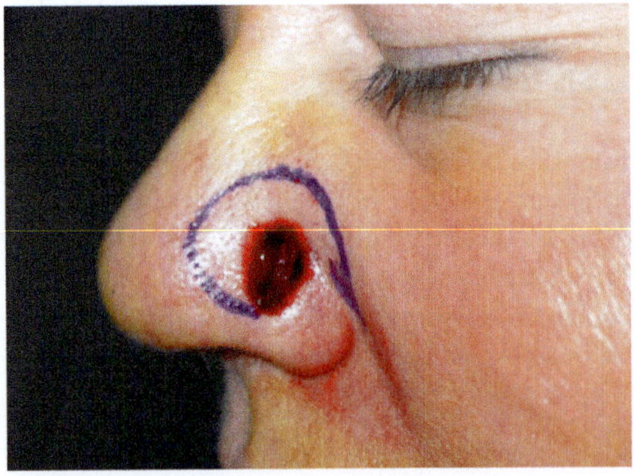

Figure 3 Outline of proposed flap. Note back cut at apex of melolabial fold.

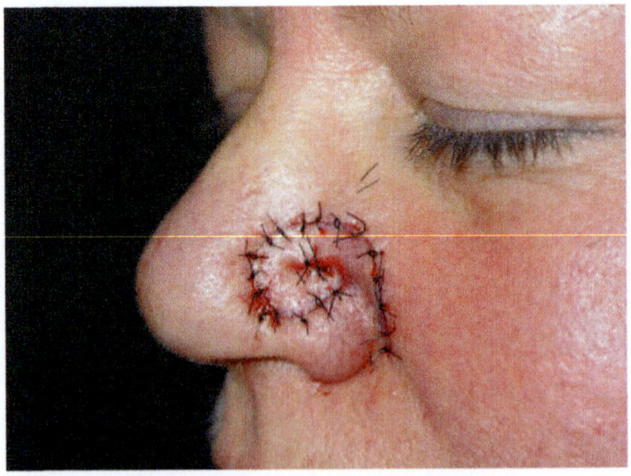

Figure 5 Flap sutured into place with minimal distortion of alar rim.

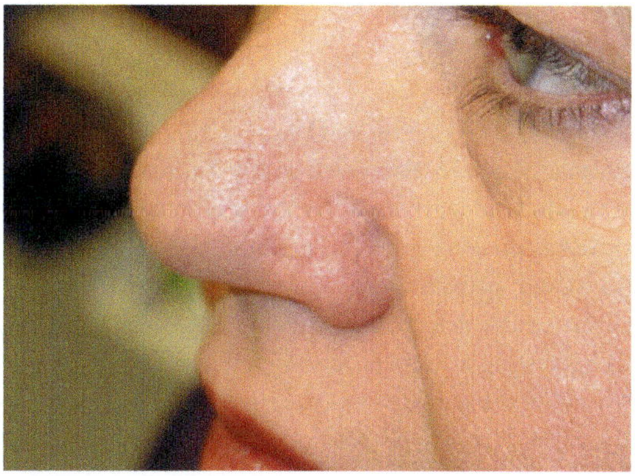

Figure 6 Scar, 1 year post–Mohs surgery, with no revision and with normal contour of alar groove.

Conundrum keys

- This flap is ideal for small- to medium-sized defects over or just lateral to the alar groove. The flap is entirely contained within the alar groove and nasal sidewall.
- The initial flap incision should parallel the alar groove and then arc around the primary defect. The width of the arc corresponds to the vertical diameter of the defect.
- The distal third of the flap should be freed, and a back cut is made at the apex of the melolabial fold to facilitate movement of the flap onto itself.
- The flap is spiraled onto itself. Small dehiscence may occur at this folding point but readily granulates. Trap-door phenomenon has not occurred.

Commentary on conundrum 12

As we have seen in other cases involving defects of the nasal ala, competence of the alar rim frequently determines the type of repair that needs to be performed. With this laterally situated defect located approximately 3–4 mm from the alar rim, the chance of developing nasal valve dysfunction or alar retraction would be considerably smaller than it would be for an alar defect situated closer to the rim (as in Conundrum 16). In some circumstances, a cartilage strut may be necessary for preservation of rim contour (Figure 10.4b). Once an auricular cartilage strut has been sewn in place, several options across a full spectrum of repairs come to mind.

There are many possible permutations of the island pedicle advancement flap in this area but for practical purposes, a simple island pedicle flap from the alar groove can work quite nicely. A recently described logarithmic spiral flap provides excellent restoration of the alar crease with a more robust vascular supply and places the entirety of the surgical scars on the nasal subunit.[1] It is important to note, however, that this flap differs in design from the more tightly spiraled flap demonstrated in this case, which is in fact a random pattern flap rather than a true island flap. An island pedicle advancement without the spiral, which intentionally leaves the superior alar groove aspect to heal by secondary intention to preserve the alar concavity, can also provide a very natural result. A small one-stage melolabial transposition flap can work as well, but it is important to place a secure periosteal tacking suture within the alar groove to minimize the risk of blunting of the alar groove (Figure 10.3). A two-stage melolabial flap can also work nicely because it avoids this risk, but obviously requires the additional surgery of pedicle takedown (Figure 12.1).

An island pedicle advancement flap from the skin superior to the defect is another possible permutation, as is harvesting a Burow's full-thickness skin graft from above along the same lines as the superiorly based island pedicle flap. A cartilage strut placed within the defect can help to reestablish some tissue volume before coverage with the skin graft. For deeper defects, however, the strut alone may not completely fill the needed volume, and a combination repair utilizing a cartilage strut, subcutaneous hinge flap, and full-thickness skin graft may be useful (Figure 10.4). Other options can also be considered, most notably placement of a cartilage strut followed by second-intention healing as has recently been described.[2]

Commentary by Dr. Cohen

References

1 Mahlberg M, Leach B, Cook J. The spiral flap for nasal alar reconstruction: our experience with 63 patients. Dermatol Surg 2012;38(3):373–80.

2 Ibrahimi O, Campbell T, Youker S, Eisen D. Nonanatomic free cartilage batten grafting with second intention healing for defects on the distal nose. J Drugs Dermatol 2012;11(1):46–50.

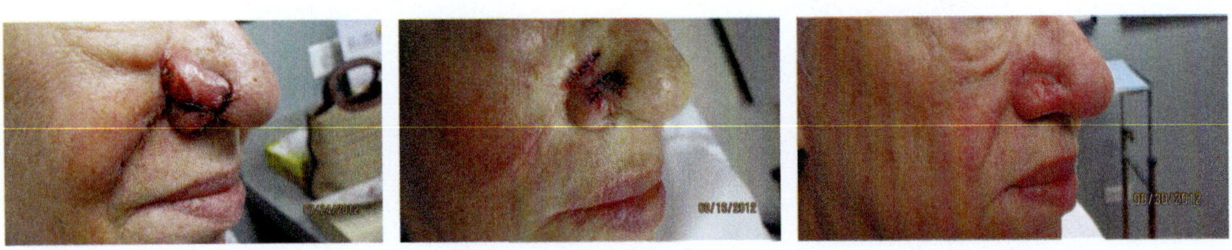

(a) (b) (c)

Figure 12.1 (a) Two-stage nasolabial transposition flap at 4 weeks. (b) Matching suture lines with nasal subunit lines at the time of pedicle division can be helpful to hide scars. (c) Two weeks later, recently sutured area blends into esthetic subunits.

13

CONUNDRUM 13

Combined Hinge Flap Full-Thickness Skin Graft for a Through-and-Through Nasal Defect

Kelly Bickle[1] *&* *Richard G. Bennett*[1,2]
[1]Department of Internal Medicine, USC School of Medicine, Los Angeles, California
[2]Department of Internal Medicine, UCLA School of Medicine, Los Angeles, California

A 60-year-old Caucasian man presented with a through-and-through nasal defect of the right anterior nasal ala. The defect was subsequent to use of an Internet-purchased "black salve" ointment applied to a self-diagnosed basal cell carcinoma. At the time of physical examination there was a 0.9 × 0.7-cm hole in the right anterior nasal ala (Figure 1), and the surrounding skin appeared shiny, telangiectatic, and sclerotic.

In addition there were multiple untreated basal cell carcinomas on the patient's forehead, cheeks, and lower right eyelid. Multiple punch biopsies were performed on the skin surrounding the nasal defect to detect any residual basal cell carcinoma that may have occurred after treatment with the black salve. The biopsies revealed scar tissue with no residual malignancy. How would you reconstruct this defect?

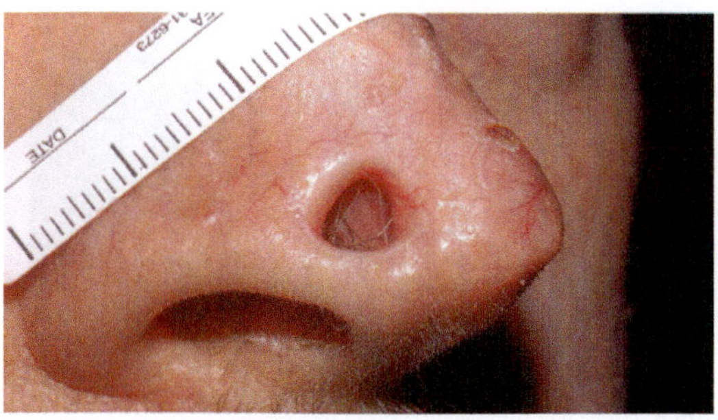

Figure 1 Full-thickness anterior nasal alar defect after self-treatment of possible basal cell carcinoma with black salve ointment.

Resolution

The nose can be thought of as a three-layer structure: skin, cartilage or fibrofatty tissue, and mucosa. For a full-thickness nasal defect, in addition to replacing the overlying skin, it is preferable that the nasal mucosa also be replaced. The intervening absent cartilage or fibrofatty tissue that acts as structural support also needs to be addressed. In our experience, the thickness of tissue that is used to replace the skin or mucosa may be sufficiently bulky to provide adequate structural support.

Repair options for a through-and-through nasal defect generally include a procedure for relining the nasal mucosa, followed by a skin flap. The repair options for reconstruction of the nasal mucosa include either a hinge flap from the nasal septum[1] or a bipedicle mucosal advancement flap from the nasal mucosa superiorly or even a full-thickness skin graft from the labial mucosa. The mucosal skin graft is subject to sloughing, however.

Reconstructive Conundrums in Dermatologic Surgery: The Nose, First Edition. Edited by Désirée Ratner, Joel L. Cohen and David G. Brodland.
© 2014 American Society for Dermatologic Surgery. Published 2014 by John Wiley & Sons, Ltd.

When this sloughing occurs and if the wound has been covered by a flap, the underside of the flap will granulate and reepidermize. This granulation tissue may result in contraction of the overlying flap. For the outside of the nasal defect, repair options include a local skin flap such as a bilobed flap or a staged pedicle flap from either the forehead or cheek. Our patient had multiple untreated basal cell carcinomas on both cheeks as well as his forehead, and he did not wish to undergo a staged procedure. Furthermore, there was little elasticity in the skin around the defect, making a local flap difficult. After reviewing the options, we decided to use the hinge flap[2,3] for our closure. This procedure would allow us to reline the nasal mucosa,[3] as well as create a recipient bed for placement of a full-thickness skin graft.[4] Local anesthetic was infiltrated into the skin, subcutaneous tissue, and mucosa around and superior to the defect. A 1.5-mm semicircular rim of tissue along the inferior defect rim was excised through and through between approximately 12 and 8 o'clock to freshen the recipient site (Figure 2). The excised tissue was examined with frozen sections to detect the presence of tumor; none was seen. Care was taken not to excise the tissue between 8 and 12 o'clock, which was the planned base of the hinge flap. The flap size and shape were carefully measured before its creation to fit the new defect. The hinge flap was created by making incisions in a semicircular shape in the mirror image of and superior to the defect (Figure 2); the flap was then developed by undermining in the mid sub-cutaneous tissue plane between 8 and 12 o'clock just superior to the planned hinge. The flap was elevated and flipped inferiorly on its intact full-thickness skin hinge. The skin

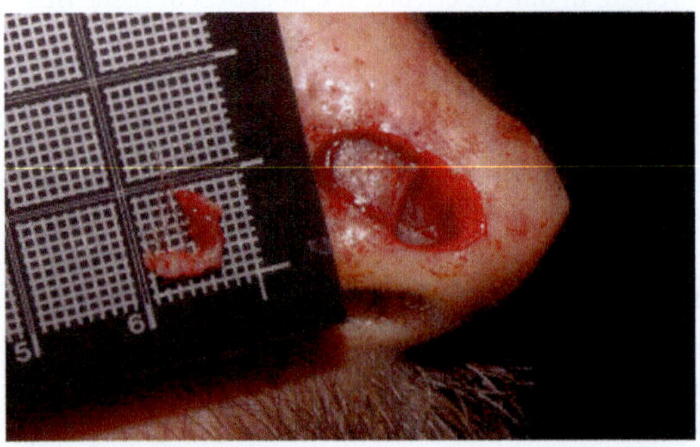

Figure 2 Full-thickness nasal defect after 1.5-mm-wide semi-circular full-thickness edge excised between 12 and 8 o'clock (shown on grid on left) and hinge flap incision made. Note that the remaining full-thickness wound edge at base of hinge flap between 8 and 12 o'clock is left intact.

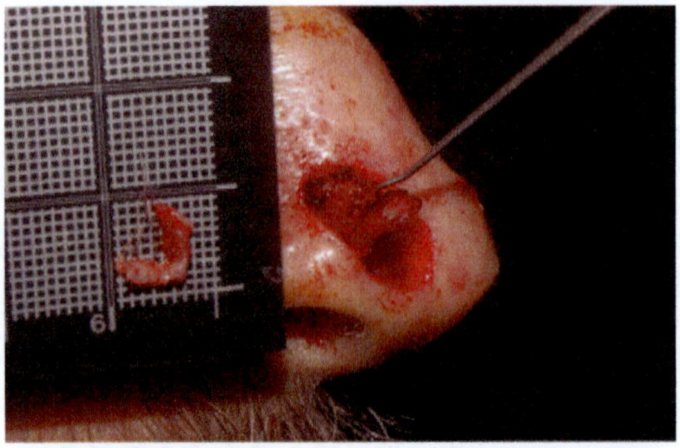

Figure 3 Hinge flap being elevated and flipped inferiorly before being placed into defect.

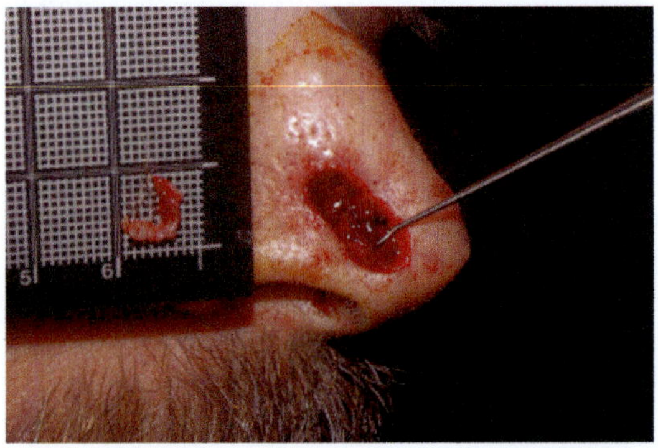

Figure 4 The hinge flap laid into place.

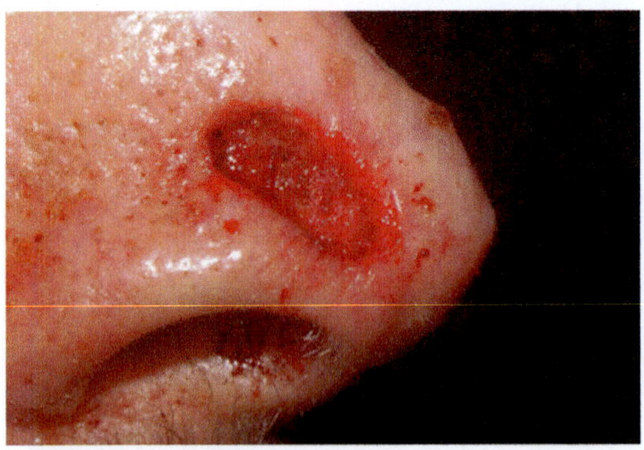

Figure 5 Hinge flap completely sutured into place.

side of the flap then became the nasal mucosal lining (Figures 3 and 4). The semicircular free skin edge of the flap was stitched to the surrounding nasal mucosa using 5-0 vicryl suture (Figure 5). Care was taken so

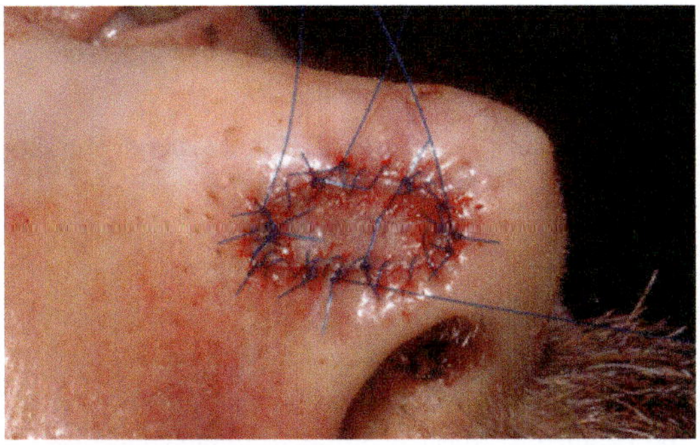

Figure 6 Full-thickness skin graft sutured into place on top of the hinge flap and its donor site.

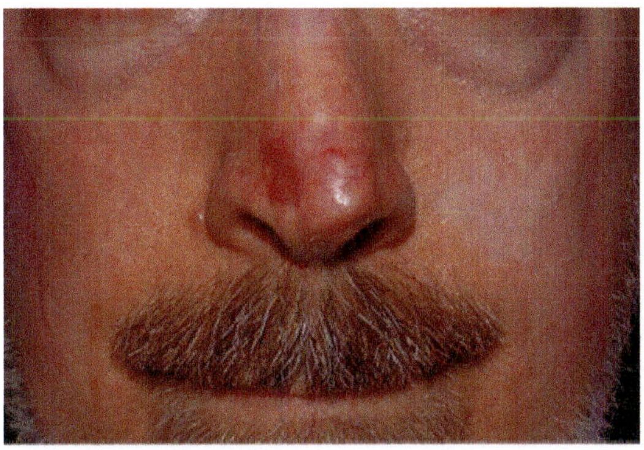

Figure 7 One month postoperation.

that there were only small gaps that could not be probed between the stitches. To reconstruct the absent nasal skin, a postauricular full-thickness skin graft was placed on the underside of the hinge flap and its donor site (Figure 6). Except for persistent erythema, an excellent cosmetic and functional result was obtained (Figures 7 and 8). We treated the erythema using a pulsed dye laser (V-Beam, Candela, Boston, MA) at 8.5 J/cm^2, pulse width 1.5 ms, and a spot size of 7 mm. There was no appreciable improvement of the erythema at 2 weeks.

The hinge flap has been described on the nose for alar rim defects or in combination with a local flap.[2,3] Our case is unique because it combines the hinge flap with a full-thickness skin graft for a nonrim defect. It fulfills the patient's desire for a simple one-stage reconstructive procedure on a rather small, tight nose.

This case provides an opportunity to alert physicians to the use of "black salves" in the community. There

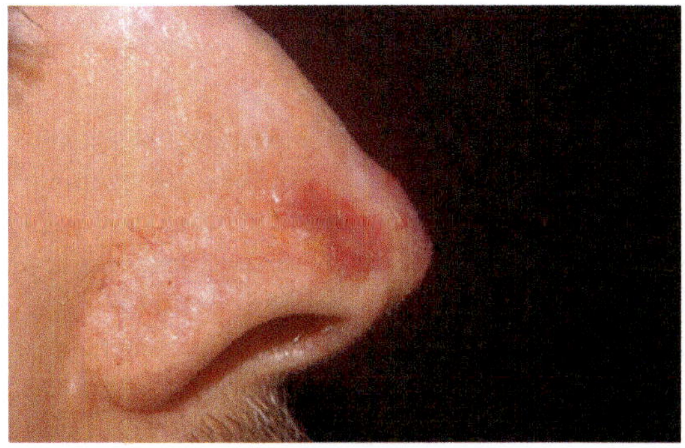

Figure 8 One month postoperation.

are numerous types of black salves that have escharotic, anticarcinogenic, antioxidant, or keratolytic activity. Common ingredients include zinc chloride, bloodroot, and other botanicals.[5]

Conundrum keys

- To repair a through-and-through nasal defect it is necessary to reconstruct a nasal lining and over-lying skin.
- Proper sizing of the hinge flap is necessary to fit the defect to be repaired.
- Careful suturing of the flipped over hinge flap to the surrounding mucosal wound edges is necessary so that no substantive gaps between stitches are identifiable.

References

1 Baker SR, Swanson NA. Local flaps in facial reconstruction. St. Louis: Mosby; 1995:215–6.
2 Lee K, Gorman AK, Swanson NA. Hinged turnover flap: a one-stage reconstruction of a full-thickness nasal ala defect. Dermatol Surg 2004;30:479–81.
3 Hosaka Y, Tsukagoshi T, Sasaki E, Yokoyama S. The use of otherwise redundant skin to provide nasal lining in the reconstruction of full-thickness alar defects by nasolabial flap repair. Br J Plas Surg 1999;52:29–32.
4 Fader DJ, Wang TS, Johnson TM. Nasal reconstruction utilizing a muscle hinge flap with overlying full-thickness skin graft. J Am Acad Dermatol 2000;43:837–40.
5 Jellinek N, Maloney ME. Escharotic and other botanical agents for the treatment of skin cancer: a review. J Am Acad Dermatol 2005;53:486–94.

Commentary on conundrum 13

The defect itself is not the only complicated problem presented here. The issue of patients literally "taking things into their own hands" and treating a self-diagnosed basal cell carcinoma with an unconventional alternative such as black salve is deeply troubling, especially given the lack of clinical trials and peer-reviewed data supporting the use of such agents. It would probably have been worth doing more than just scouting biopsies around this site to confirm that the tumor was indeed gone, particularly because the true diagnosis was uncertain. An excision around the remaining lesion could have been employed, followed by "scouting biopsies" along the wider scar, including the visible hyperkeratotic crusting on the central nasal supratip, to gain additional diagnostic information. The resulting larger defect from these additional tissue samplings could have been repaired in a similar fashion.

Another option for repair of this defect (or the larger defect from the additional excision for margin analysis) would be to consider either a staged procedure with internal lining replacement performed initially or two simultaneous flaps. The mucosal lining could be obtained by mobilizing a septal hinge flap. A cartilage strut could then be placed over this lining to provide support and fill in the defect depth, while at the same time helping to keep the vestibule patent during inspiration.[1] The cutaneous surface repair could then be performed either that same day or later.

The best options for same-day coverage would likely have been a superiorly based paranasal interpolation flap or a melolabial interpolation flap, both of which have a robust axial blood supply and would provide sufficient tissue volume to replace the deep defect and help recreate the convexity of the lateral nasal tip. However, given the anterior location of the defect, both options would require a second procedure for pedicle takedown several weeks later. For a larger and more laterally based full-thickness defect, a lining flap with a cartilage strut and a simpler one-stage melolabial transposition flap could be employed simultaneously, thus avoiding the later need for pedicle takedown. To ensure that the lining flap had demonstrated viability and the cartilage graft was doing well and in good position, a delayed closure of the cutaneous aspect of the defect could have been performe a few weeks later. Typically this approach would also decrease the size and depth of the overall defect as it healed secondarily. Similar to the authors' approach in this conundrum, a full-thickness skin graft harvested from the periauricular (pre or post) area or conchal bowl (which can often provide best tissue match for more sebaceous noses) could be utilized, with placement only after the initial lining stage was found to be successful. Even with this "delayed approach" to the surface defect,[2] the full-thickness skin graft would probably fail to fully recreate the convexity of the lateral nasal tip. An east-west advancement flap could serve as an alternative to a graft while helping to restore the convexity of the area.[3]

Commentary by Dr. Cohen

References

1 Ewanowski C, Cook J. Using cartilage and skin grafts concurrently: an alternate route to repair. Dermatol Surg 2009;35:1809–17.

2 Ibrahimi O, Campbell T, Youker S, Eisen D. Nonanatomic free cartilage batten grafting with second intention healing for defects on the distal nose. J Drugs Dermatol 2012;11(1):46–50.

3 Geist D, Maloney M. The "east-eest" advancement flap for nasal defects: reexamined and extended. Dermatol Surg 2012;38:1529–34.

14

CONUNDRUM 14

Combined Hinge and Nasolabial Transposition Flap for Repair of a Full-Thickness Nasal Alar Defect

Alisha N. Plotner & Hugh M. Gloster, Jr.
Department of Dermatology, College of Medicine, University of Cincinnati, Cincinnati, Ohio

An otherwise-healthy 53-year-old man was referred for surgical treatment of a micronodular basal cell carcinoma in the left nasal alar groove. Mohs micrographic surgery was performed, with tumor-free margins achieved after three stages. The final defect was an ovoid 1.2- × 1.0-cm full-thickness nasal defect centered at the anterior aspect of the left nasal alar groove. How would you reconstruct this surgical defect?

Resolution

Full-thickness nasal alar defects present a reconstruction challenge for the dermatologic surgeon. The nose should be thought of as a three-layer structure comprising skin, cartilage or fibrofatty tissue, and underlying nasal mucosa that lines the nasal vestibule. Repair of this nasal mucosa is critically important when there is a full-thickness nasal alar defect because second-intention healing can lead to contraction of the overlying flap, nasal distortion, and airway obstruction.[1]

Several options exist for repairing the mucosal lining of the nasal ala. Intranasal mucosa from the vestibule, middle vault, or septum may be used in an advancement flap to close the primary mucosal defect; the secondary defect is then allowed to re-epithelialize. This method requires advanced surgical skill and may not be feasible for large defects. Labial, buccal, or hard palate mucosal grafts are another option, but sloughing and contraction of the overlying flap may complicate these.[2,3] When cartilaginous support is required, a septal hinge flap consisting of mucosa and cartilage is an option, but nasal dorsum collapse may complicate this repair. When using mucosal flaps or grafts for closure of the nasal mucosa defect, cover flaps are required for correction of the cutaneous defect. These repairs are usually achieved using a nasolabial transposition flap, island pedicle flap, cheek interpolation flap, forehead based pedicle flap, or full-thickness skin graft.

Intranasal mucosa may also be repaired with skin. A variety of flaps have been designed that allow repair of the mucosal and cutaneous portions of the nasal alar defect in one- or two-step procedures. A nasolabial transposition flap rotated 180° medially on its own axis may be used for nasal mucosa repair, and a cover flap may then be used to repair the cutaneous defect.[2] When the defect involves the alar rim, the nasolabial flap may be used in a one-step repair. As described above, the medially rotated nasolabial flap is secured at the defect site to repair the nasal mucosa. The distal portion of the flap is then folded on itself to create a new alar rim and complete repair of the cutaneous defect.[4]

Cutaneous hinge flaps from the lateral nasal side-wall, also known as "turn down" flaps, are another simple option for mucosal repair. The hinge flap can also be used for correction of the mucosal and cutaneous portions of

Reconstructive Conundrums in Dermatologic Surgery: The Nose, First Edition. Edited by Désirée Ratner, Joel L. Cohen and David G. Brodland.
© 2014 American Society for Dermatologic Surgery. Published 2014 by John Wiley & Sons, Ltd.

the defect when the alar rim is involved, because like the above-described nasolabial transposition flap, the distal aspect of the flap can be folded on itself for cutaneous defect repair.[5] These flaps require meticulous debulking to prevent airway compromise but cautious undermining near the flap's narrow hinge to preserve blood supply.

When hinge flaps are used solely for mucosal repair, the triangularly shaped secondary defect must then be repaired. This may be achieved using a full-thickness skin graft[3] or a nasolabial transposition flap, which generally yields good cosmetic results. The medial cheek at the nasolabial fold is an ideal donor site for the nose, given texture and sebaceousness similar to that of the nasal ala. This combination of hinge flap and nasolabial transposition flap was the method of repair chosen for our patient (Figure 1).

A hinge flap from the superior Burow's triangle was designed to repair the nasal mucosal defect. Local anesthetic solution was injected around the defect and the superior donor site. A deep incision was made to create the triangle, with its apex oriented superiorly and base abutting the superior aspect of the primary defect. Undermining was performed in the subcutaneous plane, with care taken to preserve a 3-mm area of attachment at the triangle's base to maintain a good blood supply. Once this flap was dissected, it was rotated using a hinge maneuver so that the flap's epidermis replaced the excised nasal mucosa (Figure 2). The apex was trimmed to match

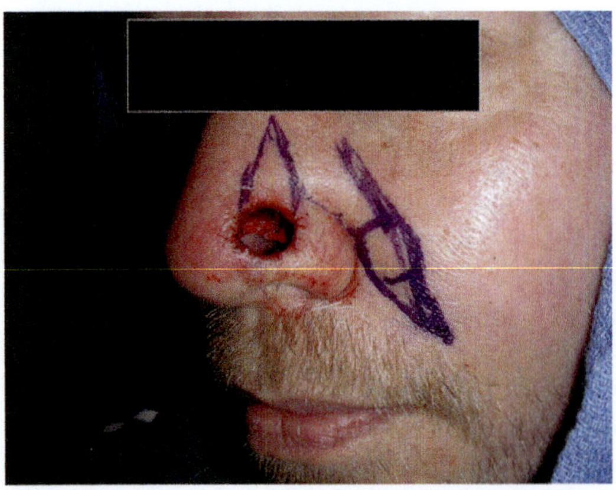

Figure 1 Combined hinge flap and nasolabial transposition flap designed to correct the primary defect.

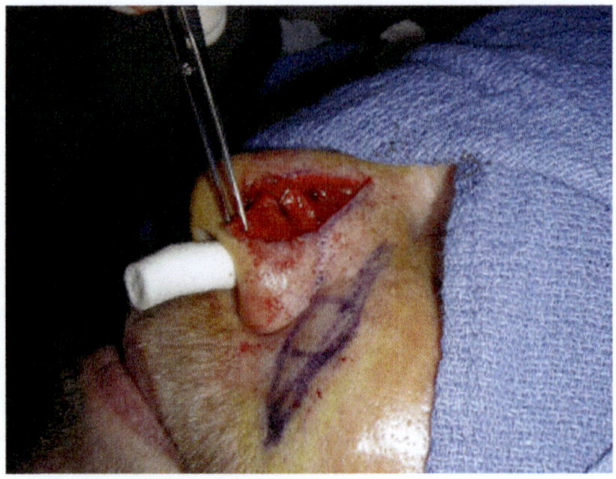

Figure 2 After careful dissection of the flap from the lateral nasal sidewall, it is rotated on its base using a hinge maneuver.

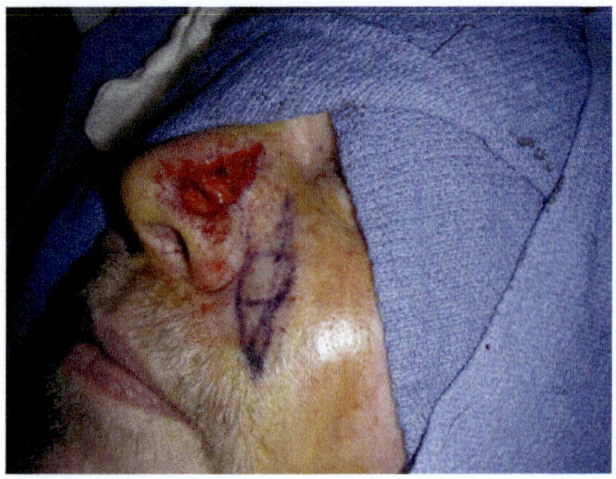

Figure 3 The hinge flap is sutured into place after trimming the apex to match the oval shape of the primary defect. Epidermis now replaces the excised nasal mucosa.

the oval nature of the defect and the flap sutured into place (Figure 3).

The newly created cutaneous defect, which included the primary oval defect centered at the alar groove and superior excised Burow's triangle, was repaired using a nasolabial transposition flap from the left cheek. The flap was designed with a high superior origin and oriented so that the final scar would lie in the nasolabial fold. Deep incisions were made in the superior and inferior limbs of the flap to the subcutaneous plane, followed

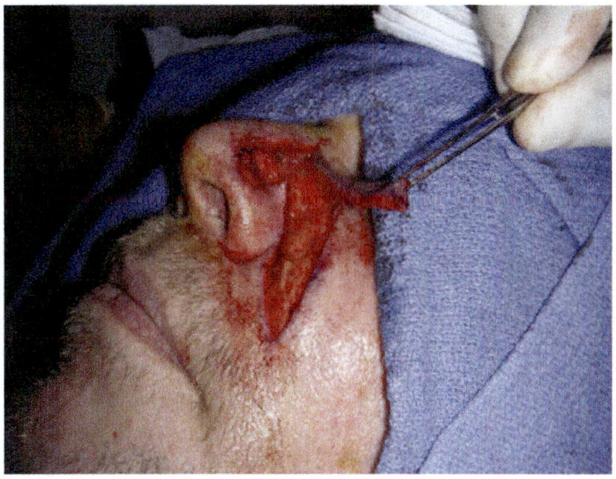

Figure 4 A nasolabial transposition flap from the left cheek is elevated and defatted to match the thickness of the defect.

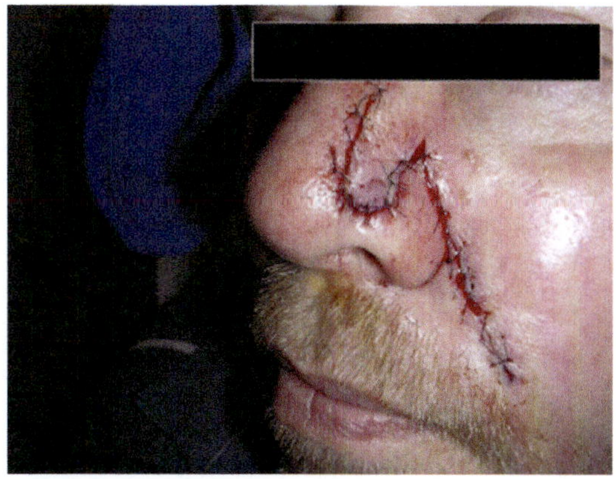

Figure 5 The flap has been trimmed and sutured into the defect. The secondary defect is repaired using a simple side-to-side closure so that the final scar lies in the nasolabial fold.

by undermining of surrounding skin. The flap was elevated and defatted to match the thickness of the defect (Figure 4). A buried 5-0 polyglactin 910 suture was placed from the flap to the periosteum of the nasofacial sulcus to avoid blunting of the sulcus. The base of the transposition flap was not tacked to the hinge flap, although this maneuver may be performed if there is concern about excess dead space or if the ala needs additional support. The remainder of the flap was closed in two layers with buried 6-0 polyglactin 910 sutures and cutaneous margin approximation with 5-0 nylon sutures. The stiffness of the hinge flap typically maintains patency of the nasal vestibule. If additional support is needed, a cartilage graft may be necessary.

The final flap measured 5.3 × 2 cm (Figure 5). The clinical outcome after 6 weeks is shown in Figure 6. The patient's left nostril is patent, and he has no difficulty breathing. He will be evaluated 10 weeks postoperatively for possible dermabrasion of the incision lines and intralesional triamcinolone acetonide if pincushioning of the flap is present.

In summary, we present the combination of nasal hinge flap and nasolabial transposition flap to repair a unilateral full-thickness defect of the nasal alar groove. This combination of flaps allows for an adequate nasal lining, creates a secondary defect that is easily repaired, and provides excellent cosmetic results.

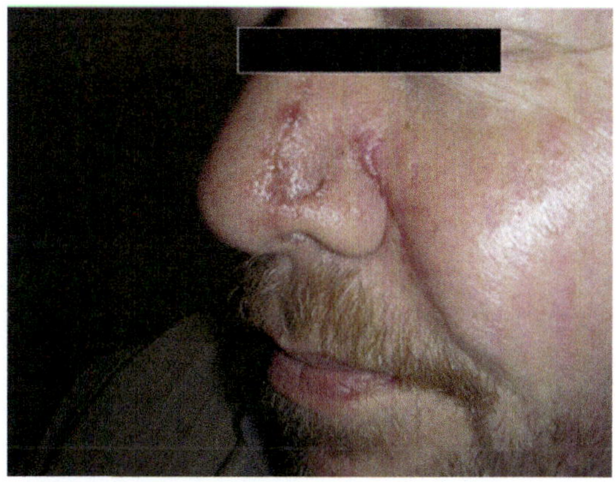

Figure 6 Six-week postoperative clinical results.

Conundrum keys

- Full-thickness nasal alar defects require repair of the nasal mucosa for optimal cosmetic results.
- The first critical step, nasal mucosa repair, can be achieved using a triangular hinge flap from the lateral nasal sidewall obtained superior to the primary defect.
- The resultant triangularly shaped defect is then amenable to repair with a nasolabial transposition flap, which can be designed so that scars are well hidden in the nasolabial fold.

References

1 Burget GC, Menick FJ. Aesthetic Reconstruction of the Nose. St. Louis: C.V. Mosby Co; 1994.

2 Humphreys T, Goldberg L, Wiemer D. Repair of defects of the nasal ala. Dermatol Surg 1997;23:335–49.

3 Bickle K, Bennett RG. Combined hinge flap full-thickness skin graft for a through-and-through nasal defect. Dermatol Surg 2008;34:389–92.

4 Skaria AM. Repair of full-thickness nasal alar defect. Dermatol Surg 2003;29:89–91.

5 Lee KK, Gorman AK, Swanson NA. Hinged turnover flap: a one-stage reconstruction of a full-thickness nasal ala defect. Dermatol Surg 2004;30:479–81.

Commentary on conundrum 14

This conundrum presents a younger patient with a through-and-through defect of the nose involving the medial ala and the lateral nasal tip. The size of this defect was a significant determinant in choosing a hinged turndown flap rather than a nasal mucosal flap.

The authors make a very important point about the need for reconstruction of missing nasal mucosa. Failure to restore this inner layer of the nasal structure will always lead to significant scar contraction and, in this location, alar distortion. In addition, the nasal valve would likely be adversely affected, leaving the surgeon with no choice but to consider a multilayered closure.

It appears that the structural integrity of the ala is preserved. We must therefore assume that the bridge of skin connecting the lateral ala and the nasal tip is sufficiently intact to obviate the need for cartilage support. In retrospect, the early postoperative results suggest slight alar retraction. If this is not corrected in longer term follow-up, delayed placement of a cartilage graft might be considered.

When faced with the need to repair nasal mucosa, the authors have nicely outlined the options to consider. The so-called bucket handle or bipedicled nasal mucosal flap is the simplest mucosal repair. However, a 1- to 1.2-cm defect is at the extreme upper end of the range of this flap. Typically, even nasal mucosal defects larger than 6–8 mm may be difficult to close with this method. The nasal septal transposition flap with its inferomedial base would be a good alternative means of covering this defect. However, the technical difficulty of working with an intranasal flap of this complexity poses a significant challenge. The challenge is not insurmountable and makes the more easily accessed turndown flap from the nasal sidewall a tempting option. The advantage of using a mucosal flap is that these flaps are generally very robust and supply a normally functioning "natural" replacement for the missing mucosa. A turndown flap is not functionally equivalent, although patients tend to tolerate the epidermal surface intranasally relatively well.

The key to successfully executing a nasal sidewall hinge flap lies in developing an adequate vascular base while mobilizing the flap so that it can rotate 180 degrees upon its base without vascular compromise. Usually, the excellent vasculature of the nose with its extensive arborization results in a viable flap. Always mindful of preserving blood supply, the final mobilization of the flap may be best carried out with a vertical spreading motion of iris scissors parallel to the blood supply to the flap base.

Once this is accomplished, a traditional nasolabial transposition flap can be executed. Harkening back to the modifications to the nasolabial transposition flap advocated by Zitelli, the superior Burow's triangle has already been "removed" in the process of performing the hinge flap.[1] The authors also mention the very important steps of wide undermining and the placement of a periosteal suture from the undersurface of the advancing base of the nasolabial flap to the periosteum of the nasofacial sulcus. This allows relatively tension-free transposition of the flap into the defect and prevents "tenting" of cheek skin lateral to the nasal sidewall. In Figure 5, the very subtle depression caused by the periosteal suture may be seen within the skin of the newly formed nasofacial sulcus.

The final step essential for optimizing the results of this flap is aggressive thinning of the distal flap. The nasolabial flap is extremely prone to pin-cushioning, largely due to its dependent nature, which can result in lymphostasis within the portion of the flap inferior to the pivot point. Defatting and appropriately thinning the distal portion of the flap, as well as undermining the recipient site, may help to minimize this phenomenon although it does not always entirely avoid it. The highlights of Figure 6 betray this phenomenon, which is even more obvious as the flap crosses over the "would be" alar crease. Six weeks postoperatively is no time to panic about flap edema. Instituting a course of aggressive fingertip massage by the patient for a period of 6–12 weeks can often improve unwanted pin-cushioning. In our office, patient massage is routinely instituted 1 month after the surgery and continues for 3–4 months or until the flap has achieved a desired appearance. In the absence of adequate improvement after 3–4 months, intralesional injections are considered, as is tangential excision and abrasive blending to improve contour. In more noticeable and refractory cases of pin-cushioning, surgical revision can be undertaken. This is performed through an incision made along a line within the desired location of the alar crease followed by defatting beneath the flap. Thereafter, undermining and lysing of the scar planes located at the flap margins further release the skin surface from tethering and results in improved smoothness. When necessary, excess skin can be trimmed and the incision lines are simply sutured back together.

Another observation in this case is the fusion of the alar skin with the medial cheek skin resulting from the loss of the concave isthmus that is the continuation of the alar crease. When possible, the initial design of nasolabial transposition flaps should incorporate an incision lateral to this 2- to 4-mm strip of skin so as to preserve the isthmus. Although this is a relatively minor anatomic structure, its loss results in noticeable asymmetry and can be avoided simply by shifting the location of the flap a few millimeters laterally.

Commentary by Dr. Brodland

Reference

1 Zitelli JA. The nasolabial flap as a single-stage procedure. Arch Dermatol 1990;126(11):1445–8.

V

PART V

Alar Groove/ Perialar Defects

15

CONUNDRUM 15

Shark Island Pedicle Flap for Repair of Combined Nasal Ala-Perialar Defects

Joseph L. Cvancara[1] *& J. Michael Wentzell*[2]
[1]Advanced Dermatology and Skin Surgery, Spokane, Washington
[2]Department of Dermatology, Deaconess Billings Clinic, Billings, Montana

Background

The combined nasal ala-perialar defect involving the concave intersection of the lateral nasal ala, nasal sidewall, cheek, and upper cutaneous lip is a problem for reconstructive surgery. During repair of combined cheek and nose defects, it is important not to blunt the alar facial sulcus. Defects involving these adjacent cosmetic units can be repaired by using combination procedures such as a flap/graft.

Objective

Our purpose is to introduce, describe, and illustrate a one-stage flap repair descriptively named the "shark" island pedicle flap (SIPF). The SIPF was developed for a specific combined nasal ala-perialar defect. This reconstruction restores the natural contours, preserves cosmetic boundaries, and eliminates the need for pexing sutures and graft/flap combinations.

Methods

The SIPF is an island pedicle flap with a superior arm that rotates 90° into the wound. This arm repairs the alar portion of the defect. The advancing island pedicle flap repairs the alar facial sulcus. The 90° rotation of the superior arm forces the alar portion of the flap to tilt 90° relative to the remaining body of the flap, forming an inverted cone of redundancy. Natural re-creation of the lateral ala and the alar facial sulcus results. Illustrative examples with a descriptive technique are provided for the SIPF.

Results

A well-planned SIPF reconstruction can provide exceptional cosmetic and functional results.

Conclusion

Cutaneous reconstructive surgeons will find the SIPF useful and reproducible in their armamentarium for single-stage aesthetic and functional repair of a specific combined lateral ala-adjacent perialar tissue defect.

Skin cancer often develops on both the lateral nasal ala and on the adjacent C-shaped "peri-alar area." These combined defects are a reconstructive conundrum. There are many cosmetic units involved, and violation of these defined units tends to cause blunting or loss of the lateral alar facial sulcus and blurring of cosmetic unit boundaries.[1] Commonly, combined contiguous cheek and nasal defects are repaired using a combination of a flap and a graft.[2] However, grafts are unsatisfactory for deeper defects, and combined procedures can be more laborious and costly.

Traditionally, the defined C-shaped perialar area includes the superior labial tissue, melolabial fold, medial cheek, and nasal tissue superior to the nasal alar crease.[3]

Reconstructive Conundrums in Dermatologic Surgery: The Nose, First Edition. Edited by Désirée Ratner, Joel L. Cohen and David G. Brodland.
© 2014 American Society for Dermatologic Surgery. Published 2014 by John Wiley & Sons, Ltd.

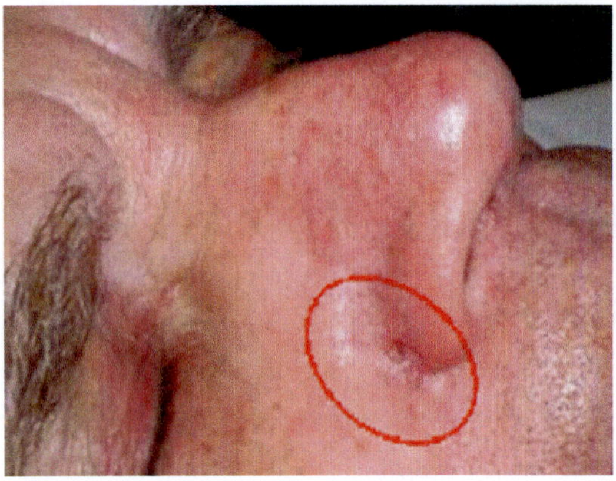

Figure 1 The location of the perialar concavity which the Shark island pedicle flap is designed to repair.

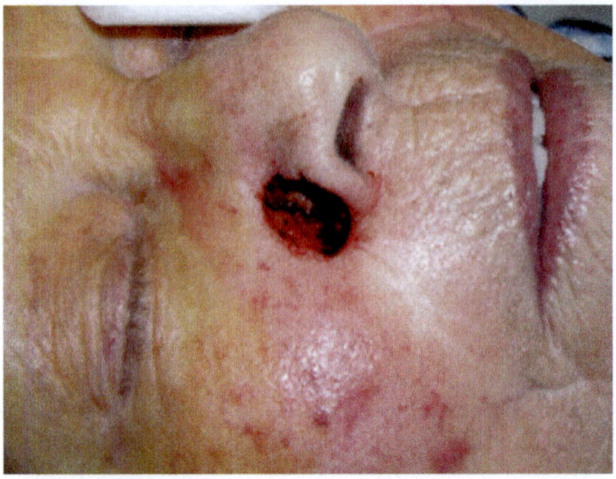

Figure 2 Common, deep oval defect in the perialar concavity created by Mohs surgery.

We present a one-stage island pedicle flap modification designed for combined repair of a specific portion of the perialar area and an adjacent deep lateral ala defect. This common, specific defect site is located in an anatomic concavity that has no descriptive name; thus, for simplicity, we have coined it the "perialar concavity (PC)." The PC is defined as the combined nasal ala-perialar region involving the concave intersection of the lateral nasal ala, nasal sidewall, cheek, upper cutaneous lip triangle directly inferior to the alar groove, and their junctional lines, which include the alar groove, nasofacial sulcus, and alar facial sulcus (see Figure 1).

This flap repair is descriptively named the "shark" island pedicle flap (SIPF) because the flap resembles a shark, with a snout and ventral mouth formed from the Mohs defect. The advancement of the SIPF with the rotational movement of the leading edge (shark's snout) spontaneously forms an inverted cone of redundancy that aesthetically re-creates the lateral alar facial sulcus and the tissues of the PC area, reestablishing normal alar contour. The "closing" of the shark's mouth reforms the lateral alar cosmetic boundary and requires no pexing, trimming, or graft placement to re-create and maintain the sulcus.

The appearance of the SIPF is similar to the popular triangularly shaped island pedicle flap (TIPF) with a rotational component. However, while the vascularity supplying the TIPF is a random pattern, the SIPF is a myocutaneous flap that derives vascularity for the "snout" from the levator labii superioris (Figures 2, 3, 4, 5, 6, 7, 8, 9, 10).[4–6]

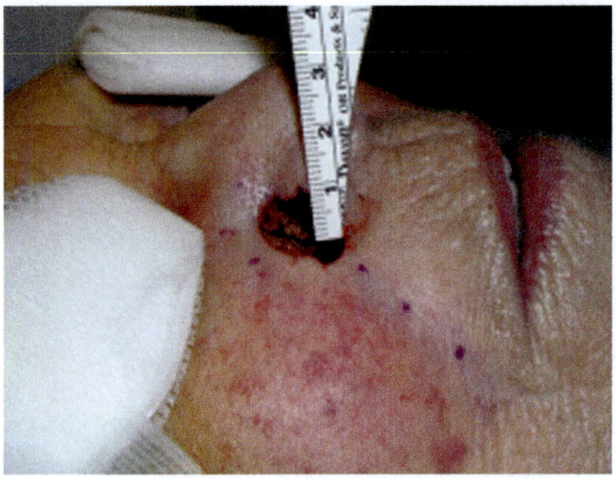

Figure 3 *Step 1*: The width of the nasal ala portion of the defect is measured from the original location of the lateral alar sulcus to the medial epithelial edge of the wound. This area will become the width of the "shark's snout."

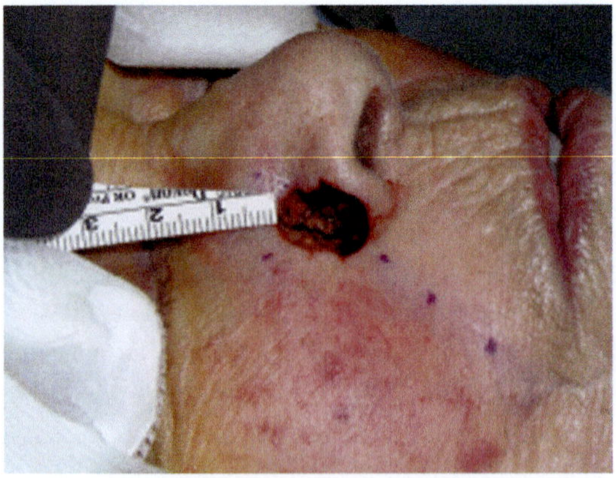

Figure 4 *Step 2*: The shark's snout is measured to be 8 mm.

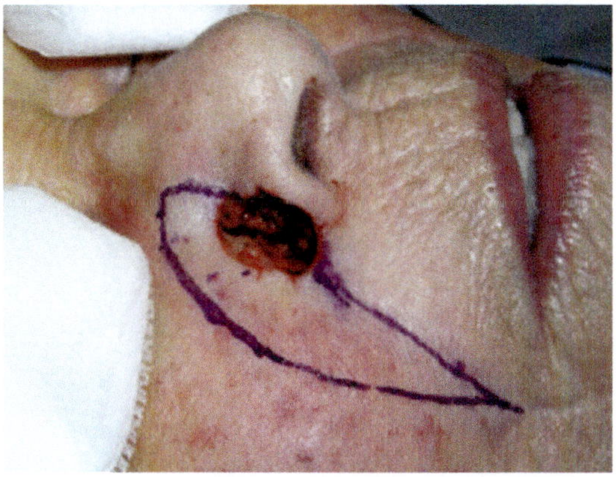

Figure 5 *Step 3*: Shark design. The pedicle has a superior long arm ("back and snout") with an inferior short arm. The Mohs defect creates the inferiorly based "open mouth." The Shark island pedicle is developed from a cheek reservoir lying in the relaxed skin tension lines. To hide the scar, the short-arm incision is placed in the melolabial fold.

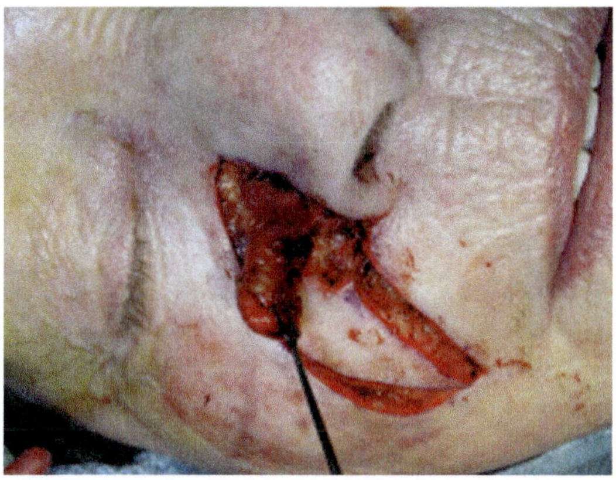

Figure 6 *Step 4*: The Shark island pedicle is a myocutaneous and random vascular flap. The hook is elevating the shark snout, illustrating the musculature beneath. Careful undermining of the shark's "snout" preserves the deep myocutaneous vascular pedicle. Additional undermining of the flap pedicle and surrounding skin may be required.

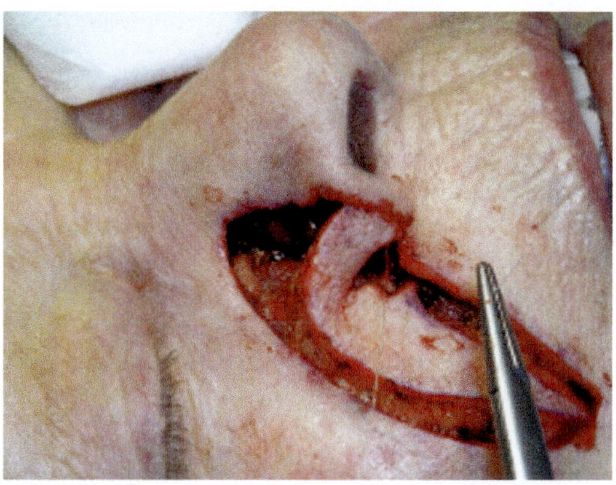

Figure 7 *Step 5*: The first key deep suture is placed in the rotated "shark's snout" and then attached to the alar rim.

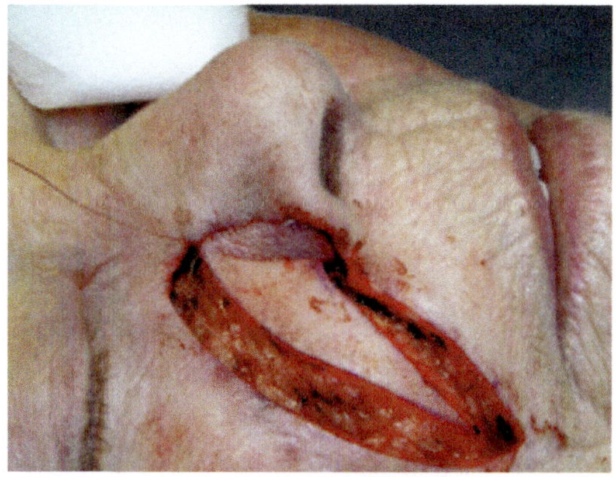

Figure 8 *Step 6*: The second key suture is a deep suture anchored to the "shark's head." This suture advances the flap and closes the "shark's jaws." As the back of the shark is pulled superomedially into position, the alar portion of the flap spontaneously tilts into a position somewhat perpendicular to the melolabial portion of the flap. The flap automatically creases along the shark's closed mouth, re-creating the sulcus and eliminating the need for pexing sutures.

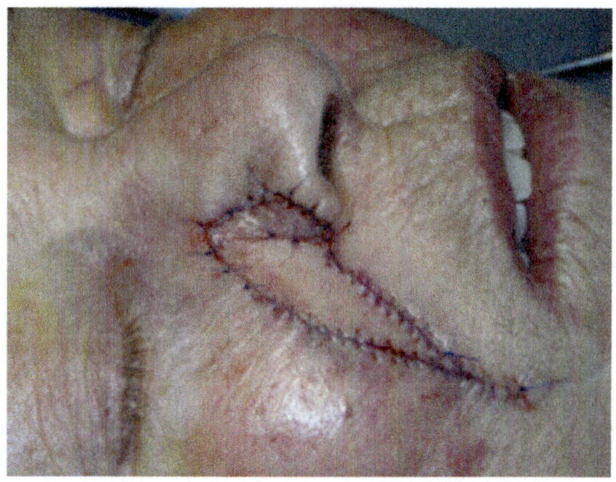

Figure 9 *Step 7*: Final suturing. No deep sutures are used for the "shark's mouth." Place between one and three very superficial 6-0 interrupted sutures across the closed shark's mouth. There is no tension at that site. Therefore, deep sutures are unnecessary and, if placed, could cause tip necrosis.

Discussion

We have used the SIPF on numerous occasions. It is a reliable one-stage repair of the cosmetically and functionally sensitive PC. The execution of the flap is uniformly reproducible and is designed specifically for repairs of deep lateral ala and perialar defects as defined by the PC. The advancement and rotation of the SIPF closes the "shark's jaws" and tilts the alar portion relative to the melolabial segment, like a book hinged on its binding. A sharply defined lateral alar facial sulcus and ala is

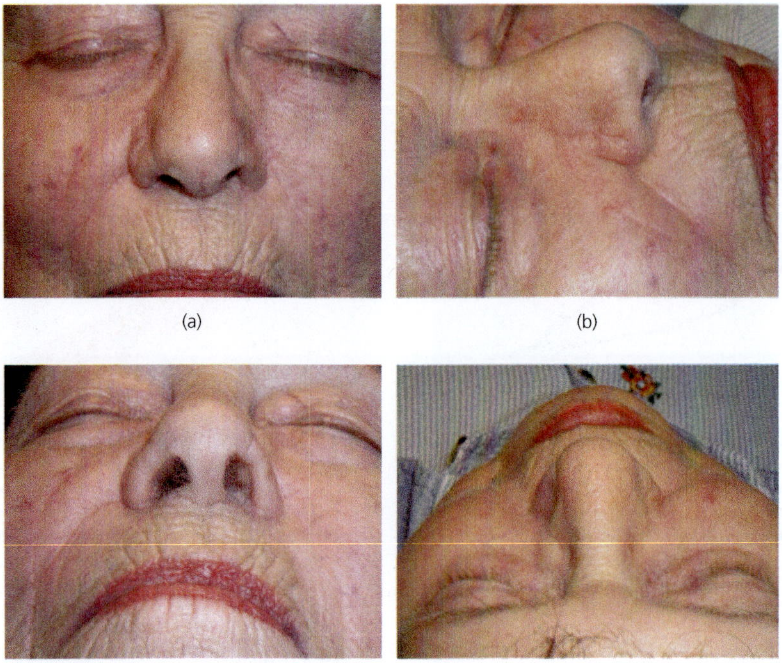

(a) (b) (c) (d)

Figure 10 (A) to (D)Two-month follow-up. Note re-creation of the right lateral alaperialar sulcus with no bridging.

spontaneously re-created without pexing sutures. The expected mild trap-dooring imparts aesthetic fullness to the re-created ala.

The SIPF relies on a myocutaneous and random subcutaneous blood supply to maintain flap viability medially. A random pattern of vascularity maintains the lateral portion of the flap. Preparing the defect as well as the pedicle is essential for movement.[7–9] Care must be taken to maintain deep myocutaneous attachments to the "snout" and to suture the "shark jaws" very superficially to prevent vascular compromise.

Conclusion

A well-planned SIPF is a useful and reproducible addition for a single-stage technique for aesthetic and functional repairs of the PC. This one flap rebuilds defects involving both the ala and the adjacent melolabial anatomy. The flap's movement spontaneously re-creates and sharply defines the lateral ala and the alar facial sulcus.

References

1 Burget GC, Menick FJ. Aesthetics, visual perception, and surgical judgment. In: Burget GC, Menick FJ, editors. Aesthetic reconstruction of the nose. St. Louis: Mosby, 1994:1–13.

2 Jewett BS. Skin and composite grafts. In: Baker SR, Naficy S, editors. Principles of nasal reconstruction. St. Louis: Mosby, 2002:95–6.

3 Levasseur JG, Mellette JR Jr. Techniques for reconstruction of perialar and perialar-nasal ala combined defects. Dermatol Surg 2000;26:1019–23.

4 Tomich JM, Wentzell JM, Grande DJ. Subcutaneous island pedicle flaps. Arch Dermatol 1987;123:514–8.

5 Rybka FJ. Reconstruction of the nasal tip using nasalis myocutaneous sliding flaps. Plast Reconstr Surg 1983;71:40–4.

6 Cvancara JL, Jones MS, Wentzell JM. The lenticular island pedicle flap. Dermatol Surg 2005;31:195–200.

7 Dzubow LM. Subcutaneous island pedicle flaps. J Dermatol Surg Oncol 1986;12:591–6.

8 Otley CC, Roenigk RK. Surgical Pearl: preparing the defect for an island pedicle flap. J Am Acad Dermatol 1997;36:257–8.

9 Chan STS. A technique of undermining a V-Y subcutaneous island flap to maximize advancement. Br J Plast Surg 1988;41: 62–7.

Commentary on conundrum 15

Combined alar-perialar defects may be tricky to reconstruct, given the need to maintain facial symmetry in this critical location, as well as to preserve the anatomic landmarks of the isthmus, apical triangle, alar crease, and nasolabial fold. The reliable vascular supply and easy availability of the nasolabial skin, as well as its excellent color match, make it a reliable source of donor skin for these defects. The anastamosing branches of the facial artery, infraorbital artery, and the dorsal branch of the ophthalmic artery contribute to its rich blood supply, making it possible to raise flaps of considerable length on a relatively narrow base, with

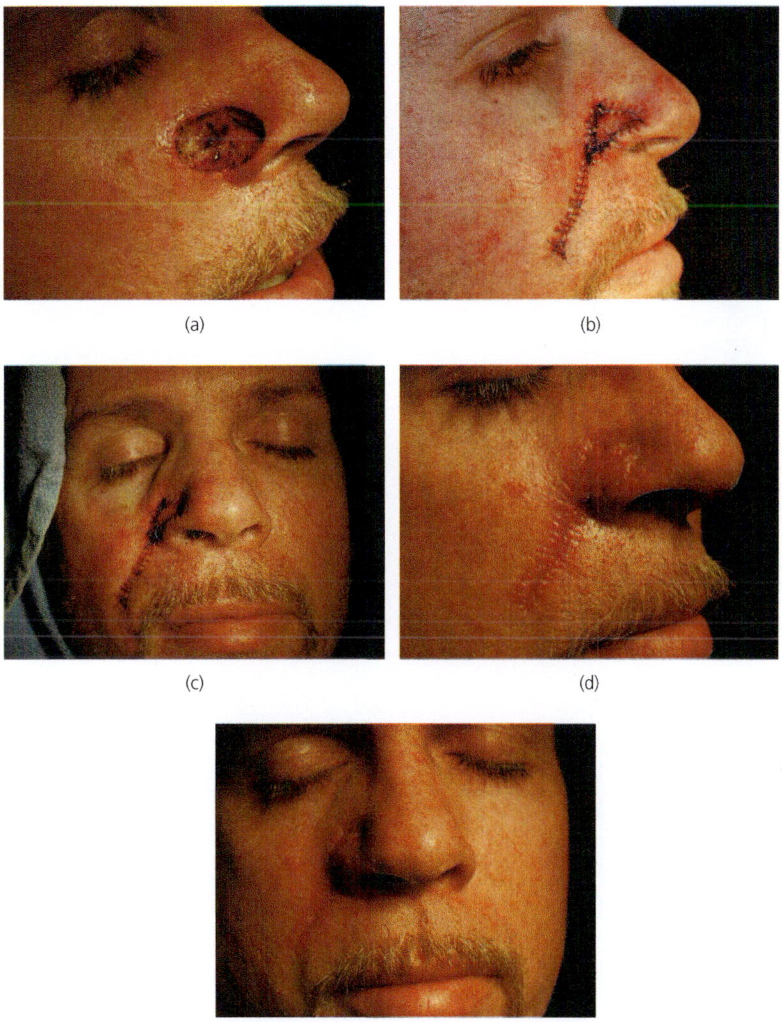

(a) (b) (c) (d) (e)

Figure 15.1 (a) Final defect involving the right perialar and alar skin. (b) Island pedicle flap was elevated, rotated 90 degrees counterclockwise, and sewn into place (side view). (c) Front view of flap sewn into place. (d and e) Suture removal. Note esthetic fullness of R nasal ala and preservation of nasofacial sulcus as well as alar crease on lateral view (d) and anterior view (e).

effective concealment of the donor site scar within the nasolabial fold.

The authors have outlined an elegant single-stage procedure that recreates and redefines the contours of the ala, including its lateral border, as well as the melolabial fold. The shark island pedicle flap is a myocutaneous flap based medially on a deep vascular pedicle derived from the levator labii superioris and also has a random pattern of vascularity that maintains its lateral portion. This flap is designed with a superior long arm and an inferior short arm ("back and snout") at its leading edge such that, when sutured into place, the flap automatically creases along the shark's closed mouth to recreate the alar crease. Mild trapdooring of the alar portion of the flap recreates the fullness that defines this cosmetic subunit, with simultaneous recreation of the lateral alar sulcus.

A similar defect is shown in Figure 15.1a, with an alternative reconstructive approach. While the shark island pedicle flap could have been used to repair this defect, a traditional island pedicle flap design was employed instead, with a slight variation in execution. Similar to the shark island flap, this flap was elevated in the subcutaneous plane, leaving a medially based deep muscular pedicle. The donor site was closed primarily within the nasolabial fold. At this point, the entire flap, and not just its distal aspect, was turned 90 degrees, trimmed, inset, and sutured into the remaining defect of the ala (Figure 15.1b). The contours of the ala, including the alar crease and lateral alar border, were thereby recreated, as seen in the frontal view (Figure 15.1c) and at the time of suture removal (Figure 15.1d and e).

In both of these cases, adjacent nasolabial skin served as an excellent donor site for repair of alar-perialar defects. A deep myocutaneous pedicle provided a reliable blood supply for both flaps. The flexibility of the tissues in this area allowed for recreation of the unique topographic features of this anatomic site in both instances, with slight variations in design and execution.

Commentary by Dr. Ratner

16

CONUNDRUM 16

"Jigsaw Puzzle" Advancement Flap for Repair of a Surgical Defect Involving the Lateral Nasal Ala

Leonard H. Goldberg, Arash Kimyai-Asadi, & Sirunya Silapunt
Houston, TX

A 69-year-old woman presented with a basal cell carcinoma on the left nasal ala. The lesion size was 0.8 × 0.8 cm. Mohs micrographic surgery was performed, and the tumor was removed with a two-stage excision. The postoperative defect measured 1.2 × 0.9 cm, and its depth was through the full thickness of the dermis (Figure 1). How would you reconstruct this defect?

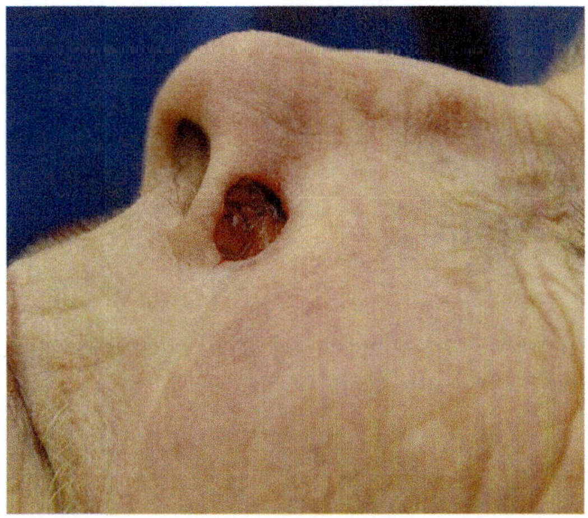

Figure 1 Defect on the lateral nasal ala.

Resolution

Nasal ala skin is unique. It is thick and sebaceous and not exactly duplicated anywhere on the body. The closest color and texture match is the conchal bowl of the ear or the adjacent cheek skin. Flaps of the nasal ala using dorsal skin from the superior skin from the nose are difficult owing to potential notching or elevation of the alar rim. Therefore, closures of the lateral nasal ala are often best achieved by full-thickness skin grafting. Full-thickness skin grafts are an excellent method of closure in this location and may provide a pleasant cosmetic result. However, full-thickness skin grafts have their own specific problems, which include the necessity of creating a second defect, not having an exact color and texture match, and lacking a primary blood supply. Second-intention healing is another good option. The healing time would be longer, and there is a danger of reduced size of the nasal ala. Moreover, second-intention healing on this area may also cause notching of the alar rim owing to scar contraction.

In cases in which the defect on the nasal skin is adjacent to the cheek, cheek skin can be used as an advancement flap. We describe a technique that demonstrates this principle. Using a template of the defect, we draw an advancement flap on the cheek with the dog-ears inferiorly along the melolabial fold and superiorly along the melonasal junction. The flap is incised and the dog-ears are excised, leaving the flap attached laterally. The underlying fat is trimmed off the flap skin. The secondary

Reconstructive Conundrums in Dermatologic Surgery: The Nose, First Edition. Edited by Désirée Ratner, Joel L. Cohen and David G. Brodland.
© 2014 American Society for Dermatologic Surgery. Published 2014 by John Wiley & Sons, Ltd.

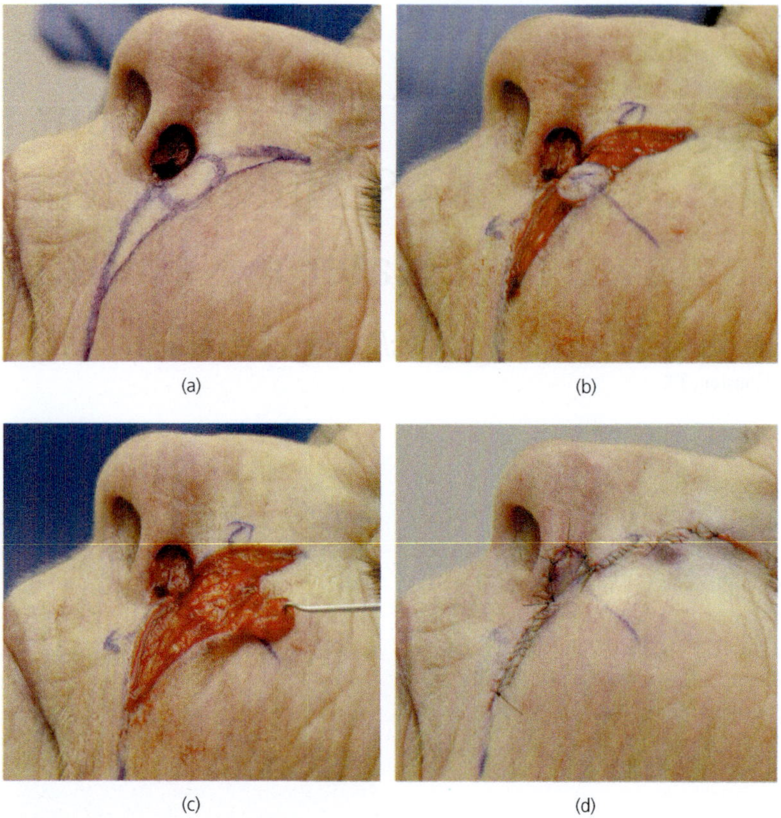

Figure 2 (A–D) Closure of the defect.

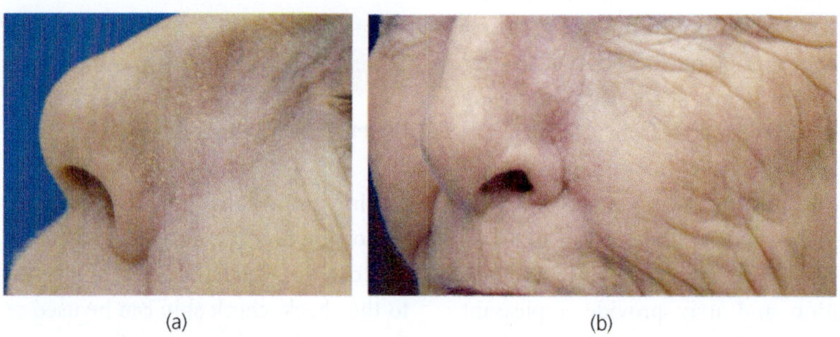

Figure 3 (A–B) At the 9-week follow-up.

defects, superiorly and inferiorly, resulting from the dog-ear excision, are closed with subcutaneous sutures from the advancing cheek skin to the periosteum of the maxillary bone. The 4-0 absorbable sutures on an FS-1 needle are used for this purpose. The flap is thus pulled downward and medially into position on the lateral nasal alar defect. The closure is completed with running cutaneous 6-0 nylon sutures. The reconstruction and follow-up photographs are shown in Figures 2 and 3.

The cheek skin adjacent to the defect was used as an advancement flap to repair the defect. This skin was selected because of its color, thickness, and texture, which are similar to those of the nasal ala. The adjacent major skin fold – the melolabial fold – was used to hide the inferior dog-ear created by the advancement of cheek skin. This major skin fold between the cosmetic units of the cheek and the upper lip is excellent for masking surgical scars. The superior dog-ear is placed vertically at the melonasal junction, which is at the angle of the nose and the cheek on the line between the cosmetic units of the cheek and nose. This angle of the skin also hides a surgical scar line well. To maintain the angle between the cheek skin and the nose, the cheek skin must be advanced in the same direction as it normally lies. To do this, the cheek skin is fixed directly to the periosteum of the maxilla in the piriform fossa with a large FS-1 needle and 4-0 absorbable sutures. If the cheek skin is fixed directly to the nose, it will tend to distort the melonasal angle. The technique of fixing the cheek skin to the periosteum demands some surgical expertise. As the cheek is pulled medially, the advancement flap itself automatically assumes the normal melonasal angle and fixes itself into position in the nasoalar defect. The shape of the advancing flap with its "head and shoulders" pattern imitates a jigsaw puzzle piece.

Owing to the narrowing of the neck of the flap between its head and shoulders, there is a reduction in blood supply and lymphatic drainage to the replacement skin. This pedicle must be carefully handled and made as wide as possible. In two of five flaps that we have performed using this technique, there was postoperative swelling of the flap, which took several months to resolve. We have had no cases of flap necrosis. The terminal branch of the facial artery (angular artery) runs on the maxillary bone deep to the location of the flap. Because the advancing cheek skin is anchored to the nasal bone periosteum underneath the nose and medial to the artery, this artery is not in danger of being pierced by the needle or ligated by the sutures.

When the defect resulting from the removal of skin cancer on the nasal ala also involves a portion of the cheek skin, this closure method remains useful. The utility of this flap is increased because two separate closure methods for two cosmetic units are not needed. The cheek defect is closed at the same time by the same flap by the advancing cheek skin as if a cheek defect had not been present. The cheek skin is moved a greater distance than if a purely nasal alar defect were closed, and the longer resultant dog-ears are removed in the same dog-ear closure lines.

Conundrum keys

- This is an advancement flap whose dog-ears are hidden in a major skin fold and a closure line between the nose and cheek cosmetic units.
- There is abundant donor skin, resulting in minimal or no closure tension.
- The advancing tissue must be anchored to the deep tissue in the piriform fossa to maintain the nose-cheek contour.
- The pedicle of the flap should not be made too narrow.
- The flap should be trimmed of all subcutaneous fat to avoid postoperative trapdoor effect.

Commentary on conundrum 16

Credit is due to the author for an unusually innovative idea in the jigsaw advancement flap. It clearly works and is actually fairly straightforward despite the name suggesting a level of complexity comparable to that of a jigsaw puzzle. The final result shown in Figure 16.1b does appear to have some blunting of the alar groove, which could be modified with a simple excision within the groove to recapitulate the concavity, which could then either be sutured or better yet left to granulate. Perhaps a simpler repair for this defect would be to use the same

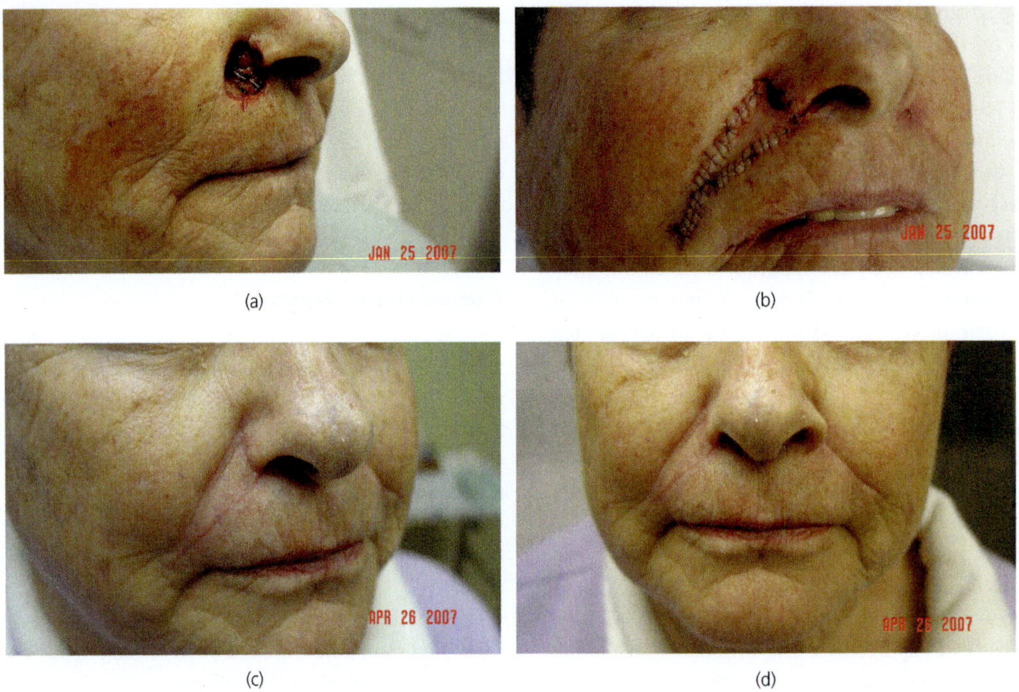

Figure 16.1 (a) Deep alar Mohs surgical defect extending to the alar rim and involving apical triangle. (b) Island pedicle advancement flap utilized to close majority of defect. Remaining alar defect left to heal by secondary intention to recapitulate alar groove concavity. (c) Follow-up at 3 months (lateral view). (d) Mild asymmetry seen on anterior view.

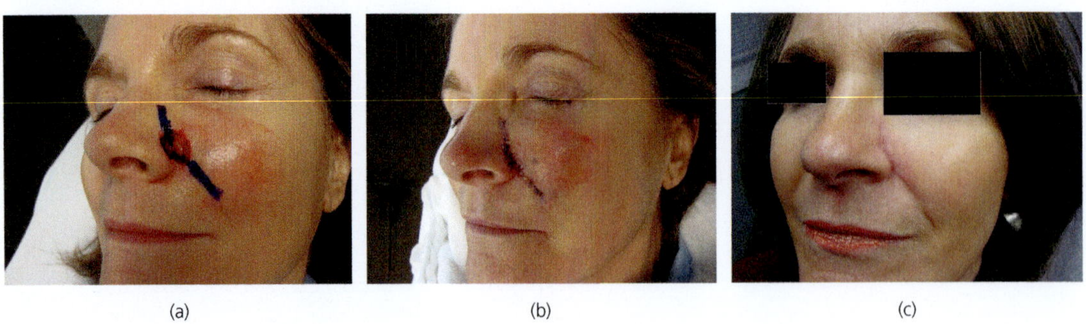

Figure 16.2 (a) Mohs surgical defect involving the alar sidewall and medial cheek. Cosmetic subunits demarcated with gentian violet. (b) Linear closure of cheek portion of defect. Burow's triangle from superior standing cone used to repair remaining lateral alar defect. (c) Three-month follow-up showing recapitulation of alar groove and good tissue match of Burow's graft with alar skin.

linear cheek advancement without the jigsaw leading edge with a Burow's triangle graft (either the superior or inferior standing cone of the linear closure) for the alar subunit (Figure 16.1). To replace the alar volume of a deeper defect, a subcutaneous hinge flap can be performed along with the cheek advancement, followed by a Burow's full-thickness skin graft of the alar subunit (Figure 16.2).[1]

An alternative option for repair of the original defect would have been simply to allow the remaining defect on the ala to heal by secondary intention (Figure 16.3) – as exemplified in this V to Y advancement flap with the remaining alar subunit defect left to granulate. However, allowing this type of defect to granulate can result in asymmetry that is visible from the front or swimmer's view (Figure 16.3g).

Another possibility would have been to undermine the cheek defect between 2 and 5 o'clock, using an absorbable suture thereafter to close virtually the entire cheek aspect of the defect while preserving the alar groove concavity

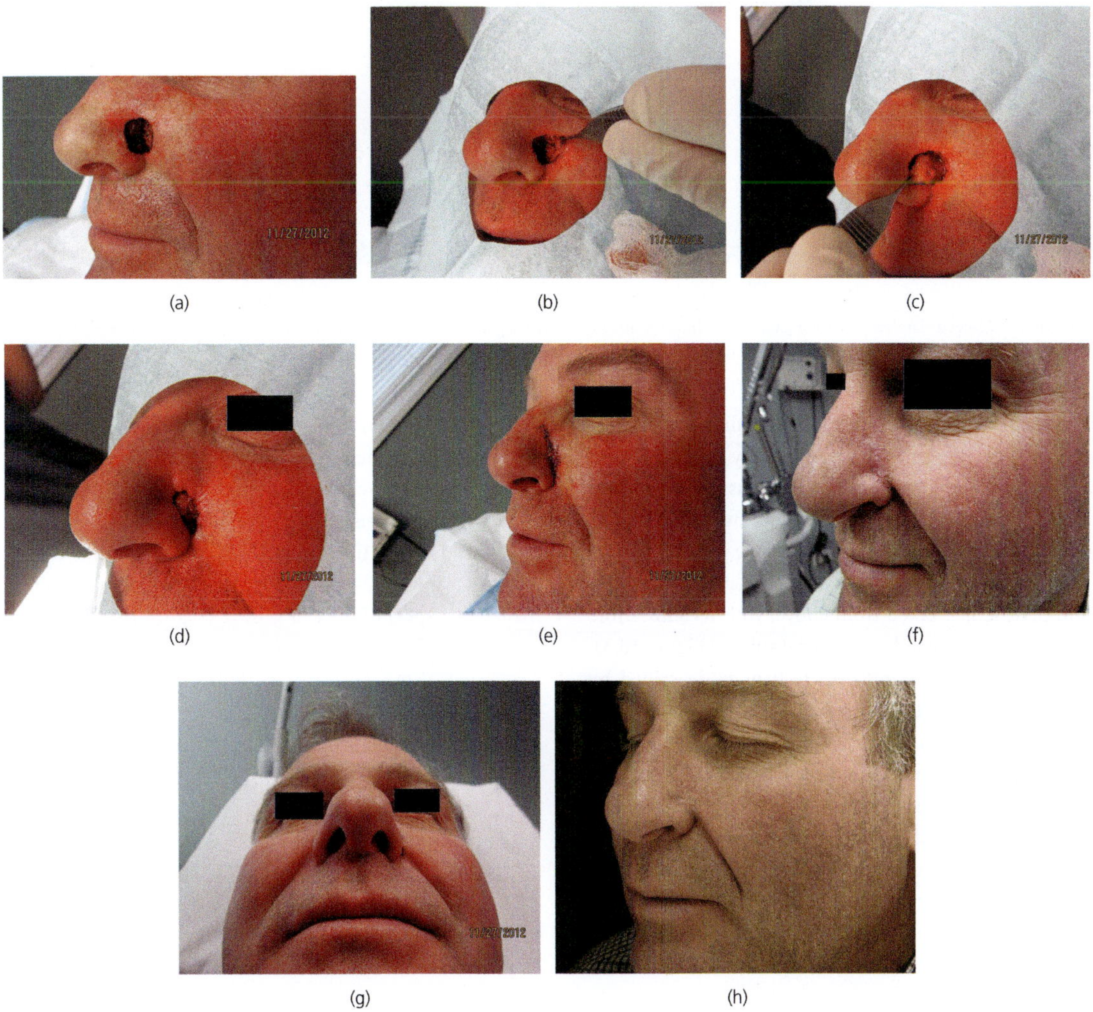

Figure 16.3 (a) Deep Mohs surgical defect extending from lateral alar skin onto the medial cheek. (b) Subcutaneous hinge flap mobilized from the cheek. (c) Hinge flap positioned as though turning the page of a book to decrease defect depth. (d) Plication sutures decreased the remaining defect size. (e) Cheek defect was repaired along the nasofacial sulcus. Remaining defect was resurfaced with Burow's graft from superior triangle. (f) Lateral view at 4.5 weeks. (g) Swimmer's view at 4.5 weeks. (h) Lateral view at 6 months.

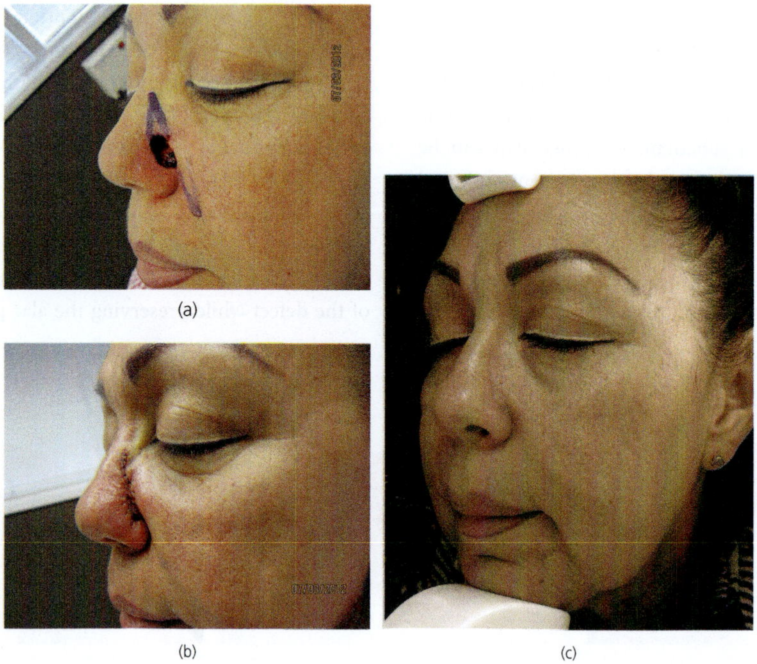

Figure 16.4 (a) Lateral alar defect extending to, but not into, the alar groove. (b) Superiorly based island pedicle flap. (c) Follow-up view at 3.5 months. Scar could benefit from some focal resurfacing to blend and minimize the scar.

with a periosteal tacking suture. The remaining alar defect could then be repaired with a superiorly based rotation flap designed along the nasofacial sulcus with a medial back-cut, which places the eventual Burow's triangle directly along the line of the alar groove. An alternative to the rotation flap portion of this repair could be an island pedicle flap taken from above, with its suture line similarly placed along the nasofacial sulcus (Figure 16.4).

Finally, the shark-island pedicle flap, as described by Cvancara and Wentzell,[2] is a variation on the island pedicle flap that involves a rotational component to recreate the peri-alar crease and could have been considered here. Although this flap has improved vascularity compared to the graft options discussed here and provides volume restoration of the lateral ala, its superior aspect does not fall within a cosmetic boundary, rendering its suture lines more prominent.

Despite the blunting of the alar groove, the "jigsaw advancement" as described here is indeed novel and certainly an alternative to consider in this setting, especially when repair options are limited. However, it might best be utilized when the defect does not cross into other anatomic subunits, so as to minimize the risk of blunting the lateral aspect of the alar groove (Figure 16.4).

Commentary by Dr. Cohen

References

1 Braun M, Cook J Hinge flaps in facial reconstruction. Dermatol Surg 2007;33(2):213–21.

2 Cvancara J, Wentzell M Shark island pedicle flap for repair of combined ala-perialar defects. Dermatol Surg. 2006;32(5):726–9.

17

CONUNDRUM 17

Dog-Ear Island Pedicle Flap for Repair of Ala and Nasal Wall Defects

Priya Zeikus[1], Mollie MacCormack[2], & Suzanne Olbricht[2]
[1]Department of Dermatology, UT Southwestern Medical School, Dallas, Texas
[2]Department of Dermatology, Lahey Clinic, Burlington, Massachusetts

The nasal ala has a unique architecture, and its integrity must be maintained during alar reconstruction for optimal functional and cosmetic results. It is well defined and framed by the alar crease superiorly, the nasofacial sulcus and upper cutaneous lip triangle laterally, and the alar rim inferiorly. Distortion of any of these structural boundaries can produce an unnatural appearance to the ala and may prevent proper inspiration. In general, there are limited options for the reconstruction of larger defects on the ala and nasal sidewall.

A 71-year-old woman was referred for Mohs micrographic surgery for a nodular basal cell carcinoma on the right alar crease. Complete excision of the tumor required three stages, resulting in a defect measuring 1.5 × 1.4 cm (Figure 1). How would you reconstruct this defect?

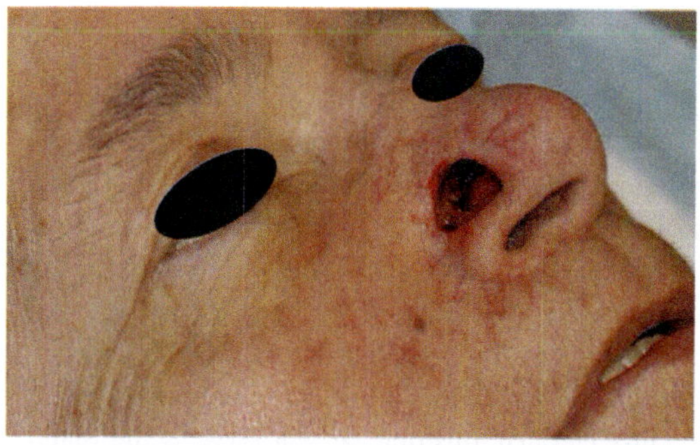

Figure 1 Patient with a partial-thickness alar defect after Mohs surgery measuring 1.5 by 1.4 cm.

Resolution

Standard reconstruction options for large defects that involve the ala and nasal sidewall include the cheek advancement flap,[1] dorsal nasal flap,[2] bilobed flap,[3] nasolabial flap,[4] full-thickness skin graft, interpolated flaps, and subcutaneous hinge flaps, but there are many limitations associated with these conventional reconstructions, including blunting of the alar crease, distortion of the nasal architecture, trapdooring, bridging of the nasofacial sulcus, poor nasal contour, and poor color and texture match. A closure that would preserve the alar architecture and its boundaries would be ideal. We describe a novel combination flap for the repair of alar and nasal wall defects that preserves the integrity of the ala. This flap individually repairs the two nasal subunits, distinguishing the nasal sidewall from the ala.

The dog ear island pedicle flap is designed for partial-thickness alar defects that involve the alar crease and defects in the nasal side wall (Figure 1). This technique can be used to repair defect sizes ranging from 1.0 to 2.0 cm in diameter. This repair combines two flaps: a cheek advancement flap and a rotated island pedicle flap

Reconstructive Conundrums in Dermatologic Surgery: The Nose, First Edition. Edited by Désirée Ratner, Joel L. Cohen and David G. Brodland.
© 2014 American Society for Dermatologic Surgery. Published 2014 by John Wiley & Sons, Ltd.

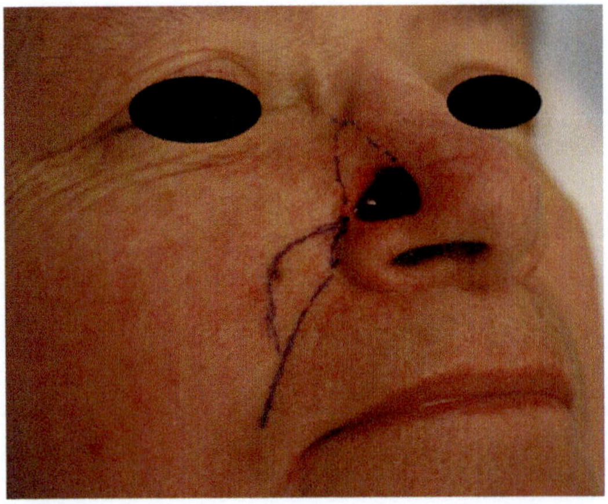

Figure 2 The dog ear island pedicle flap is a combination flap consisting of a cheek advancement flap and a rotated dog ear island pedicle flap.

(Figure 2). The island pedicle flap is derived from the superior dog ear or Burow's triangle created during the movement of the cheek advancement flap. Traditionally, the superior dog ear associated with this flap has been discarded or saved and used as a full-thickness skin graft.[5]

The procedure is performed under local anesthesia. As a first step, the cheek advancement flap is designed, and the superior dog ear is predicted. The first incisions are made directly superior to the defect to delineate the dog ear. Once elevated, this dog ear will serve as the island pedicle flap (Figure 3). It is carefully dissected so that the pedicle is at the medial edge of the flap. The pedicle is based on the nasalis muscle, which provides a robust blood supply. Once elevated, the island pedicle flap is

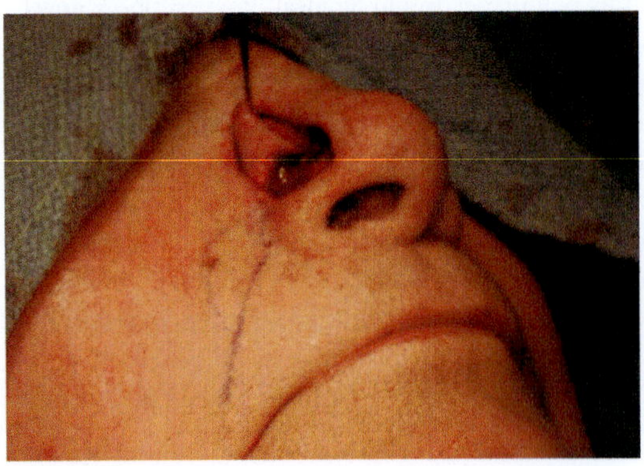

Figure 3 The superior dog ear created during the cheek advancement flap serves as the island pedicle flap.

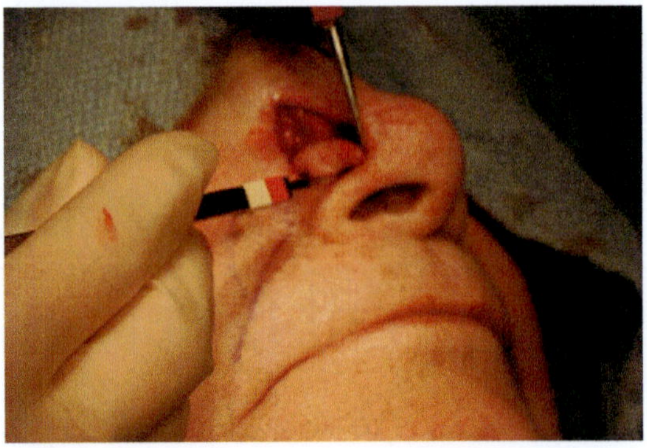

Figure 4 The dog ear island pedicle is rotated and transposed to fill the alar defect.

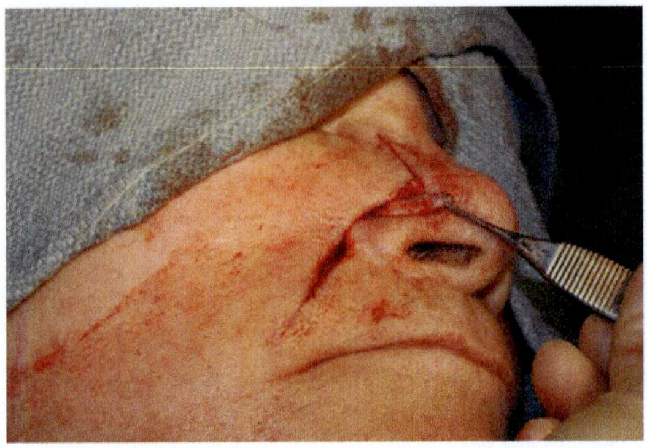

Figure 5 The cheek is advanced to cover the nasal wall defect.

rotated and transposed to fill the alar defect and recreate the convex contour (Figure 4). Next, the cheek advancement flap is elevated and advanced under minimal to no tension to cover the nasal wall defect (Figure 5); 5-0 absorbable suture is used to secure the flaps into place, and 6-0 non-absorbable sutures accurately align the epidermal edges to complete the repair. The junction of these two flaps meets and recreates the alar crease (Figure 6). Immediate, 1-week, and 2-month postoperative results are shown (Figures 7, 8 and 9).

Discussion

Large surgical defects involving the ala and nasal sidewall present a unique challenge to the reconstructive surgeon. The contour and boundaries of the ala must be respected,

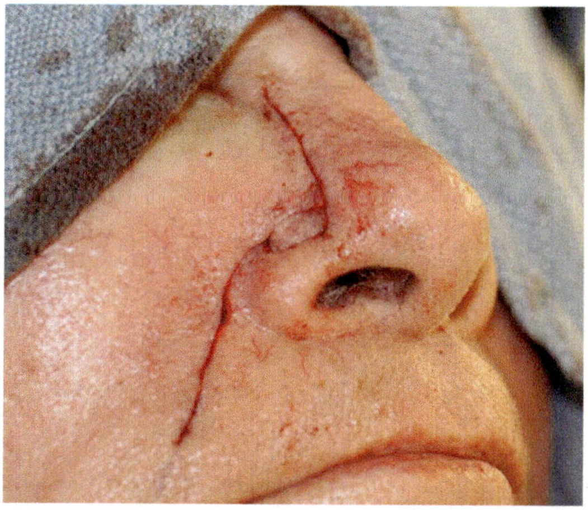

Figure 6 The alar crease is recreated at the junction of the two flaps.

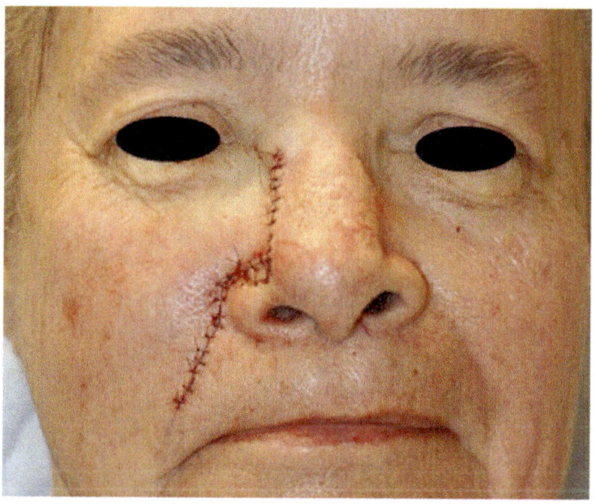

Figure 7 Immediate postoperative results. Mild depression of the ala is noted.

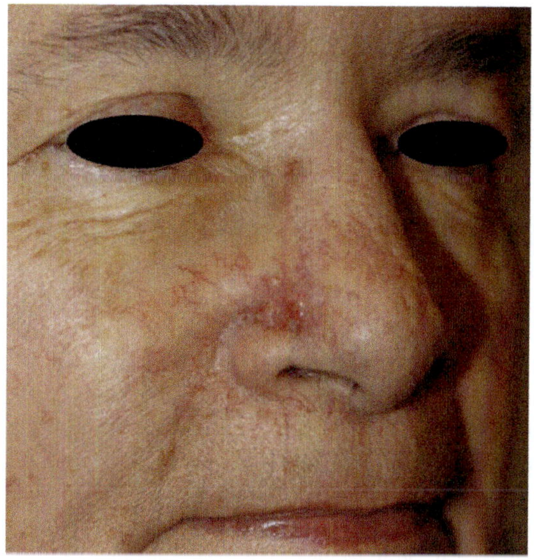

Figure 8 One-week postoperative results. Position of the ala and alar contour is excellent.

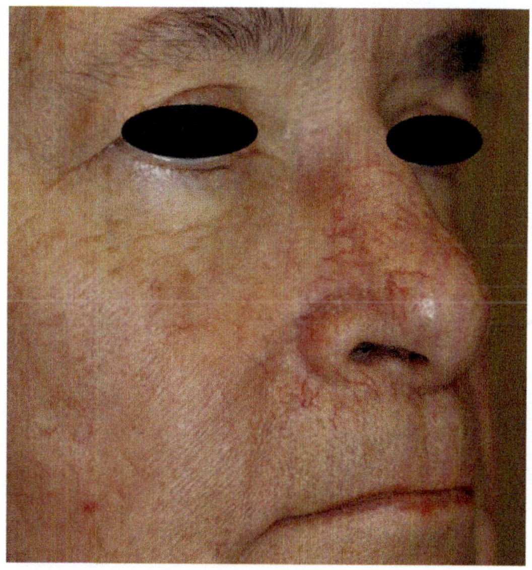

Figure 9 Two-month postoperative results.

because even minimal blunting of the alar crease or naso-facial sulcus becomes cosmetically obvious. Standard reconstructions include the dorsal nasal flap, bilobed flap, nasolabial flap, or cheek advancement flap. The dorsal nasal flap and bilobed flap both provide excellent tissue match and limit the repair to the nasal cosmetic subunit, but limitations include risk of trapdooring, scars that do not fall in natural cosmetic unit boundary lines, and loss of the alar crease.[6] Similarly, although the nasolabial flap is a reliable repair, it is associated with a high risk of trapdooring and blunting of the naso-facial sulcus.[7] The trapdoor effect can be seen when proper suspension sutures are not used. Limitations of the cheek advancement flap include blunting of the alar crease, loss of the upper lip cutaneous triangle, and potential blunting of the nasofacial sulcus.[8] A closure that individually repairs and distinguishes the two nasal subunits would be ideal.

The combination flap described in this article is an ideal repair because it combines two different flaps to repair the ala and nasal sidewall individually. This repair has several advantages over other methods of reconstruction. It is a one-stage procedure that preserves the contour and appearance of the ala. The flap lines and the scars are well camouflaged in the patient's natural skin lines, and most importantly, the alar crease is preserved. Finally, this flap also maintains the natural skin tone and texture of the nose. Blunting of the nasofacial sulcus and trap-dooring are not a concern with this repair. Potential limitations of this flap include loss of the island pedicle flap, because the dog ear is rotated about the pedicle, which may restrict blood flow to the flap. Necrosis of the island pedicle flap has not been seen in any of our patients. Also, the movement of the island pedicle has a slightly vertical component that can push the ala down immediately postoperatively. However, in our case the ala returned to its normal position by the 1-week postoperative visit (Figures 7 and 8). There was no difficulty experienced in movement of the island pedicle flap, although limitations may exist for larger alar defects. Although a cheek advancement flap and full-thickness skin graft would be an acceptable combination flap in this location,[5] we have found that the dog ear island pedicle combination has greater success and shorter healing times. An additional potential limitation of this flap, also seen with cheek advancement flaps, is asymmetry of the nasolabial fold. This was not significant in our patients. This complication is minimized with this dual flap because the upper flap triangle is preserved. Finally, in the repair of larger alar defects, one must be careful not to constrict the nasal valve. For these larger alar defects, a cartilage graft inserted in the ala becomes necessary. None of the patients experienced decreased patency of the nasal valve with this repair.

The authors have performed this repair in five patients and have had excellent cosmetic and functional outcomes with their patients.

References

1 Yoo SS, Miller SJ. The crescentic advancement flap revisited. Dermatol Surg 2003;29:856–8.

2 Bray DA, Eichel BS, Kaplan HJ. The dorsal nasal flap. Arch Otolaryngol 1981;107:765–6.

3 Zitelli JA. The bilobed flap for nasal reconstruction. Arch Derm 1989;125:957–9.

4 Zitelli JA. The nasolabial flap as a single stage procedure. Arch Derm 1990;126:1445–8.

5 Kim KH, Gross VL, Jaffee AT, Herbst AM. The use of the melolabial Burow's graft in the reconstruction of combination nasal sidewall-cheek defects. Derm Surg 2004;30:205–7.

6 Dinehart SM. The Rhombic flap for nasal reconstruction. Derm Surg 2001;27:501–4.

7 Drisco BP, Baker SR. Reconstruction of nasal alar defects. Arch Facial Plast Surg 2001;3:91–9.

8 Svedman P. Advancement flaps for alar reconstruction. Ann Plast Reconstr Surg 1990;25:502–7.

Commentary on conundrum 17

Defects of the nasal ala extending onto the nasal sidewall are exceedingly common in surgical practice. Each patient's individual anatomy and tissue laxity, as well as the size, configuration, and depth of the individual defect, helps to determine the optimal choice of repair. In this reconstructive conundrum, the authors closed the sidewall and alar aspects of the defect with separate, but integrally related, repairs, using the superior dog-ear of a cheek advancement flap as an island pedicle flap to repair the alar portion of the defect. Advantages of this technique include preservation of facial symmetry and maintenance of the contour and boundaries of the ala, sidewall, and nasofacial sulcus without blunting of the alar crease.

When devising a reconstructive approach to repair defects of the nasal ala and sidewall, it is important to assess the available tissue laxity as completely as possible. At this location, the cheek skin lateral to the defect can often be used as a donor site for a superolaterally based transposition flap. Alternatively, nasal supratip and sidewall skin may at times be used to perform a rhombic or bilobed transposition flap, usually when the alar defect is more medially located, with concealment of the dog-ear within the lateral alar crease. Either of these types of repairs could have been performed for this particular alar defect.

The defect shown in Figure 17.1a, while comparable in terms of its location on the lateral nasal ala well

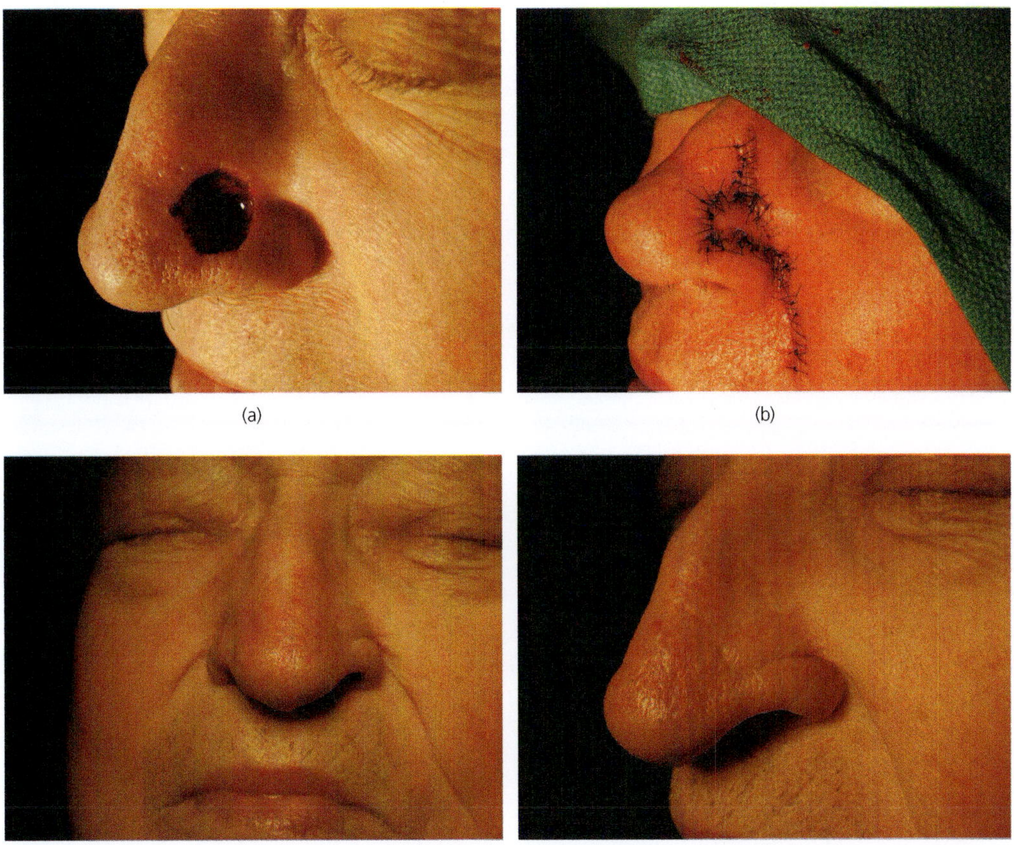

(a) (b) (c) (d)

Figure 17.1 (a) Defect of the nasal ala extending onto the lower portion of the nasal sidewall, with obliteration of alar crease. (b) Superolaterally based rhombic flap used for repair. (c and d) Follow-up view at 4 months showing persistent slight trapdooring of flap anteriorly (c) and laterally (d).

above the alar rim, was approached differently. As in the reconstructive conundrum case, the alar crease was nearly obliterated because of extension of the defect onto the nasal sidewall. A dog-ear island pedicle flap with a cheek advancement flap would certainly have been doable. In this instance however the reservoir of lax skin present superolaterally at the junction of the nasal sidewall and medial cheek was used to perform a transposition flap, with concealment of the incision line superiorly within the nasofacial sulcus and extension of the dog ear inferiorly along the lateral alar crease (Figure 17.1b). In this way, as in the reconstructive conundrum case, the alar crease was recreated, with preservation of the alar contour, and the incision lines were camouflaged within the patient's own facial lines (Figure 17.1c and d).

Commentary by Dr. Ratner

VI

PART VI
Alar Rim

18

CONUNDRUM 18

Repair of an Alar Defect

Joel Cook

Department of Dermatology, Medical University of South Carolina, Charleston, SC

A healthy, 44-year-old white man was referred for Mohs micrographic surgery of a biopsy-proven basal cell carcinoma of the left ala. At presentation, the patient had a nodular plaque measuring 0.6 × 0.5 cm with ill-defined clinical borders of the left ala. Given the critical anatomic location and ill-defined borders, Mohs micrographic surgery was indicated. The tumor was subsequently extirpated in two stages using the Mohs technique producing a surgical defect measuring 1.4 × 1.0 cm in greatest dimension. The resultant surgical defect extended into the subcutaneous tissue of the left ala but did not perforate into the nasal vestibule (Figure 1). Reconstructive options considered included second intention healing, full-thickness skin graft, composite graft, island pedicle flap, and a two-stage interpolation flap. As a dermatologic surgeon, how would you address this patient's surgical defect to yield the optimum functional and aesthetic restoration?

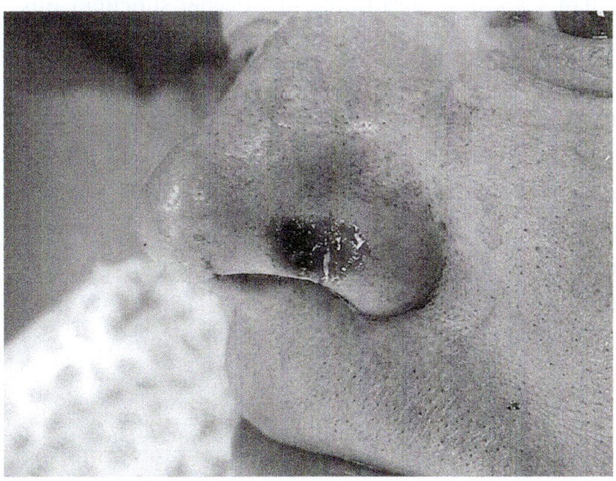

Figure 1

Resolution

After tumor extirpation in which accurate surgical margins have been assured to be negative, the dermatologic surgeon is frequently confronted with soft-tissue defects of the nasal ala. The paramount reconstruction goal includes restoring function if lost or preserving function if maintained. This must be allied with a reconstructive option that produces elegant cosmetic results with concomitant little morbidity in a cost-effective fashion.

The topographic complexity of the nasal ala has frequently challenged the dermatologic surgeon. In this particular instance, the defect was rather small and was not full thickness. However, the close proximity to the free alar margin has produced a surgical defect of moderate complexity. The reconstructive surgeon must clearly understand the aesthetic importance of this area of the nose and the poor tolerance for alar movement in achieving excellent cosmetic results. If the ala is displaced upward, suboptimal results and patient dissatisfaction may result. The reconstructive surgeon must also consider the anatomy of the nasal valve and the patency of the nasal airway when reconstructing defects in this anatomic location.

Although second intention healing may produce nice results in the more concave areas of the ala (around the alar groove), it is not a viable option in this case.

Reconstructive Conundrums in Dermatologic Surgery: The Nose, First Edition. Edited by Désirée Ratner, Joel L. Cohen and David G. Brodland.
© 2014 American Society for Dermatologic Surgery. Published 2014 by John Wiley & Sons, Ltd.

Predictable wound contraction would undoubtedly produce elevation of the free alar margin and a poor end cosmetic result. The close proximity of the caudad margin of this surgical defect to the free alar rim must be carefully considered. In my opinion, a full-thickness skin graft obtained from a suitable donor site (e.g., the conchal bowl) would in this case prove not only inadequate to fill the contour defect but also may allow for cephalic alar retraction. A composite graft of skin and perichondrium or skin, perichondrium, and cartilage may have been used to reconstruct this surgical defect. A composite graft may yield less retraction during a postoperative period. A composite graft containing an underlying strut of cartilage may have been harvested from the conchal floor to repair this surgical defect. However, in my experience, the viability of the composite grafts for alar defects is significantly less predictable than that of random pattern cutaneous flaps.

For surgical defects of this type, random pattern flaps prove unsurpassed in matching the qualities of missing skin and soft tissue and their ability to restore the complex topography of this anatomic subunit. Local flaps obtained from the lower nasal sidewall or lateral portion of the ala (bilobed transposition flapmedial base and island pedicle flap, respectively) would prove difficult in this particular situation. These flaps rely on some degree of secondary movement to achieve surgical closure and would place an inordinate risk on distortion of the alar margin. For this reason, I thought that the best reconstructive option was a two-staged interpolation flap (Figure 2). This is a random pattern cutaneous flap that is based somewhat on the vasculature of the angular artery, a branch of the facial artery. These interpolation flaps, if done with surgical precision, are typically robust flaps. The cheek interpolation flap traditionally has a donor site at or near the midpoint of the melolabial fold. This allows the result of the donor scar to be placed carefully within the melolabial fold, assisting in scar camouflage. However, this is problematic for several reasons. In men, the interpolation flap may frequently transpose course terminal hair onto the ala, resulting in an obvious cosmetic problem. Secondary ablative procedures or laser-assisted hair removal may improve the cosmetic results but add yet another stage to the reconstructive efforts. Furthermore, for larger alar defects, the harvesting of the melolabial flap from the cheek as traditionally described may result in conspicuous flattening of the cheek and subtle asymmetry of the melolabial folds, an aesthetic result that some patients may find displeasing. For these reasons, I chose to change convention and place the donor site along the paranasal cheek at the junction of the aesthetic subunits of the lateral nasal dorsum and medial cheek. The resultant donor scar will hide carefully in this aesthetic boundary. This flap lacks the coarse terminal hair of the lower face, and the donor site may be easily closed by advancing the cheek to fill the surgical defect.

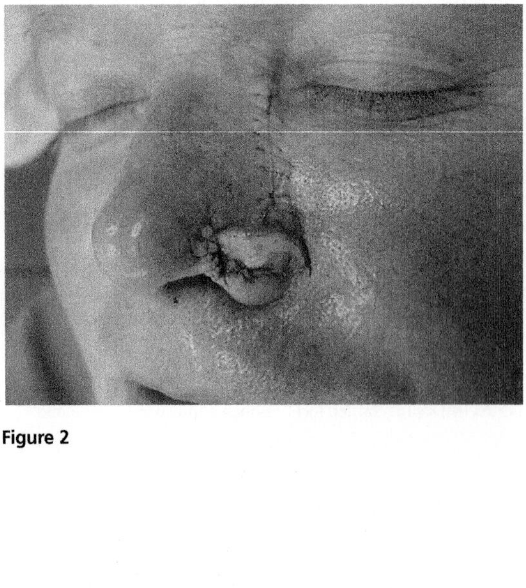

Figure 2

When performing this flap, it is of paramount importance to preserve the vascular integrity at the base of the flap. Careful undermining in a deeper subcutaneous plane will preserve this vascular pedicle. The flap is then trimmed to meet the size of the surgical defect of the ala and sutured into place. The donor site is appropriately closed in this case, as noted by sliding the cheek medially to the border of the aesthetic subunit. Sutures are removed in 5 days, and the flap is allowed to mature for 3 weeks from the date of the initial surgery. At this time, the pedicle is transected. The flap skin is then thinned and inset to fill the surgical defect and is sutured into place. The reconstructive surgeon at this point may wish to extend the surgical defect to encompass the entire remnant of the aesthetic unit. Sutures from the secondary procedure are removed at 7 days. The patient is then followed carefully to observe for any postoperative complications, although they rarely occur with this particular flap. In this case, the end aesthetic result was nice, and no additional surgical procedures were performed (Figure 3).

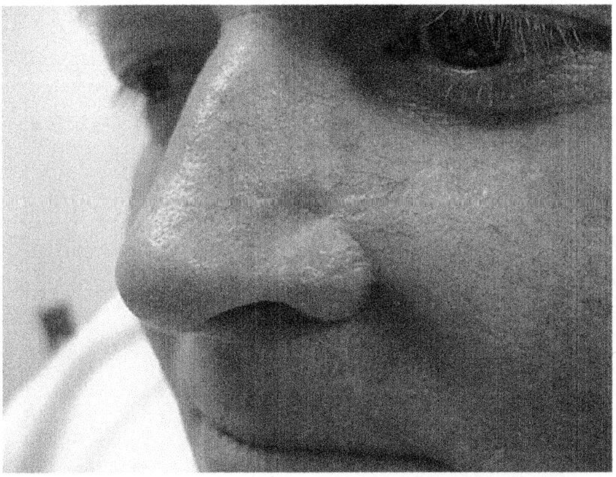

Figure 3

Conundrum keys

· Care must be taken to maintain or restore alar function and form.

· Two-staged interpolation flaps offer the advantages of closely matching skin, contour restoration, and avoidance of scarring and distortion caused by incorrectly designed adjacent flaps.

· The inferiorly based paranasal cheek interpolation flap has the advantage of avoiding transfer of terminal hair to the nose and distortion of the lower cheek and is easily camouflaged at the border of the aesthetic units of nasal sidewall and cheek.

Commentary on conundrum 18

Defects involving the free margin of the alar rim can be challenging to repair. As the author points out, repair of such defects must focus on avoidance of upward rim displacement and preservation of the alar contour. A full-thickness skin graft alone, even from a carefully matched donor tissue, would likely contract over the course of natural healing, leading to a suboptimal cosmetic result. A two-stage interpolation flap offers the advantages of contour restoration and closely matching skin. The inferiorly based donor site for the flap, in this case, is an excellent choice given the absence of coarse terminal hairs in the donor tissue as well as the ability to camouflage the donor suture line within the nasofacial sulcus. However, two operative visits are still required to complete the procedure, which some patients may be unwilling or unable to undergo.

A single-stage alternative to this defect would be to place a cartilage strut along the alar rim, followed by a full-thickness skin graft. This approach stabilizes the alar rim and consistently produces excellent cosmetic and functional results. In the accompanying series of photos, a partial-thickness nasal defect is shown, similar to the one shown in the reconstruction conundrum, whose inferior margin extends close to the alar rim (Figure 18.1). Rim stabilization was therefore a key element in the successful repair of this defect. A cartilage graft was harvested from the posterior conchal bowl, placed along the inferior margin of the nasal defect, and interlocked with pockets undermined in the soft tissue on either side (Figure 18.2). A 5-0 polyglycolic acid suture was used as an additional means of securing the graft to the underlying soft tissue. A full-thickness skin graft taken from the preauricular region was then placed over the cartilage graft and secured peripherally with 6-0 fast absorbing gut sutures (Figure 18.3). A bolster was sewn over the graft and left in place for 1 week. The result at the time of suture removal shows preservation of the alar contour following this

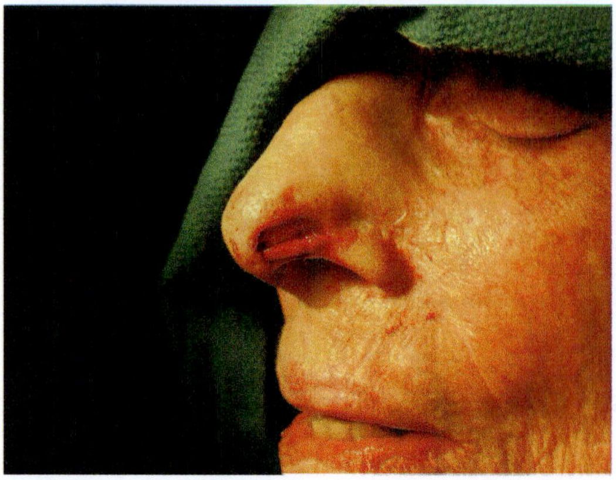

Figure 18.2 Cartilage graft in place. Soft tissue pockets have been undermined on either side of the defect into which the graft ends have been inserted.

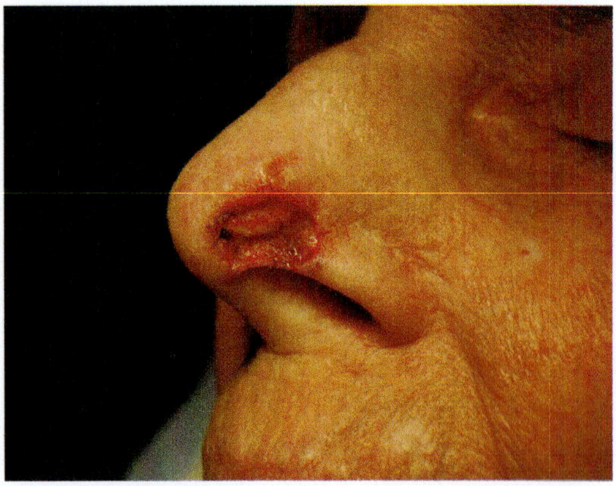

Figure 18.1 Partial-thickness defect of left ala with inferior margin extending along the alar rim.

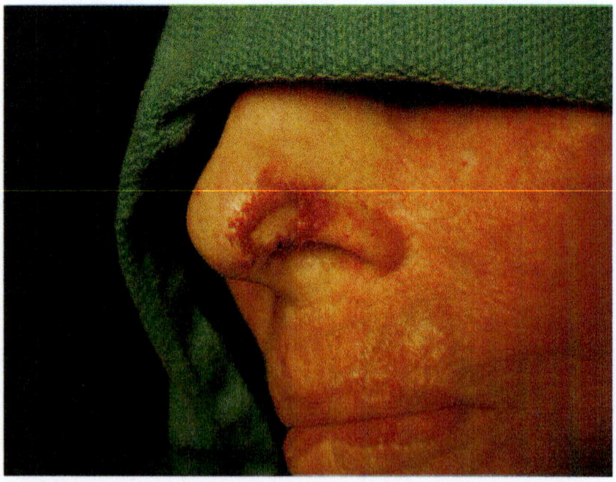

Figure 18.3 Preauricular full-thickness skin graft sewn into place over cartilage graft with 6-0 fast absorbing gut sutures.

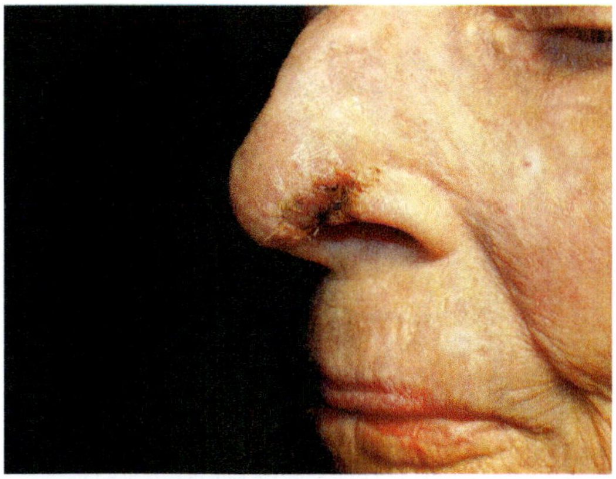

Figure 18.4 Graft at the time of suture removal showing 100% graft take and preservation of alar rim contour.

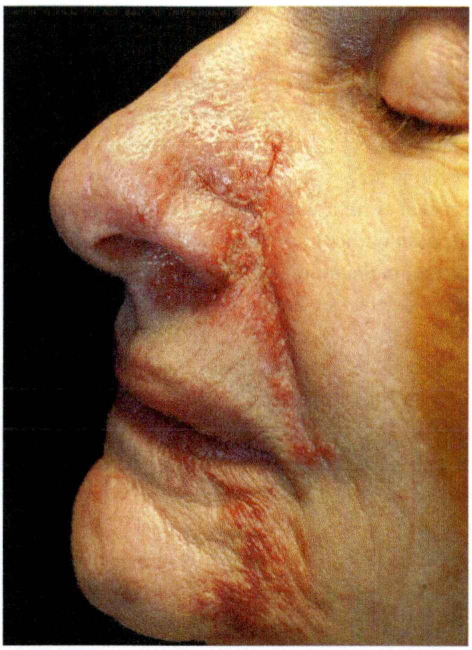

Figure 18.5 Patient underwent another surgical procedure 6 months later for basal cell carcinoma (BCC) of the left nasofacial sulcus. Surgical site of the left medial alar rim shows good alar contour and tissue match.

single-stage procedure (Figure 18.4), with an excellent cosmetic result 6 months later (Figure 18.5).

Each surgeon will inevitably have unique preferences regarding donor site selection and techniques for graft harvesting and placement. Some surgeons use antihelical cartilage for structural support, as they find it more flexible and easier to handle than curved conchal cartilage, as well as less prone to fractures. While larger auricular cartilage grafts are more easily harvested from the antihelix via an anterior approach, I tend to use the posterior conchal bowl as the donor site of choice for narrow cartilage struts to stabilize the alar rim. Grafts 3–4 mm in width and 1–1.5 cm in length are straightforward to harvest from this location. While fracture can occasionally occur, a second cartilaginous strip can be quickly harvested as a replacement if needed. Furthermore, the posterior donor site is easy to close, with an invisible donor site scar tucked behind the ear. I tend to "lasso" the cartilage with an absorbable polyglycolic acid suture to secure it to the underlying soft tissue, rather than suturing through it, because of the attendant risk of fracture and also interlocks the ends of the strut with soft tissue pockets undermined on either side of the defect to minimize the risk of graft displacement.

While postauricular skin can be an excellent source of donor tissue, postauricular skin may at times be thinner, less sebaceous, and less sun damaged than the nasal skin that it replaces, resulting in a less than perfect match. Careful attention must be paid to all aspects of the donor tissue and recipient sites when performing skin grafting on the nose, including sebaceous quality, skin thickness, skin vascularity, extent of sun damage, color, and texture, to ensure an optimal match. This author tends to use preauricular skin more consistently for nasal full-thickness grafts because I find that it tends to provide a better match than postauricular skin for patients with thicker, more sun-damaged nasal skin (Figures 18.6, 18.7 and 18.8). Conchal bowl skin may also serve as a good match particularly for sebaceous noses. It is important to recognize the gradations in color, texture, and sebaceous quality that exist within the preauricular skin itself as it extends from the hairline to the lobule, which can be helpful in optimizing donor tissue match for nasal defects requiring full-thickness skin graft coverage.

Despite the fact that some studies have questioned the effectiveness of bolsters in enhancing the survival of skin grafts, I routinely bolster all of the grafts with a very high survival rate. The bolster stays in place for 1 week. After it has been removed, patients continue wound care for the next 1–2 weeks with several applications of petrolatum daily and, for larger grafts, daily reapplication of xeroform gauze as well.

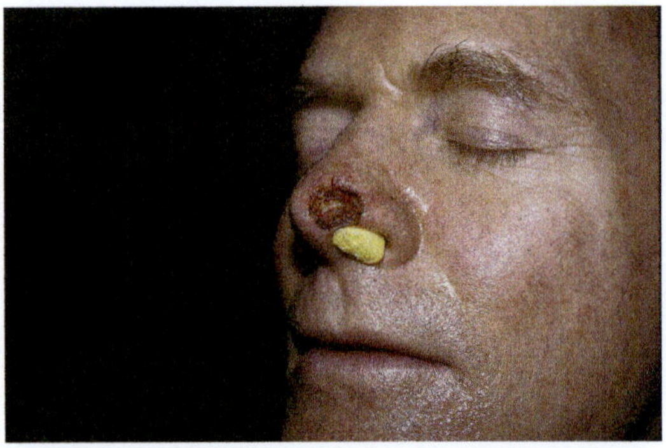

Figure 18.6 Mohs surgical defect of the left nasal tip and soft triangle extending close to the alar rim.

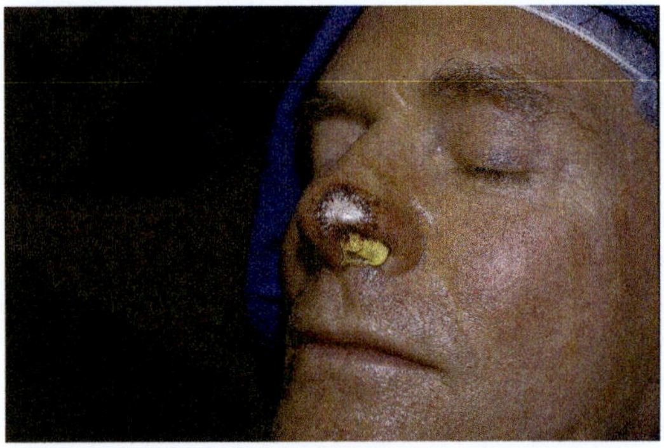

Figure 18.7 A cartilage strut was placed beneath a preauricular full-thickness skin graft to stabilize the alar rim.

I have found that the rate of necrosis with combined grafts is not higher than that of traditional full-thickness skin grafts and is significantly lower than that of composite grafts. Extrusion of the absorbable sutures used to anchor the cartilage grafts can occur, and all patients are therefore seen several weeks after surgery to remove any protruding suture fragments. Mild hypertrophic scarring, which at times manifests itself as thickening of the entire graft, or merely the inferior aspect of the graft beneath the cartilage strut, can be easily managed with small doses of intralesional triamcinolone, generally 10 mg/mL every 3 weeks after surgery for the first 3–4 months and tends to resolve completely.

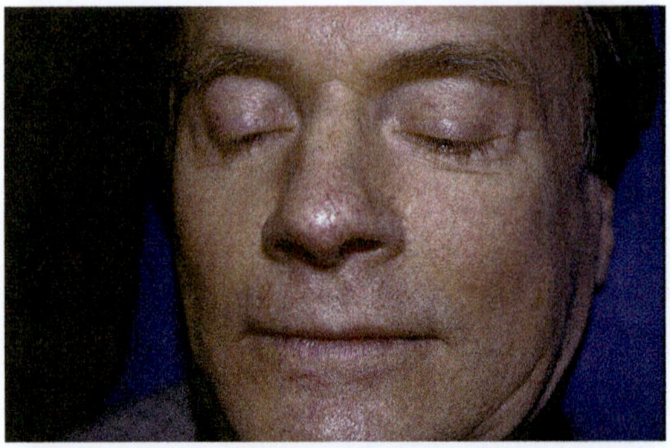

Figure 18.8 Alar rim in perfect position 6 months after surgery. The graft shows good color and texture match with the surrounding nasal skin.

The goal of esthetic surgical repair is to achieve the best possible cosmetic and functional result. Ultimately, there is always more than one way to close any defect. For this type of nasal defect, an interpolation flap with a paranasal cheek donor site, as illustrated in this conundrum, a more traditional melolabial interpolation flap, or a free cartilage graft with full-thickness skin graft coverage, when properly performed, can achieve that goal, but it is critical that the surgeon carefully assess the available donor tissue and options for scar camouflage to determine the best option for each patient.

Commentary by Dr. Ratner

19

CONUNDRUM 19

Reconstruction of a Full Thickness Soft Triangle Defect

Galen H. Fisher

Laser and Skin Surgery Center of Richmond, Richmond, Virginia

An 84-year-old white woman presented with a full-thickness defect of her soft triangle, medial alar rim, and partial thickness defect of the left lateral columella.

Defects of the soft triangle present a challenge to the reconstructive surgeon. The suspended web of the soft triangle needs to be reconstructed on the anterior and posterior surface. This challenge has been met with many different approaches. How would you close this defect of the soft triangle?

Options for closure of full-thickness soft triangle defects of the nose include an interpolated melolabial flap, interpolated paramedian forehead flap, nasalis muscle-based turnover flap with full-thickness skin graft, columellar turnover flap with a full-thickness skin graft, and a composite graft containing cartilage to offer maximal structural support.

Grafts are an excellent option for nasal reconstruction in patients whose skin tends to be somewhat hypopigmented, but in many cases grafts will fail to adequately match with regard to color, texture, and contour. With a full-thickness defect such as this, there are two methods that would allow for the use of a graft closure. The first is to supply a vascular bed using a turnover flap based on the nasalis muscle or the columella. The second graft-based reconstructive option is a classic composite graft containing cartilage and skin, frequently derived from the crux-helix. Both of these graft-based approaches can be rewarding, but with the sebaceous nature of our patient's nose, we felt that a graft would not maximize final cosmesis, regardless of donor site. Furthermore, composite grafts have less reliability than other methods of closure, especially when trying to span larger defects such as the example shown in this case.

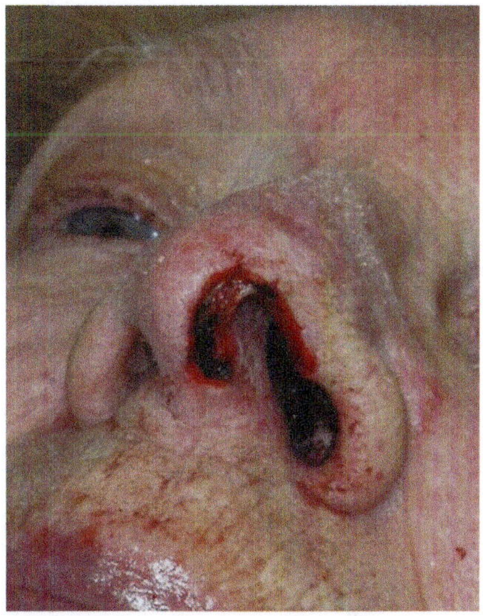

Figure 1 Defect after Mohs extirpation of a basal cell carcinoma of the soft triangle.

Interpolation flaps offer a method of reliably transferring well-vascularized tissue from a discontiguous donor site into the defect. The lush vascularity of axial and random pattern interpolation flaps allows successful transfer of full-thickness dermis and subcutis, facilitating contour restoration and precluding development of the hypopigmentation and shiny texture that is often seen

Reconstructive Conundrums in Dermatologic Surgery: The Nose, First Edition. Edited by Désirée Ratner, Joel L. Cohen and David G. Brodland.
© 2014 American Society for Dermatologic Surgery. Published 2014 by John Wiley & Sons, Ltd.

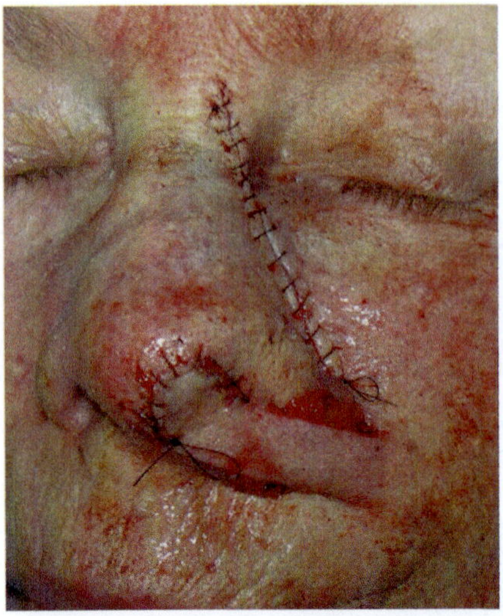

Figure 2 Paranasal flap in place and donor site closed.

with graft reconstruction. Although offering maximal final cosmesis, there are several matters to be considered before choosing to use an interpolation flap. As Cook recently highlighted, the melolabial interpolation flap can produce cheek asymmetry.[1] A forehead flap avoids the issue of centrofacial asymmetry but results in significant patient-perceived morbidity and is possibly judiciously saved for a larger nasal defect than the one shown in this case example. The interpolated paranasal flap offers the advantages of the traditional interpolation flaps with regard to tissue match and contour restoration but sidesteps the concerns mentioned above with the melolabial and forehead interpolation flaps.[2,3] This reconstruction was therefore pursued using an interpolated paranasal flap (Figure 2).

Technique

Before using the interpolated paranasal flap, the patient's upper nasal sidewall was evaluated to ensure adequate tissue match and local donor site generosity. Next the flap was designed with sufficient width, centered along the nasofacial sulcus near the proximal origin of the flap, and carried onto the nose toward the distal end of the flap at the nasal root. The flap was incised to the subcutis and undermined with care to preserve a vascular pedicle at the origin. The distal flap was thinned and carefully sutured into place in the defect. Three weeks later, the flap was divided, thinned, cleared of excess granulation tissue on the posterior aspect, and folded back on itself to give lining to the posterior aspect of the soft triangle (Figure 3). The folding of the flap helps to recreate the desired rim contour. During the insetting process, we used the contralateral side as a reference to guide in contouring. One month after suture removal, manual dermabrasion was used to further optimize cosmesis (Figure 4).

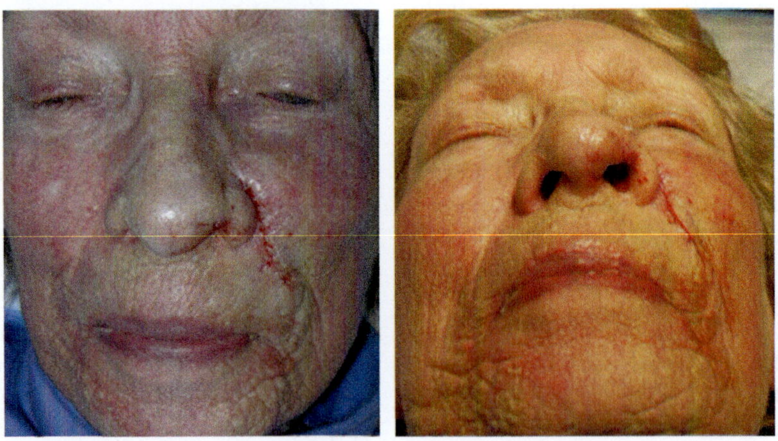

(a) (b)

Figure 3 At 3 weeks, the flap is separated and the donor site repaired.

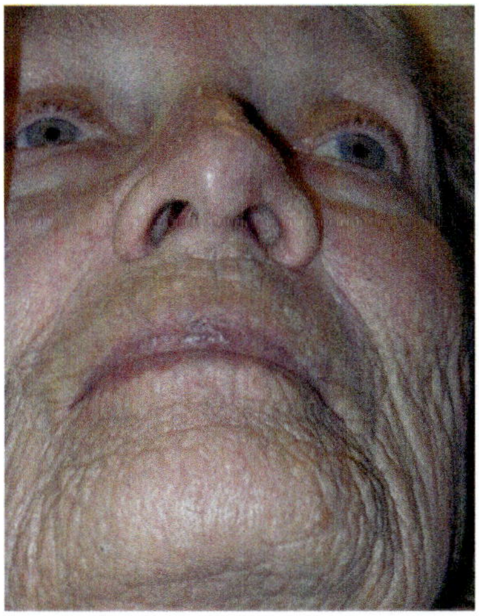

Figure 4 Final result.

Conundrum keys

· In this patient, the upper nasal sidewall was a good match for her missing skin.

· The interpolated paranasal flap offers robust vascularity, allowing for transfer of discontiguous skin.

· The location of the pedicle donor site along the naso-facial sulcus preserved cheek symmetry.

· Patients seem to experience less morbidity with an interpolated paranasal flap than a forehead interpolation flap or a superiorly based melolabial flap.

· Sufficient donor site laxity is a necessity for this flap; it may not be feasible in patients who lack redundancy in the donor site area.

· Sufficient flap width prevents distortion; rotational shortening must be accounted for during the process of flap design.

· Further refinement such as dermabrasion may be helpful to optimize final cosmesis.

References

1 Cook JL. The undesirable influence of reconstructive procedures on the symmetry of the nasolabial folds. Dermatol Surg 2005;31 (11 Pt 1):1409–16.

2 Fisher GHaC, Joel W. The interpolated paranasal flap: a novel and advantageous option for nasal-alar reconstruction. Dermatol Surg 2009;35:656–61.

3 Cook J. Repair of an alar defect. Dermatol Surg 2003;29: 1089–91.

Commentary on conundrum 19

To say that reconstruction of the nasal soft triangle is a challenge is an understatement. The soft triangle is unique in that it consists of a free margin of skin without a rigid nasal infrastructure. The skin is draped between the cartilage of the nasal tip and the fibro-fatty structure of the mid and lateral ala. Minor injury and scar contraction can irreversibly induce distortion of this very delicate structure. One can argue that the lip is similar in that it has no rigid infrastructure and consists of skin, muscle, and mucosa. However, if orbicularis oris muscle function is preserved, a skilled surgeon can reconstruct the lip with minimal distortion and maintain function. Furthermore, the inherent elasticity of the lip makes it a forgiving material to work with; such elasticity is not a feature of the soft triangle. While the soft triangle has no critical function, it is located in the midfacial area and as a result, perceived asymmetry creates an unavoidable esthetic distraction even after the most miniscule injury.

Reconstructive options presented in this case include variations on full-thickness skin grafts, turnover flaps, composite grafts, and interpolation flaps from the forehead or medial cheek. This is not a complete list of options, as variations on bilobed flaps and dorsal nasal flaps have also been successfully used for soft triangle defects. I completely agree with the authors that well-executed flaps provide the most predictable closure option both from the standpoint of flap survival and esthetic results as compared with full-thickness grafts. However, I would admonish the reconstructive surgeon to always consider grafting in this location not only because grafts often provide results equal to those of flaps but also because they are usually much easier for the patient to tolerate.

One must remember that although a graft results in a sutured wound distant from the surgery site, flaps involve more incisions, undermining, and potential for tissue distortion, the morbidity of which should not be taken lightly. While a full-thickness skin graft may not have been the best closure option in this instance, it is readily apparent that the patient underwent an incision the entire length of her nose with advancement of the cheek medially to close the donor site. Prior to takedown of the flap the patient had to live with an undeniably peculiar appearance. Furthermore, the exposed pedicle of interpolation flaps has a relatively high rate of early postoperative bleeding. Only the patient knows the inconvenience of living with a strip of skin and soft tissue attached from cheek to nose for 3 weeks. Meanwhile, a successful graft will be essentially healed within a few weeks without the more prolonged social and physical inconveniences of an interpolation flap.

The point is that, while the cosmetic results of a full-thickness skin graft are less predictable than those of the average flap, the results of skin grafting can be excellent. The authors' portrayal of full-thickness skin grafts as always falling short of flaps as a reconstructive option ignores the reality that there are pros and cons for each closure option.

For the soft triangle defect, the turndown or turnover flap based either laterally on the nasalis muscle or medially on the columella can be a simple and elegant way to re-establish the normal contour of the soft triangle. The biggest challenge is in preventing accidental avulsion of the graft or flap during the critical first 4 weeks after reconstruction. The soft triangle is in such a prominent part of the face, and is so frequently bumped and rubbed, that the prevention of early postsurgical avulsion is particularly challenging. The use of a turndown flap and a full-thickness graft can be a relatively risky technique because of blood supply issues. Overall, the size of this defect argues strongly against the use of any turndown flap.[1]

The authors correctly describe the reliability and excellent vascularity typically associated with the interpolation flap. However, this flap has potential vulnerabilities as well. Because of the prominence of the mid portion of the face which, as mentioned earlier, is often bumped and rubbed, the risk of accidental flap avulsion is not negligible. Furthermore, according to studies quantifying the pain of various flap types, pain is a significant feature of interpolation flaps.[2] Postoperative bleeding is also a concern and, not uncommonly, a problem requiring further consultation and sometimes even intervention by medical personnel.

An excellent point made by this case is that the inferiorly based interpolation flap is a useful option, especially for distal nose and alar rim defects. This is because of the delicate characteristics of the flap skin harvested from the upper nasofacial sulcus or, as in this case, the nasal root. This delicate skin more closely matches the inferior surface of the nose and is also more conducive to folding upon itself to recreate the normal thickness of the alar rim. As indicated by the authors, there is the additional benefit that the melolabial sulcus is less altered when inferiorly based than when the flap is superiorly based.

The authors report that 1 month after suture removal, the wound edges of the repair were dermabraded. This raises an interesting question that has not yet been definitively answered. It has been suggested that the abrasive injury created during the early wound healing phase induces a more complete and imperceptible camouflage of the surgical scars, and early abrasion has been reported to provide superior results.[3] Although this has not been unequivocally proven, there is no doubt that earlier treatment of scars may result in unnecessary surgery. Many scars which are visible in the first month or two after surgery can resolve nearly entirely within a few more months. It is arguable that because of wound healing physiology and the timing of scar remodeling, it may be judicious to defer dermabrasion for at least 3–4 months in order to allow the natural wound healing processes to be completed and to give abnormal contours a chance to improve spontaneously. After scar remodeling has progressed, if there continues to be a contour irregularity, its correction becomes a simple matter of replaning and smoothing the surface of the skin with abrasion techniques. There are undoubtedly valid arguments for both early and delayed abrasive blending, but the important fact is that abrasion is a very important adjunctive modality for cutaneous surgeons in optimizing the final cosmetic result. With lasers, there is some preliminary evidence that early intervention with ablative fractional lasers at the time of surgical repair (after the deep sutures but before the epidermal sutures) may be most beneficial.[4]

The single view provided of the long-term results would suggest a good cosmetic result, although from this angle it is difficult to tell whether the height of the soft triangle is symmetric with that of other side. The use of cartilaginous struts to support these flaps can always be considered when reconstructing the soft triangle, both to maintain symmetry and to prevent free margin contraction. This can be done either at the time of the initial reconstruction or at the time of flap takedown and insetting. Placement of a cartilage graft can counteract the tendency for scar contraction to distort an otherwise well-positioned and well-restored soft triangle repair.

Commentary by Dr. Brodland

References

1 Zitelli JA. Repair of the soft triangle of the nose. J Dermatol Surg Oncol 1994;20(12):839–41.

2 Merritt BG, Lee NY, Brodland DG, Zitelli JA, Cook J. The safety of Mohs surgery: a prospective multicenter cohort study. J Am Acad Dermatol 2012;67(6):1302–9.

3 Harmon CB, Zelickson BD, Roenigk RK, Wayner EA, Hoffstrom D, Pittelkow MR, Brodland DG. Dermabrasive scar revision: immunohistochemical and ultrastructural evaluation. Dermatol Surg 1995;21:503–84.

4 Ozog DM, Moy RL. A randomized split-scar study of intraoperative treatment of surgical wound edges to minimize scarring. Arch Dermatol 2011;147:1108–10.

CONUNDRUM 20

A Tunneled and Turned-Over Nasolabial Flap for Reconstruction of Full-Thickness Nasal Ala Defects

Chris Kearney[1], Adam Sheridan[1], Carl Vinciullo[2], & Tim Elliott[3]
[1]Sydney Specialist Dermatology, Bondi Junction, Australia
[2]Oxford Day Surgery and Dermatology, Perth, Western Australia
[3]South Perth Specialist Skin Cancer Centre, South Perth, Western Australia

A 56-year-old man presented with a biopsy-proven squamous cell carcinoma of the right ala nasi. Mohs micrographic surgery was performed, and clear margins were obtained after three stages of surgery. The defect was full thickness through the alar rim, although the lateral alar groove was preserved (Figure 1). The defect measured 2 × 2 cm. How would you reconstruct this defect?

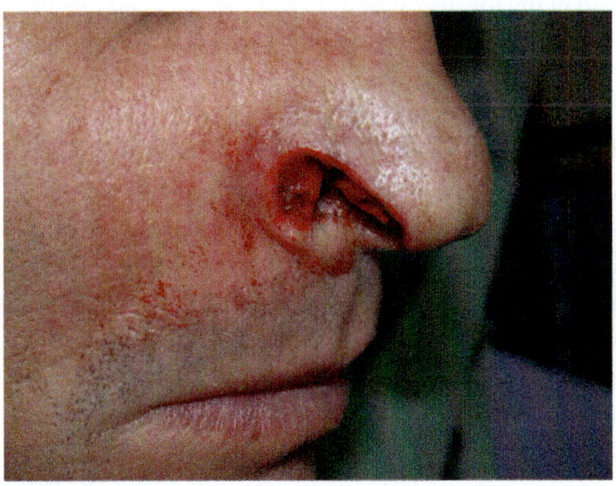

Figure 1 Case 1: Full thickness alar rim defect.

Resolution

A tunneled nasolabial turnover flap was designed (Figure 2). One of the most challenging reconstructions for the dermatologic surgeon is that of a full-thickness alar rim defect. The alae nasi, including the alar groove

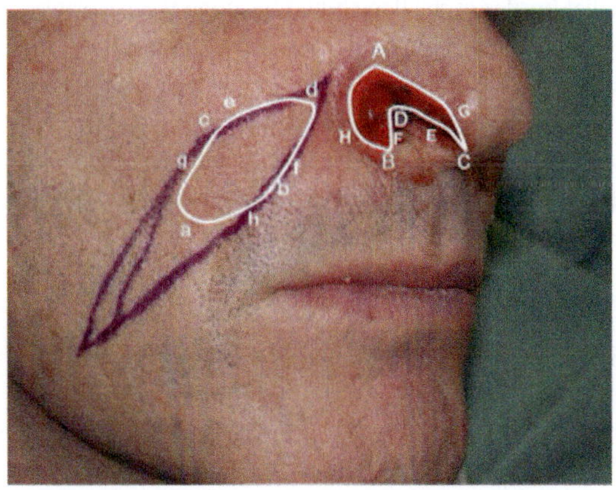

Figure 2 Case 1: Full thickness alar rim defect and tunneled nasolabial turnover flap design. Point a will ultimately be sutured to point A, point b will be sutured to point B, etc.

Reconstructive Conundrums in Dermatologic Surgery: The Nose, First Edition. Edited by Désirée Ratner, Joel L. Cohen and David G. Brodland.
© 2014 American Society for Dermatologic Surgery. Published 2014 by John Wiley & Sons, Ltd.

and alar rim, are complex structures with great cosmetic importance. Their three-dimensional contours are particularly difficult to re-create without distortion, vascular compromise, and functional disturbance of the nasal airway. The single-stage turnover nasolabial flap described by Spear and colleagues is an elegant technique for reconstruction of full-thickness alar rim defects involving loss of the lateral alar groove.[1] We have modified this flap to reconstruct a full-thickness alar rim defect where the lateral portion of the ala and the adjacent lateral alar groove has been preserved during excision of tumor. The key feature of the technique described here is the tunneling of a nasolabial flap beneath the lateral alar groove and then use of a turnover technique similar to that described by Spear and colleagues.[1]

The flap is designed by fashioning a template of the tissue required at the recipient site and using this template to design a fusiform nasolabial flap of adequate width and length at the donor nasolabial fold. It is important that the width of the flap at its widest point (c-b in Figure 2) be 125% of the width of the defect (C-B in Figure 2). This excess width will allow the flap to bow outward naturally, re-creating the normal convexity of the ala nasi. The apex of the donor site flap should be approximately 3 mm lateral to the lateral alar groove. The medial border of the flap should lie along the nasolabial and melolabial fold. Care should be taken to ensure that primary closure of the donor site will be possible without excessive tension. The flap is undermined at the level of the superficial subcutaneous fat from the most inferolateral point to within 5 mm of the superomedial end of the drawn template (d in Figure 2). The residual triangle of tissue on the fusiform nasolabial flap proximal to the template apex (d in Figure 2) is removed at the supramuscular level and discarded. At this stage, a tunnel beneath the lateral alar groove in a plane above muscle and deep to subcutaneous fat beneath the lateral alar groove is fashioned using blunt dissection. This tunnel should be approximately 75% of the width of the widest point of the donor flap. As part of the same maneuver, the proximal end of the flap is mobilized using wide blunt superficial subcutaneous dissection of the surrounding skin laterally and deeper blunt subcutaneous dissection to the level of muscle until there is enough movement to enable it to be passed beneath the alar groove without excess tension. The flap is folded forward and medially on itself "like the page of a book,"[1] so that the adipose tissue of the flap is facing anteriorly and passes beneath the alar groove (Figure 3). The mucosal lining of the ala nasi defect is repaired first by suturing the proximal apex of the flap (d in Figure 2) to the internal apex of the defect (D in Figure 2) with fast-absorbing suture material such as cat gut. The flap is sutured to the entire internal lining of the defect in this fashion. It is important that the width of the portion of the flap that closes the mucosal side of the alar defect (e-f in Figure 2) be equal to the width of the mucosal defect (E-F in Figure 2) and that the portion of the flap that closes the external cutaneous side of the alar defect (g-h in Figure 2) be 125% of the width of the cutaneous defect (G-H in Figure 2). This width difference causes the reconstructed ala to bow outwards naturally, re-creating the natural convexity of the ala nasi and increasing rigidity of the flap, helping prevent nasal valving. The flap is then turned forward and superiorly on itself to re-create the alar rim and the external ala nasi. At this stage, the bulk of the recreated alar rim is assessed. The alar rim should be approximately twice the thickness of the contralateral rim to allow sufficient bulk and rigidity of the new alar rim to give a satisfactory outward curvature. If deemed excessively bulky, the flap may be carefully thinned, although excessive thinning of subcutaneous fat may compromise vascularity of the flap. The external component of the flap is secured using deep absorbable sutures and a combination of 5/0 and 6/0 nonabsorbable cutaneous sutures. Finally, the distal end of the flap is trimmed to the required length to place the

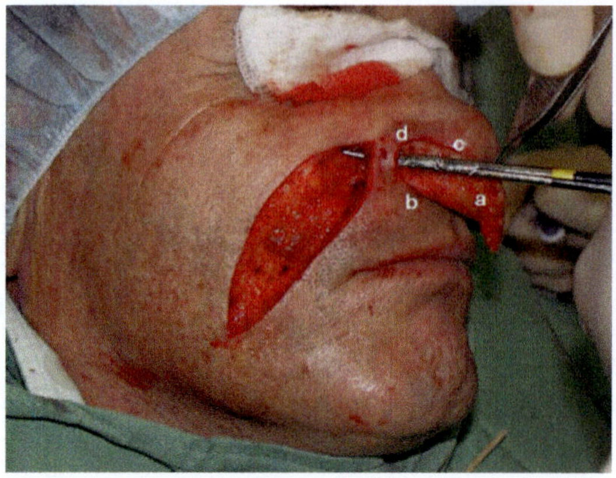

Figure 3 Case 1: Nasolabial flap folded anteriorly and supero-medially and tunneled beneath the lateral alar groove.

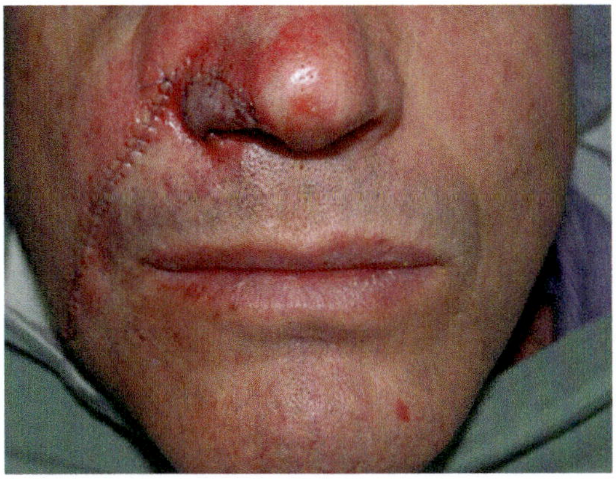

Figure 4 Case 1: Immediate post-operative appearance.

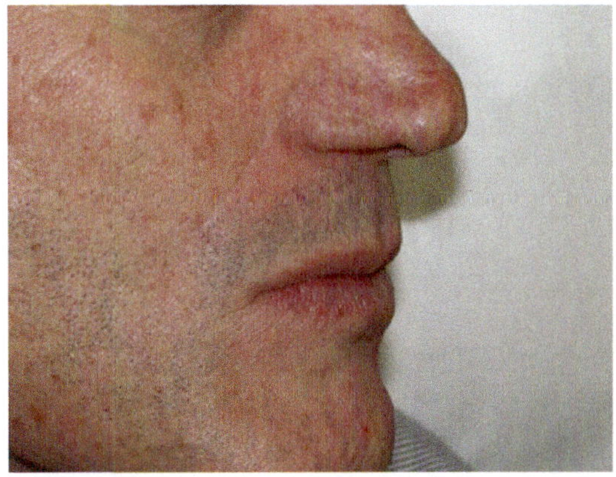

Figure 6 Case 1: Six months post-operative appearance (lateral view).

new alar rim at a vertical height equal to that of the contralateral side, avoiding alar rim elevation or depression. The donor site is closed primarily, with tension carefully directed perpendicular to the oral commissure (Figure 4). The elliptical shape of the donor site excision allows for minimal tension at the superomedial end adjacent to the alar groove. The ipsilateral nasal cavity is packed, and a firm compression dressing is applied externally to prevent venous congestion of the flap. The flap is inspected at 24 hours for viability.

In this case, sutures were removed from donor and recipient sites at day 6. The suture lines were treated with fractional 1,550 nm erbium fiber laser resurfacing (Fraxel Re:store, Solta Medical Inc., Hayward, CA) at postoperative days 6, 20, and 34. The reconstructed ala nasi was initially bulky but spontaneously thinned

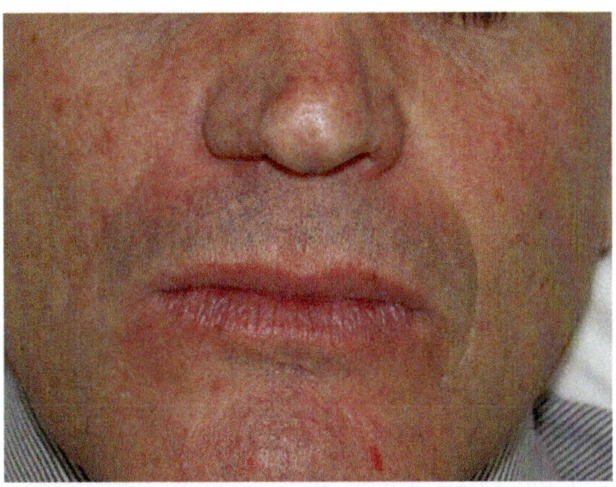

Figure 5 Case 1: Six months post-operative appearance (AP view).

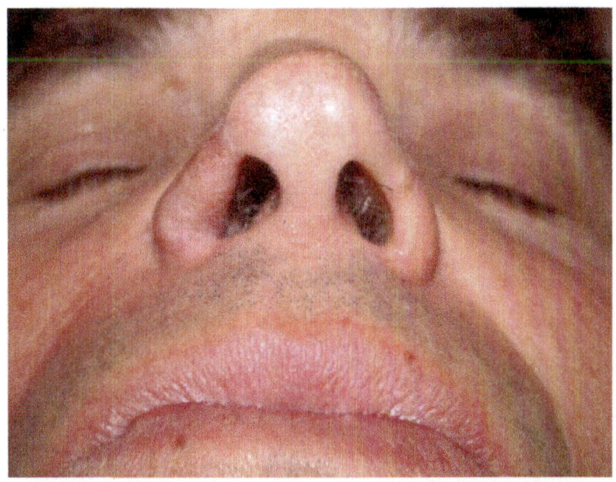

Figure 7 Case 1: Six months post-operative appearance (inferior view).

significantly over the following 6 months (Figures 5 and 6). The final alar rim was somewhat less rigid than the natural structure, although there was no functional nasal valve restriction or occlusion (Figure 7). The patient was offered placement of a cartilage baton and a small elevation of the alar rim to improve the appearance, but he was happy with the outcome and declined the offer of further surgery.

A second, similar case is illustrated in Figures 8, 9, 10 and 11. A 74-year-old man underwent Mohs surgery for an infiltrating basal cell carcinoma of the left ala nasi. A full-thickness defect of the alar rim resulted, with preservation of the lateral alar groove (Figure 8). The defect measured 25 × 18 mm. A tunneled nasolabial turnover flap was performed (Figure 9) in an identical fashion to that described above. The final flap was slightly bulky;

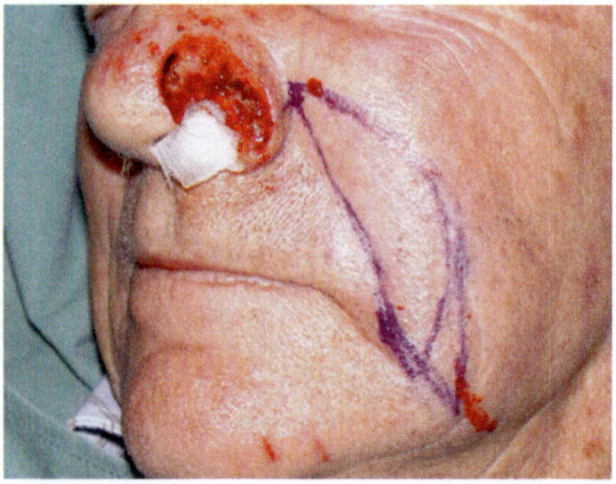

Figure 8 Case 2: Full thickness alar rim defect and tunneled nasolabial turnover flap design.

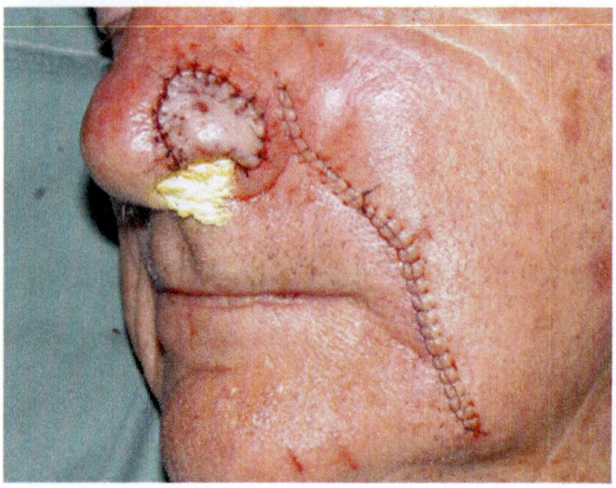

Figure 9 Case 2: Immediate post-operative appearance.

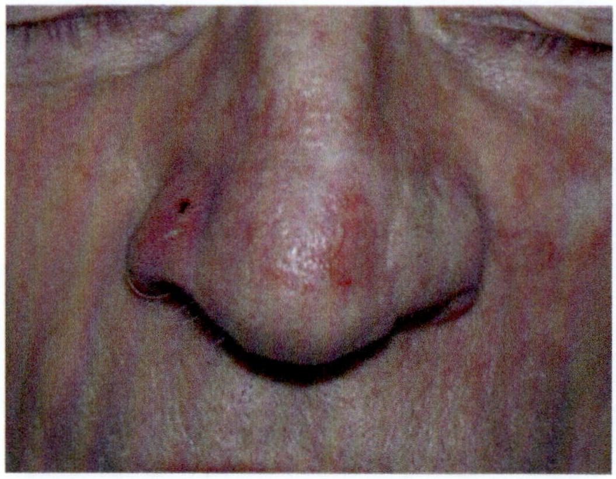

Figure 10 Case 2: Six months post-operative appearance (AP view).

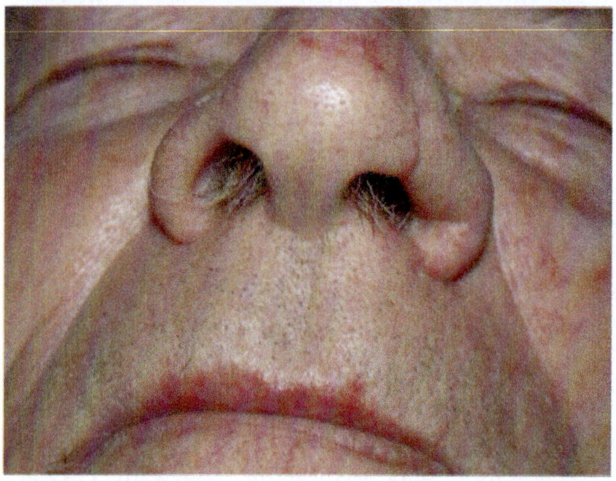

Figure 11 Case 2: Six months post-operative appearance (inferior view).

however, the patient declined the offer of a small revision procedure (Figures 10 and 11).

Discussion

An alternative to tunneling of this flap is to sacrifice the lateral alar groove and perform a standard Spear flap,[2,3] and this can produce a satisfactory result, but a reconstructed alar groove is never as good as the intact original, and perhaps the most difficult and unpredictable part of a traditional Spear flap is re-establishing and maintaining proper position of the lateral alar groove. Thus, preserving the lateral alar groove if it is not lost during tumor excision, rather than sacrificing it to perform a traditional Spear flap, should result in a superior cosmetic outcome. Another alternative for repairing such a defect is a composite cartilage graft;[4,5] however, this has a high risk of graft failure due to vascular compromise and is usually limited to defects no wider than 1.5 cm. Nasolabial or median forehead interpolation flaps may be useful in this situation but are multistage procedures.

Krishnan and colleagues have described tunneling of a nasolabial flap to repair defects on the ala nasi but not full-thickness defects of the alar rim as described here.[6]

An important feature in design of this closure is ensuring that the width of the donor flap is slightly greater than that of the defect, or more specifically that the external portion of the turnover flap is slightly oversized and the internal portion of the flap is matched for size with the defect. This will help the reconstructed ala nasi to bow outward naturally, re-creating the natural convexity. The reconstructed alar rim will be a degree more bulky than the contralateral alar rim. It is partly this bulkiness that helps create the convexity of the reconstructed ala. In our patients, the width discrepancy has been unnoticeable from the usual social anterior-posterior (AP) or lateral view of the nose and is noticeable only from an inferior view. If the bulky rim bothers the patient, it could be thinned in a later procedure. We would recommend waiting 6 months to allow spontaneous thinning of the flap and consideration of the use of deep intralesional cortisone before a surgical revision for thinning. If surgery is deemed necessary, placement of a cartilage baton of length greater than the width of the flap to promote outward bowing of the ala nasi is recommended. As with the Spear flap, there may be coarse terminal hair growth on the reconstructed ala nasi, particularly in men. This can often be avoided by careful design of the position of the nasolabial flap. In our cases, there was some initial bulkiness of the medial cheek below the tunnel containing the flap pedicle, but this diminished steadily with massage within the first 2 postoperative months. The development of a nasal valve is a potential complication; however, none of our patients who have undergone this procedure have experienced this. We have seen it with one of our patients treated with a traditional, nontunneled Spear flap, and this was successfully corrected with placement of a cartilage baton. The dermatologic surgeon may consider placing a cartilage baton within the folded flap along the reconstructed alar rim at the time of initial repair in wider defects to provide extra rigidity to the alar rim. This will inevitably result in a bulkier reconstructed alar rim. We recommend initial reconstruction without placement of a cartilage baton and performing this as a later procedure only if a nasal valve develops. As with the traditional Spear flap, the nasolabial flap described here appears to be reliable in terms of vascular supply. The flap is based on a broad muscular pedicle and is often deceptively short in length from pedicle (beneath d in Figure 2) to tip (a in Figure 2).

A drawback shared by all of the variations of the nasolabial flap is the asymmetry that results between the depths of the melolabial folds due to removal of tissue from the flap donor site,[1] but this asymmetry tends to result in cosmetic disfigurement of minor significance in comparison with the asymmetry between the alae nasi. The described flap sacrifices some asymmetry of the nasolabial and melolabial folds to preserve symmetry of the alae nasi.

Although this flap is specifically for use when the lateral alar groove has not been lost during excision of tumor, the authors believe that there are some features of the design that are useful modifications applicable to any traditional Spear flap, that is, even when the lateral alar groove has been lost. In particular, for our tunneled and traditional nontunneled turnover nasolabial flaps, we use an elliptical design of the donor site, with an apex point at the lateral margin of the defect (medial end of the donor site) rather than a broad medial end as Spear and colleagues originally described. This requires removal and sacrifice of the dermis and subcutaneous fat from the medial few millimeters of the flap but allows easy closure of the donor site without elevation of the lip, a common difficulty with the original Spear flap. This makes the flap somewhat longer, although we have not experienced any problems with vascular supply with even the longest of our Spear flaps. One could consider using this modification of tunneling for Spear flaps even when there is loss of the alar groove. When there is loss of the lateral alar groove, the lateral margin of the defect will usually still need to be advanced medially to recreate the alar groove in a good position, although there may be less tendency for the new lateral alar groove to move laterally if a tunnel is used rather than crossing the lateral defect margin with an excision.

The described flap has several advantages over alternative reconstruction options for full-thickness alar rim defects: it provides good color, texture, and contour match; completely preserves the lateral alar groove; allows the donor site scar to be hidden in a cosmetic junction line; has a reliable vascular supply; and is executed as a single-stage procedure.

Conundrum keys

- Where possible, preservation of the lateral alar groove is highly desirable because this is a difficult structure to reconstruct. The described flap preserves the lateral alar groove by tunneling beneath it.
- The flap based on muscle deep to the lateral alar groove and medial cheek is highly vascular and mobile, supporting long flaps easily.

· The width of the external portion of the flap should be slightly oversized, and the width of the internal component of the turnover flap should be matched for size with the defect. This creates an outward bowing of the flap, re-creating the natural convexity of the alar.

· The donor site is designed as an ellipse, and the medial supramuscular portion of this ellipse is sacrificed. This requires the flap to move a greater distance than a traditional Spear flap but allows closure of the medial end of the donor site under minimal tension, avoiding elevation of the upper lip.

References

1 Cook JL. The undesirable influence of reconstructive procedures on the symmetry of the nasolabial folds. Dermatol Surg 2005;31:1409–16.

2 Cook JL. Reconstruction of a full-thickness alar wound with a single operative procedure. Dermatol Surg 2003;29:956–62.

3 Goldman GD. One-stage reconstruction following complete alar loss. Dermatol Surg 2006;32:418–22.

4 Cherpelis BS, Carls JL. One-stage reconstruction of a full-thickness nasal defect involving the alar rim. Dermatol Surg 2007;33:1361–4.

5 Hendi A. Reconstruction of an alar rim defect. Dermatol Surg 2006;32:1179–80.

6 Krishnan RS, Clark DP, Donnelly HB. Tunneled transposition flap for reconstruction of defects of the nasal ala. Dermatol Surg 2007;33:1496–501.

Commentary on conundrum 20

This conundrum represents a common and complex situation, in which the full thickness of the alar rim has been removed. This defect requires a vascularized flap and is most often addressed with a pedicled flap closure. Two-stage flaps, such as a forehead flap or nasolabial interpolation flap, are effective; however, the option presented has the potential advantage of being a single-stage closure and uses the same principles as the renowned "Spear flap." It would be advisable to be intimately familiar with the traditional Spear flap before attempting this closure.

The primary goal for this case is to recreate the rolled, hemicylindrical, convexly curved structure of the alar rim. Once this has been accomplished, re-establishment of the structural integrity of the rim is addressed. All of this entails a keen sense of planning for a three-dimensional structure. The uniqueness of this repair is that, unlike the traditional Spear flap, the entire flap is passed through a subcutaneous tunnel and delivered to the defect site. Preservation of the alar base is very important whenever possible and was accomplished in this case. When the alar base is surgically absent, the best way to re-establish the anatomic junction between the nose, cheek, and upper lip is the traditional Spear flap. However, with preservation of this junction, the fundamentals of the Spear flap are still useful, and the flap can be passed through the tunnel to achieve a comparable result. If for some reason this cannot be accomplished, an alternative closure would be a two-staged nasolabial interpolation flap.

It is important to designate the exact placement of the pedicle base in advance. This area, which also serves as the pivot point for the flap, should be located as close to the defect as possible. In this case, the most effective location of the pedicle is near the area labeled "d." Developing the pedicle elsewhere will necessitate a longer reach and result in an unnecessary risk of vascular compromise.

The diagram in Figure 2 nicely illustrates the eventual location of the flap while in vivo. The preoperative planning described in this conundrum is also an excellent guide to estimating the flap's dimensions. The suggestion for the width of the flap to be 125% of the width of the widest point of the defect illustrates the importance of considering the three dimensions of this closure. If the flap is created at a 1:1 width ratio, it does not take into account the fact that the alar rim is convex in nature. The author's recommendation to make the mucosal side of the flap proportional with the defect in a 1:1 ratio assures that the greater width of the external surface of the flap will result in a convex configuration rather than a flat or concave shape. Although not indicated in this case, the measurements of the flap should be taken while the donor site skin is gently stretched. This assures that, when sutured into place, the flap will be under the ideal state of tension, resulting in a more natural appearing skin surface.

The next key to this closure is the development of the pedicle. Lateral to the donor site, the bulk of undermining can be done sharply. When "untethering" the pedicle itself, blunt dissection is preferred. When attempting to "lengthen" its reach, carefully spreading with tissue scissors perpendicular to the direction of the vasculature of the pedicle is least likely to compromise the blood supply. As the pedicle is developed, it should be stretched in the direction of the defect and while under tension, the "tap test" should be done to identify the remaining tethering impediments. The tap test is performed with scissors or skin hooks by simply tapping on the pedicle as it is being stretched. The most tightly stretched tissue will be apparent based on the tactile feedback from the restraining tissue. This allows the surgeon to dissect selectively to further mobilize the flap. This process should be carried out incrementally and cautiously so that adequate "reach" is achieved without compromise of the pedicle's vasculature.

Another key point mentioned in this conundrum is the tunnel. It is essential to develop a tunnel that will not compromise the vasculature of the subcutaneous pedicle. If the tunnel is too constrictive, particularly at the point where it abuts the inferior alar groove, it can result in vascular congestion and even flap hypoxia. It may therefore be necessary to excise some of the subcutaneous tissue lining the tunnel to make room for the pedicle. This also helps to diminish the bulkiness and visibility of the pedicle subsequently. While this bulkiness does tend to decrease with time, debulking is sometimes needed to optimize the long-term esthetic results.

The authors elected not to include a cartilage batten, although if the donor site is unusually thin or lacks substance, a cartilage graft can be conveniently incorporated into this flap. Interestingly, the thickness and rigidity of the cartilage used for this purpose is less important than one might expect. Even when soft flexible cartilage such as that found at the anterior helical rim is used, as long as there is intranasal support of the flap in the early postoperative period, cartilage grafts bestow an impressive rigidity to the alar rim. Regardless of whether a cartilage graft is used, it is important to provide intranasal support postoperatively to hold the flap in the optimal position. The use of nasal packing, such as a round dental roll, replaced every few days or a rigid intranasal cast for 2 weeks maximizes the chance for an ideally shaped alar rim.

The essence of this flap is careful, three-dimensional planning and development of a well-vascularized pedicle that reaches the defect with minimal tension. This is a slightly more advanced procedure than the traditional two-stage pedicle flap. It would therefore be advisable to have experience with pedicle development in a two-staged flap before attempting a tunneled pedicle flap. Having said that, as shown by the excellent results of these cases, this technique affords the convenience of a single-staged flap and at the same time yields a beautiful cosmetic and functional outcome. This discussion beautifully outlines many of the pitfalls of tunneled flaps and provides many subtle tips on how to optimize execution of this complex repair.

Commentary by Dr. Brodland

21

CONUNDRUM 21

Reconstruction of an Alar Rim Defect

Ali Hendi
Department of Dermatology, Mayo Clinic, Jacksonville, Florida

An 80-year-old woman underwent surgery to treat primary basal cell carcinoma on the right nasal ala. The tumor measured 0.9 × 0.4 cm and appeared to involve the nasal lining (Figure 1). Tumor-free margins were obtained after the first stage of Mohs micrographic surgery. A 1.3 × 0.6-cm defect involving 2 mm of the nasal lining remained (Figure 2). How would you reconstruct this defect?

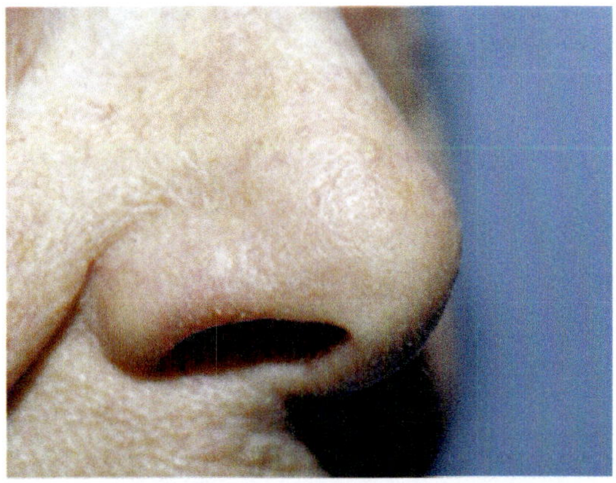

Figure 1 Basal cell carcinoma on the nasal ala.

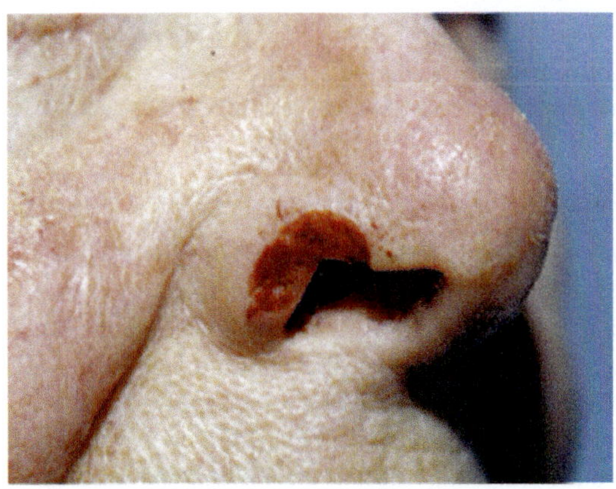

Figure 2 Alar rim defect involving the nasal lining.

Resolution

Defects of the alar rim can be challenging to reconstruct. Distortion of the alar rim leads to asymmetry of the central face and often is unacceptable to the surgeon and patient. The alar rim consists of fibrofatty tissue that varies in thickness among patients. Large alar defects may require recreation of the lining and structural support, that is, a cartilage graft. Smaller defects are best repaired using a full-thickness skin graft,[1] but this procedure may produce suboptimal results (notching of the alar rim). Any distortion of the normal anatomy of the nose is conspicuous because the nose, along with the lips and eyes, is a fixation point in visual perception of the face. Our eyes "consciously 'see' the unexpected" and "'assume' the expected."[2]

The patient's alar rim was repaired by a full-thickness skin graft in combination with a small-wedge excision of the anterior alar rim to ensure a smooth transition from the edge of the recipient skin to the graft (Figures 3 and 4).

Reconstructive Conundrums in Dermatologic Surgery: The Nose, First Edition. Edited by Désirée Ratner, Joel L. Cohen and David G. Brodland.
© 2014 American Society for Dermatologic Surgery. Published 2014 by John Wiley & Sons, Ltd.

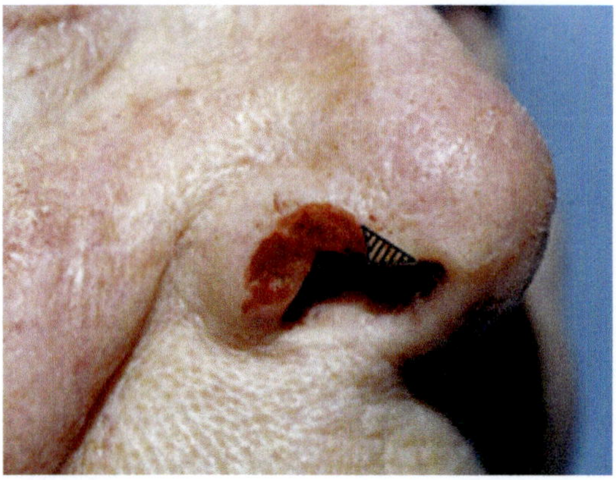

Figure 3 Artist's depiction of the wedge of skin excised from the anterior alar rim to recreate a normal contour.

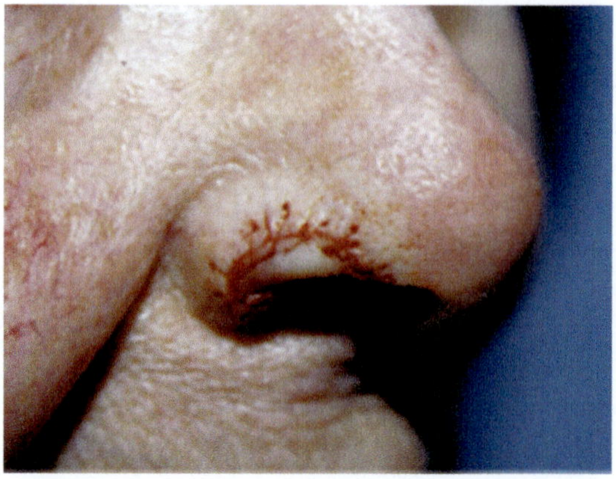

Figure 5 Immediate postoperative photograph. The full-thickness skin graft and secondary defect are sutured with absorbable sutures.

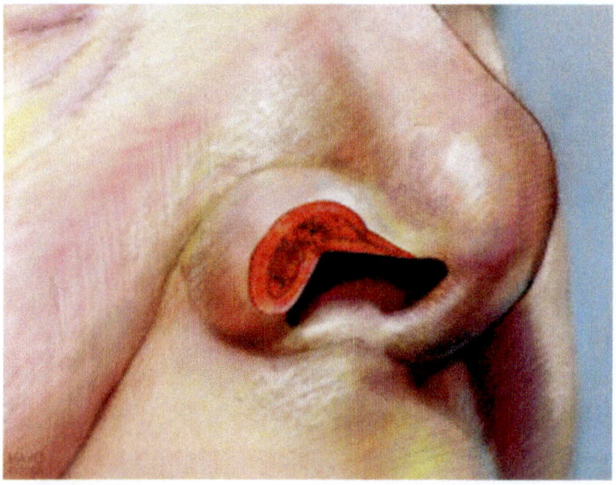

Figure 4 Artist's depiction of the primary defect and the defect created by the small excision of the anterior alar rim. (Reprinted by permission of Mayo Foundation for Medical Education and Research.)

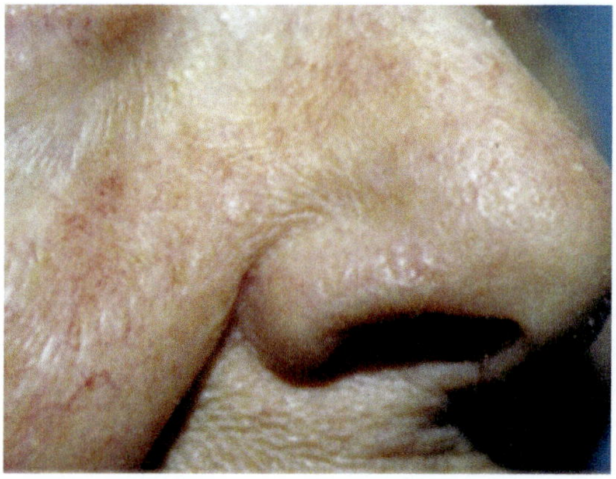

Figure 6 Three-month postoperative photograph. Note the normal alar rim contour.

The excised wedge measured 0.5×0.3 cm. The defect created by the small-wedge excision was sutured primarily using absorbable running sutures. A full-thickness skin graft, which included the perichondrium, was harvested from the ipsilateral conchal bowl with the aid of a template made from the suture package foil. The graft was sutured onto the remaining defect of the alar rim and nasal lining (Figure 5). A bolster dressing was sutured onto the cutaneous alar rim. The 3-month follow-up photograph (Figure 6) shows that the normal contour of the alar rim was maintained. The symmetry of the ala was also maintained (not photographed).

Conundrum keys

- Normal facial contours are important in our perception of what is normal and should be maintained in the course of reconstructive surgery.
- Small defects of the alar rim are best repaired with a full-thickness skin graft.

· The conchal bowl is a good donor site for defects of the nasal ala and tip. In most patients, the conchal bowl has a high density of sebaceous glands, similar to those of the nasal ala and tip.

· In the reconstruction of small alar defects, a natural contour can be recreated by a small-wedge excision and primary closure.

References

1 Zitelli JA, Fazio MJ. Reconstruction of the nose with local flaps. J Dermatol Surg Oncol 1991;17:184–9.

2 Burget GC, Menick FJ. Aesthetic reconstruction of the nose. St. Louis: Mosby, 1994:p. 11–2.

Commentary on conundrum 21

This defect, as with all defects involving a portion of the alar rim, is one that requires reconstruction of the convex, hemicylindrical, and smoothly curved rim in addition to maintaining nasal symmetry. Function is an important issue and is inextricably associated with form. A poorly functioning nostril (i.e., one that collapses on inspiration) will be as unesthetic as it is lacking in functionality. It can be generally stated that the reconstructive surgeon's primary concern should be in maintaining function, followed closely by optimization of esthetics. As is pointed out by the authors and has long been espoused by Burget and Menick in their Aesthetic Reconstruction of the Nose, "our eyes consciously see the unexpected and assume the expected." The paramount feature in achieving an esthetic appearance for the ala is symmetry.

The decision to close this defect with a full-thickness skin graft is a bold one. Grafts on free margins are often tenuous and can be unpredictable in appearance. However, as this case beautifully illustrates, the experienced and attentive surgeon can accurately identify and execute successful reconstructions that may be relatively simple to perform and easier for patients to tolerate. Selecting a simple but effective closure is an important goal and could be argued to be a duty of the surgeon.

The subtype of full-thickness skin graft used is the so-called "perichondrial full-thickness skin graft." The inclusion of perichondrium has long been advocated as having advantages over nonperichondrium-containing grafts. The potential benefits attributed to inclusion of perichondrium in a graft include enhanced survivability, decreased postsurgical contraction, improved turgor and improved retention of normal texture, and color. All of these characteristics would make this the ideal type of graft for this defect.

The greatest practical risk in using a full-thickness skin graft on a free margin such as the nostril is the risk of graft avulsion during healing. The susceptibility of a graft to this risk diminishes only slightly after the first week. It is not uncommon for accidental shearing forces to avulse a part or all of the graft during week 2 or 3, and sometimes even week 4 postoperatively. A bolster provides a rigid, protective, shell-like structure and is therefore ideal for these types of closures. A plastic-molded cast of the free margin should be considered. Thermoplast (Aquaplast PS Thermoplastic Nasal Splints, WFR/Aquaplast Corporation, Avondale, PA 19311, United States) is an ideal way of creating a "bolster" that provides a rigid support and protection needed for the free margin as well as compression, which assures contact of the graft with the wound base during the critical graft period of inosculation. Our regimen is to suture the Thermoplast bolster to the surrounding skin and to leave it in place for 1 week. At 1 week the "cast" of the ala is removed, washed, and then reapplied over an occlusive bandage such as a thin duoderm dressing, glued with mastisol or tincture of benzoin or taped into place, and left for one more week. Thereafter, the patient is instructed on cleansing the "cast" daily as well as how to use it as a protective device for the first month postoperatively. After 1 month, the graft is durable enough to withstand normal accidental bumps and shearing forces. The use of this type of bolster can also be helpful with flaps. However, flaps are typically not as fragile 1–2 weeks after reconstruction.

The results of this case are elegant and would be difficult to improve upon with any local or two-stage flap. When properly executed, full-thickness skin grafts can be very effective for the repair of carefully selected defects.

Commentary by Dr. Brodland

CONUNDRUM 22

Island Pedicle Flaps for Repair of a Nose, Cheek, and Lip Defect

Richard A. Krathen[1], *Daniel Behroozan*[2,3], *&*
Leonard H. Goldberg[2]
[1]Department of Dermatology, Baylor College of Medicine, Houston, Texas
[2]DermSurgery Associates, Houston, Texas
[3]Division of Dermatology, David Geffen School of Medicine at UCLA, Los Angeles, CA

A 72-year-old woman presented with a basal cell carcinoma of the left lateral nasal ala measuring 1.0 × 1.3 cm. The tumor was excised with Mohs micrographic surgery. Two stages were required to clear the tumor, resulting in the full-thickness defect pictured below, measuring 1.9 × 1.5 cm (Figure 1). How would you repair this defect?

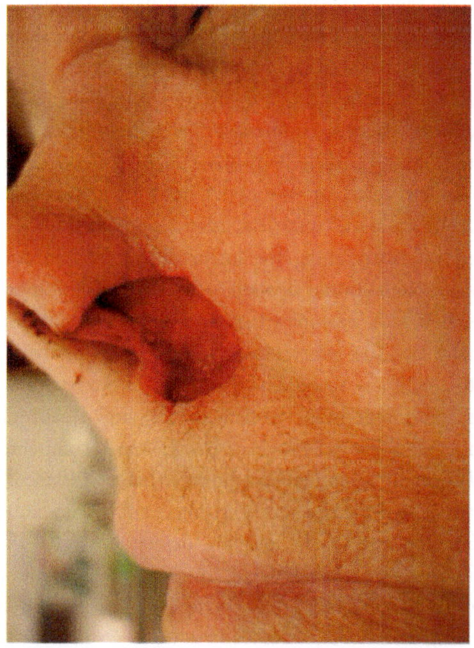

Figure 1 Surgical defect after two stages of Mohs micrographic surgery.

Resolution

This defect involved three cosmetic subunits: the lateral nasal ala including the alar rim, the upper lateral cutaneous lip, and the medial cheek at the nasolabial fold. Thus, the repair required reconstruction of portions of all the involved cosmetic subunits while attempting to reconstitute the normal anatomic boundaries between them.

The nasolabial fold is an important facial sulcus, which anatomically defines the border between the cheek and the lip. When distorted, the resulting facial asymmetry is readily noted by others. The nasofacial sulcus that separates the nose from the cheek is likewise an important part of normal facial anatomy. Blunting of this normal structure from surgical repair is best avoided if possible. Longstanding tenets of reconstructive surgery dictate that the repair of a defect within a cosmetic unit or subunit should produce a superior cosmetic result. In addition, surgical scars should preferably be hidden within the boundaries between cosmetic units. Defects resulting after Mohs surgery, however, may cross the boundaries between cosmetic units, as in this case, creating a more difficult repair.

Reconstructive Conundrums in Dermatologic Surgery: The Nose, First Edition. Edited by Désirée Ratner, Joel L. Cohen and David G. Brodland.
© 2014 American Society for Dermatologic Surgery. Published 2014 by John Wiley & Sons, Ltd.

A number of options for repair were considered at the time of surgery. Healing by second intention in this area would likely have caused retraction of the ala, narrowing of the nostril, and possibly upward retraction of the upper cutaneous lip. This option would not have been cosmetically acceptable. A full-thickness skin graft was another option. This might have caused blunting of the nasolabial fold and alar groove, however. In addition, this defect involved more than just alar skin. A skin graft would not have given a good cosmetic result, as alar skin has unique textural and color characteristics distinct from those of the nearby lip and cheek. One graft over the entire area would surely not have blended in well with the surrounding skin. A third option was a nasolabial interpolation flap. This is a two-stage procedure, however, requiring an intermediate step where the pedicle is divided and may also have caused blunting of the nasofacial groove. A fourth option was a paramedian forehead transposition flap, but this is also a two-staged procedure, excessive for a defect of this size.

A closure using a combination of two random-axis adjoining island pedicle flaps was designed. We decided to close the defect on the upper lip with a flap from the same cosmetic unit. An island pedicle flap was incised inferiorly along the lateral lip. This skin was advanced medially and upward to reconstruct the upper lip as a V-to-Y closure where the alar groove would normally lie. The inferior aspect was closed primarily and the flap was sutured in place with both subcutaneous absorbable monofilament suture, poliglecaprone (Monocryl, Ethicon, Cincinnati, OH) and cutaneous nonabsorbable monofilament sutures (nylon; Figure 2). This flap closed the cheek and lip defect and significantly reduced the size of the original defect; however, the nasal alar defect still remained. The nasolabial fold was preserved and the alar groove was partially recreated at this point.

Closure of the lateral alar defect was accomplished with a slightly modified island pedicle flap from the medial aspect of the nasal ala and dorsum, where the leading edge of the flap involved the medial aspect of the alar defect and the trailing apex ran horizontally across the dorsal nose (Figure 3). A small portion of the superior border of this flap was not incised (Figure 4). This small portion of skin is actually cheek skin. This allowed a small degree of rotation of the flap, which made the new ala smaller inferiorly and enabled a more natural shape to the recreated ala. In addition, this also gave the flap another pedicle for vascular flow. Although mobilization of flaps on the nose may be challenging due to fibrofatty tissue, this is more easily accomplished on the medial

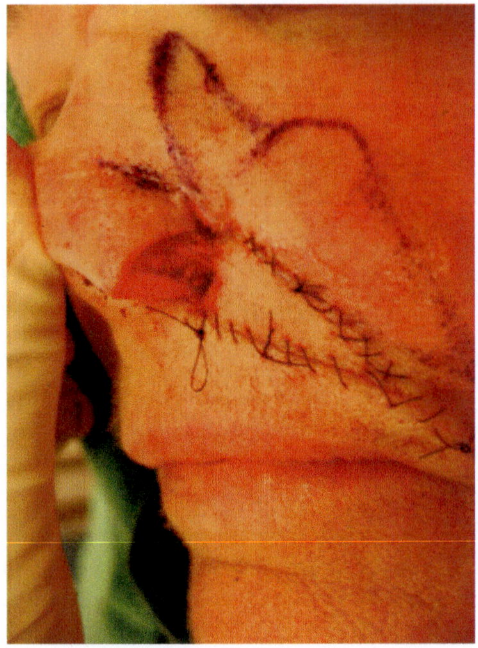

Figure 2 Inferior island pedicle flap sutured in place.

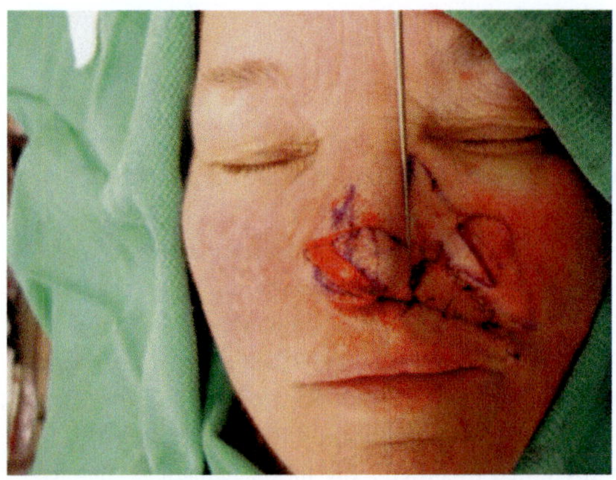

Figure 3 Incision of the nasal island pedicle flap.

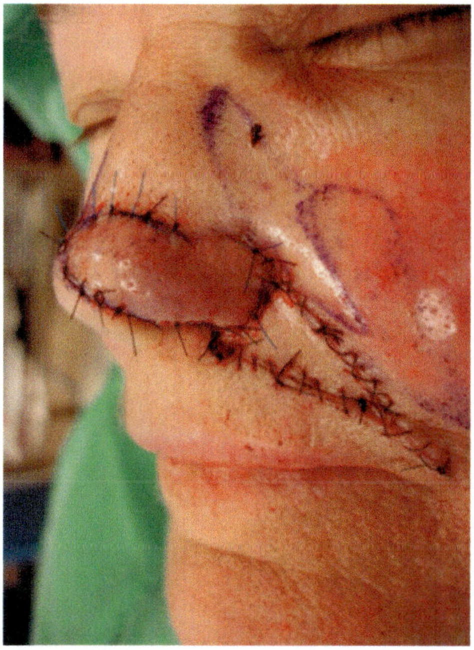

Figure 4 Both island pedicle flaps sutured in place, lateral view. Note the small portion of cheek skin superiorly not incised.

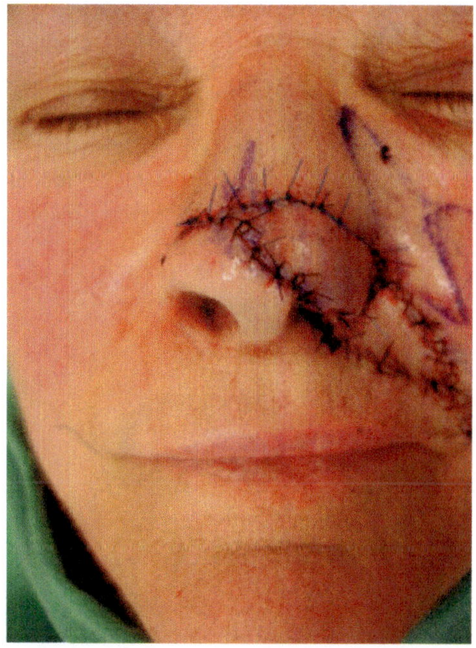

Figure 5 Both island pedicle flaps sutured in place, anterior view.

aspect of the nose, especially where there is underlying musculature. This flap was more medially based, allowing adequate movement and closure of the defect. Primary closure of the tail of this flap was performed in the usual fashion without distortion of the nose. At the nasal point where the nasal flap was attached to the cheek/lip repair flap, the lip flap was deepithelialized to the upper dermis, so that dermis was sutured to dermis. The remainder of the flap was sutured in place using absorbable monofilament suture, poliglecaprone (Monocryl) and nonabsorbable monofilament suture (polypropylene and nylon; Figures 4 and 5). This second island pedicle flap completed recreation of the alar groove at the point where the two flaps meet. The postoperative course was uncomplicated and sutures were removed 1 week later with a very satisfactory cosmetic outcome seen at 2 months (Figure 6). This closure did not require a two-staged procedure, as is necessary in a nasolabial transposition flap or paramedian forehead transposition flap. The island pedicle flap is a random-axis flap that allows more diverse reconstructive options, as opposed to the pedicled forehead and interpolation flaps that rely on a single arterial supply. Interpolation flaps are larger and more complicated and require the patient to undergo an additional procedure to take down the pedicle in addition to more complicated wound care in the extended interim period. These adjoining island pedicle flaps enabled reconstruction of a difficult defect

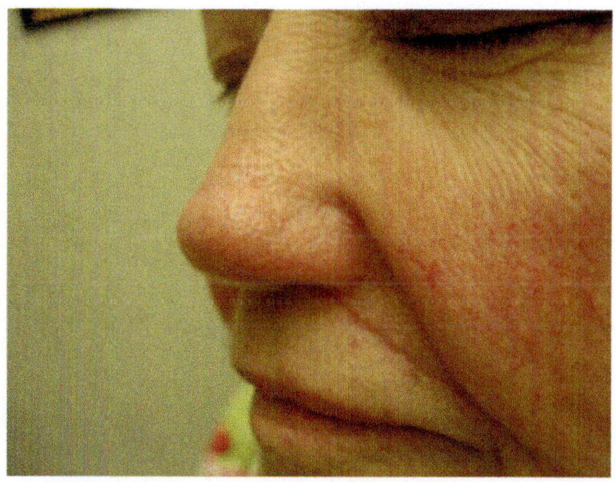

Figure 6 Postoperative follow-up at 2 months.

involving three cosmetic subunits in a single procedure with an excellent cosmetic and functional outcome.

Conundrum keys

· This defect involving multiple cosmetic subunits required a two-step closure to better recreate normal anatomic boundaries.

· The use of adjoining island pedicle flaps allowed movement of adjacent skin for the best possible color and texture match.

· Each anatomic defect was closed using skin from the same cosmetic subunit.

· Preservation of the alar groove and nasolabial fold was of utmost importance in this repair to retain a normal appearance.

Commentary on conundrum 22

Defects straddling multiple cosmetic units on the central face can be extremely challenging to repair and often need to be divided into their constituent parts for optimal reconstruction. The use of adjoining island pedicle flaps to repair such defects is a clever way of solving this problem. Advantages of this type of repair, as highlighted by the authors, include the movement of adjacent skin from the nasal and lip cosmetic units for the best possible color and texture match, with preservation of the alar groove and nasolabial fold. One disadvantage of using island pedicle flaps is their tendency to trapdoor, at times visibly highlighting any lines that do not fall within the patient's pre-existing facial contours (Figure 6). While intralesional corticosteroid injections may be helpful in eliminating the scar tissue that can arise in the early phases of healing, the visible flap lines do not always camouflage well but can be made less prominent with laser or other technologies which blend those demarcation lines. In certain patients, it may therefore be worth considering an alternative reconstructive approach for defects involving the lateral ala, the upper lateral cutaneous lip, or apical triangle, and the medial cheek.

The defect shown here (Figure 22.1) is a defect similar to the one shown in this case, which involves the lateral nasal ala and alar rim and extends onto the upper cutaneous lip and medial cheek. The approach to repair was similar in that the cosmetic units were dealt with separately so as to conceal the inevitable incision lines to the greatest degree possible. The alar portion of the defect required a hinge flap from the soft tissue of the adjacent cheek to decrease its depth (Figure 22.2). The cheek portion of the defect was repaired by advancing the upper cheek skin medially, concealing the incision line within the nasofacial sulcus. The upper lip defect was repaired by advancing and rotating the cutaneous lip skin upward, with an incision made along the nasolabial fold. A redundant standing cone was removed medially

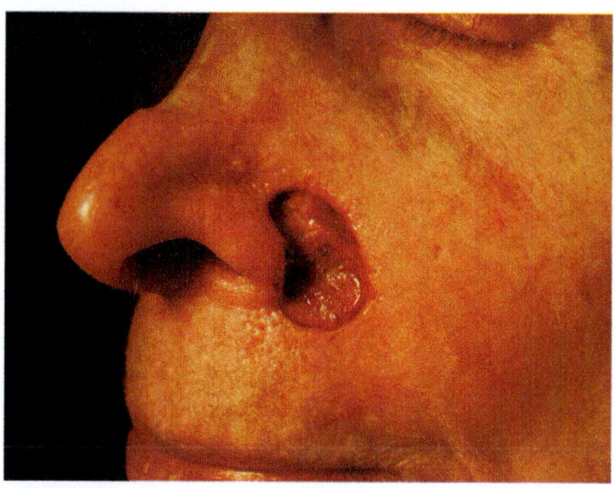

Figure 22.1 Defect involving left nasal ala, cutaneous upper lip, and medial cheek.

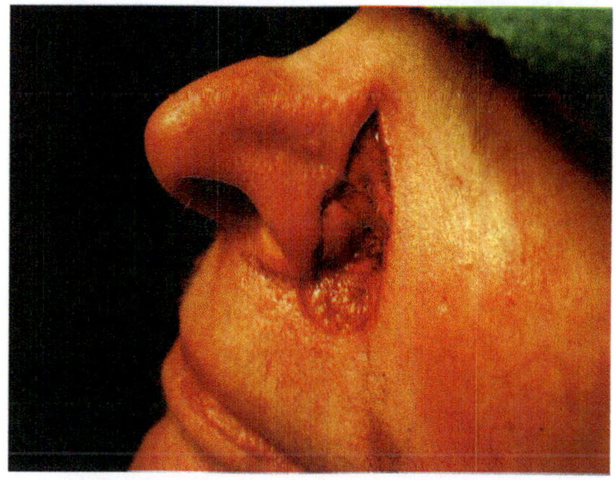

Figure 22.2 Repair with hinge flap composed of subcutaneous fat from medial cheek, based on a muscular pedicle.

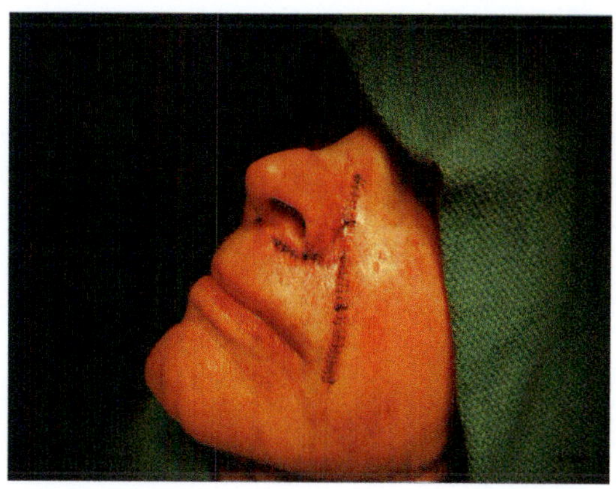

Figure 22.3 Repair with lip advancement/rotation flap to recreate the apical triangle, cheek advancement flap with suture line camouflaged in nasofacial sulcus, and Burow's full-thickness skin graft.

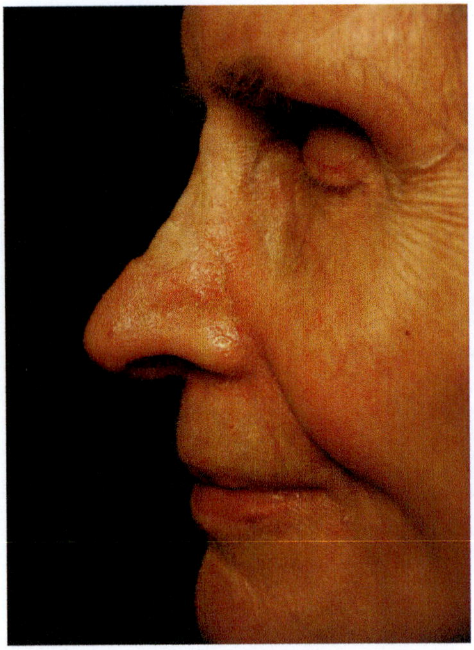

Figure 22.4 Follow-up view at 2 months.

along the nasal sill, thereby concealing the incision line beneath the nose. A Burow's full-thickness skin graft taken from the nasal sill dog-ear was then used to repair the remaining alar defect (Figure 22.3). A follow-up view taken 2 months after surgery illustrates the way in which the incision lines have blended into the patient's natural contours (Figure 22.4).

Both defects shown here involve multiple cosmetic subunits. In each case, adjacent skin was mobilized to the greatest degree possible, both for the best possible color and texture match, and to maintain the normal anatomic boundaries and contours. While the use of adjoining island pedicle flaps was utilized in this conundrum, sliding flaps from the adjacent cheek and lip skin can also be employed to recreate those anatomic subunits, along with a hinge flap and Burow's graft to recreate the natural contours of the nasal ala.

Commentary by Dr. Ratner

23

CONUNDRUM 23

Revisionary Technique for Alar Rim Notching: The Stair-Step Flap

Brian C. Leach[1] *& Joel Cook*[2]

[1]Colorado Springs Dermatology Clinic, Colorado Springs, Colorado

[2]Departments of Dermatology and Dermatologic Surgery and Otolaryngology, Medical University of South Carolina, Charleston, South Carolina

"Measure Twice, Cut Once."

Norm Abram

This Old House

Perhaps these words are more befitting the facial reconstructive surgeon than the master carpenter, for revision of the sequelae of improperly designed flaps or untoward reconstructive outcomes are some of the most challenging cases in a surgeon's career. Undoubtedly, adherence to this adage, with careful preoperative planning and performance of repairs, will minimize unfavorable outcomes, but invariably all surgeons at some point will be the recipient of such a conundrum.

Of the potential complications following surgical reconstruction, one of the most vexing for the surgeon and patient is that of excessive alar elevation or alar rim "notching." Alar notching may occur after rim defects are allowed to heal via secondary-intention healing, after flap reconstruction that approximates the nasal rim with inadequate cartilaginous support, or as a result of a failed flap or graft survival.

Many techniques have been described for the repair of alar elevation, but the majority of these require cartilage batten grafting, two stages of repair, or distant tissue donor sites.[1–7] Composite grafts, although used to repair rim defects, are in our experience highly variable in their outcome, and it is difficult to obtain reproducibly reliable results in their use.

Originally described by Dreyer in 1984, the stair-step flap was proposed as a repair for the reconstruction of alar defects allowed to re-epithelialize by secondary intention after standard surgical tumor extirpation. The initial operative or traumatic defect was allowed to heal and contract, rotating the alar skin internally to the mucosa and the lateral rim to granulate superiorly to resemble the rim, albeit malpositioned. Once healed, the stair-step flap was performed in a delayed fashion for defect repair and alar reconstruction.[8]

Within our practice, we have found equal utility for the stair-step flap in the correction of alar notching and undesired rim elevation as sequelae of wound healing or reconstructive failure.

A case report and operative technique will be described herein.

Methods

A 91-year-old man was referred in February 2008 to the Dermatologic Surgery Unit for evaluation and revision of excessive alar elevation of the right nasal ala. Two years before, the patient underwent excision of a basal cell carcinoma on the ala and sidewall, with notching subsequent to a reconstructive procedure done elsewhere. The defect was reconstructed using a single-stage nasolabial transposition flap without cartilage batten grafting for support.

On presentation, the patient's primary concerns were functional, not aesthetic; he complained of persistent difficulty with nasal inspiration, mucosal sicca, and a

Reconstructive Conundrums in Dermatologic Surgery: The Nose, First Edition. Edited by Désirée Ratner, Joel L. Cohen and David G. Brodland.
© 2014 American Society for Dermatologic Surgery. Published 2014 by John Wiley & Sons, Ltd.

taut, pulling sensation radiating into the lower lid and medial canthus. Collectively, these were bothersome to the patient, and he desired revision of the former flap and reconstructed ala.

On examination, the patient was noted to have coarse, sebaceous nasal skin with multiple hypopigmented sclerotic scars from prior treatments with cryotherapy and electrodesiccation. This contributed to limited tissue laxity and mobility. The right nasal sidewall and ala revealed a well-healed nasolabial transposition flap (Figure 1), although poor flap design had resulted in the bridging of four cosmetic subunits, to include the right ala nasi, perialar concavity, nasal sidewall, and medial cheek. The contractile tension vectors from this reconstruction had resulted in a notching of the lateral alar rim (due to rim proximity and lack of cartilaginous support), decreased size of the nasal vestibule (due to nasal valve collapse), and taut webbing of the caudal flap margin (secondary to flap contracture across cosmetic subunits). The nasolabial flap and resultant notching are diagrammed in Figure 2.

The patient requested revision for symptomatic relief only, and he was presented with a variety of revisionary

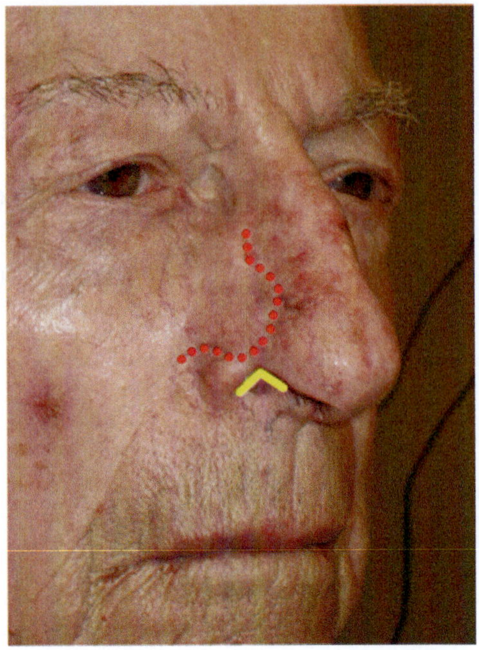

Figure 2 Diagrammatic outline of the nasolabial transposition flap (dotted red line), obscuring the perialar concavity with resultant alar notching (yellow angle) due to rim proximity without adequate cartilage support.

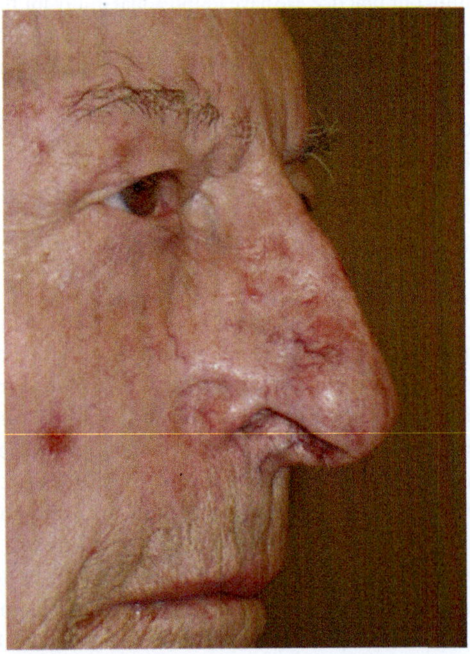

Figure 1 Preoperative lateral view of the patient's nose and well-healed nasolabial transposition flap. Note the coarse, scarred, cutaneous nasal skin.

options. After this discussion, the patient strongly preferred a single operative procedure without placement of a cartilage alar batten graft. An appropriate stair-step flap of the right nasal ala combined with a z-plasty of the medial cheek web was designed and executed.

Discussion

Although Dreyer originally described the stair-step flap for delayed reconstruction of alar rim defects after traditional excision, the technique has equal utility in the correction of postreconstructive alar notching and elevation. The original design of the stair-step flap from Dreyer's article is demonstrated in Figure 3a, and the flap movement is demonstrated in Figure 3b.

This technique may be adapted for the correction of alar notching simply by the development of an additional anterior rim "step" to facilitate flap advancement.

Flap design consists of the formation of running z-plasties or "steps" (Figure 4). Placement originates at the anteriormost edge of the alar notch and is carried

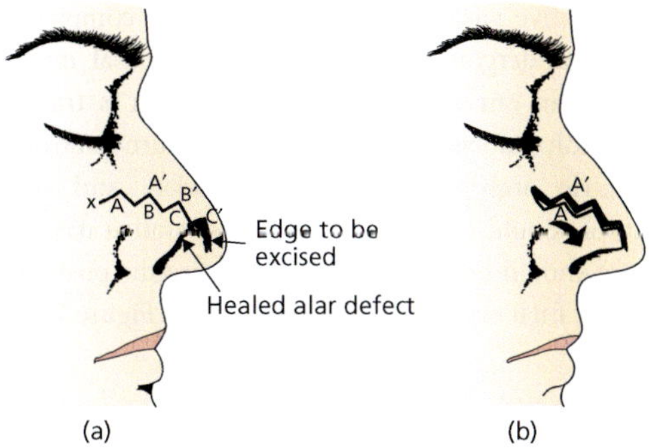

Figure 3 (a) Illustration of the stair-step flap design from Dreyer's article, with demonstration of the development of running z-plasties or "stair-steps," originally described for delayed reconstruction of a healed alar defect after traditional tumor extirpation. (b) Demonstration of the full-thickness flap cut and flap rotation and advancement. Each stair-step "walks down" into the defect created below it. (Figure 3a and b reprinted with permission from Dreyer, TM. The stair-step flap for nasal alar reconstruction. Plast Reconstr Surg 1984;74(5):704–5.)

superiorly and posteriorly to facilitate flap rotation and advancement. Two or three steps are initially used, but more can be added, in the manner of a backcut, to reduce tension and facilitate mobility.[8]

After flap demarcation, the surgical site is anesthetized with 1% lidocaine with 1:100,000 epinephrine and prepared aseptically. A vacuum-based suction apparatus should be available because of the significant hemorrhaging associated with surgery of the nasal mucosa, for better operative visibility and preservation of the patient's airway.

In our patient, before initiating the stair-step flap, we first performed a z-plasty to the caudal nasolabial flap margin. This released the excessive upward– outward tension on the lateral ala by shortening the web length and redirecting the lateral nasolabial flap tension. This minor revision additionally served to facilitate ease of rotation of the stair-step flap.

For performance of the stair-step flap, a through-and-through full-thickness cut is then carried through the skin, cartilage, and mucosa using a #15 or #11 blade. Protection of the underlying septal mucosa is assisted by insertion of the flat end of a forceps handle into the nasal vestibule during the incision. Once performed, this incision will result in the ala and lower nasal sidewall "falling open" laterally (Figure 5).

At this point, mobility may be assessed, and an additional superior step or backcut may be used to facilitate

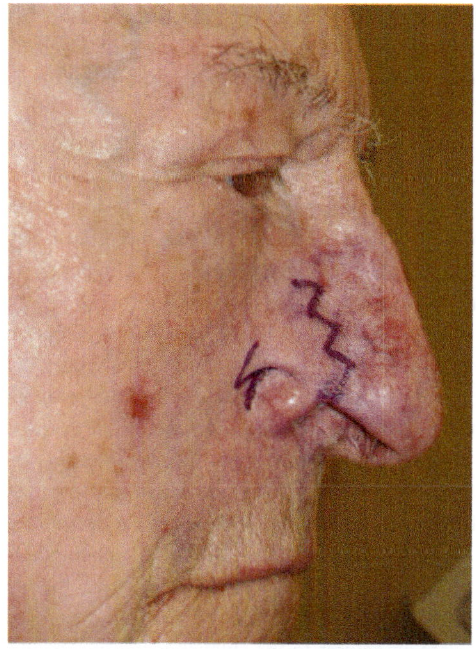

Figure 4 Design of the stair-step flap, originating at the anterior edge of the alar notch with three initial "steps" directed superiorly and posteriorly. The additional z-plasty of the caudal webbing of the nasolabial flap is also demarcated.

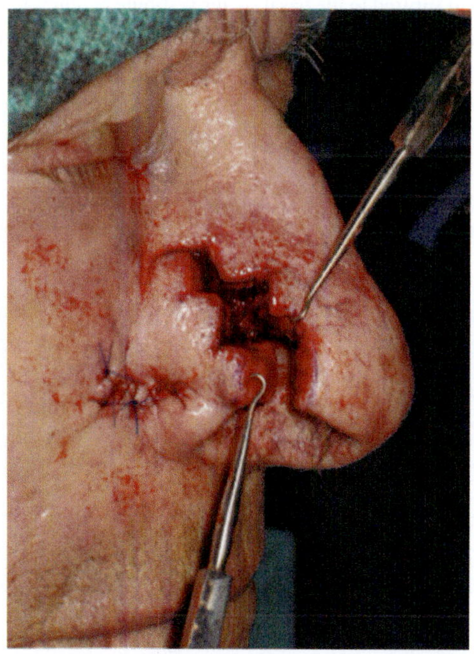

Figure 5 A full-thickness cut is made through skin, cartilage, and mucosa to permit flap movement. The steps are advanced and rotated anteriorly to assess final rim placement.

rotation or advancement. For this same reason, the authors prefer to remove the recipient step anteriorly only after this assessment of mobility and final alar rim placement has been made.

Once this final step has been removed from the anterior alar rim, the flap is then rotated into place, with each stair-step "walking down" into the defect below it. The lowest stair fits into the medial alar rim defect flush with the residual rim. The defect from where the upper step is taken closes upon itself after rotation.[8]

Suturing is best accomplished with initial placement of chromic gut sutures to close the mucosal edges, followed by absorbable polyglactin buried vertical mattress sutures for flap approximation and wound edge eversion. This is particularly important at the alar margin, and eversion at this site should be exaggerated to compensate for contraction during healing and prevention of further alar notching. Finally, external closure should be accomplished with chromic gut sutures across the alar margin to facilitate ease of removal and non-absorbable monofilament sutures to the cutaneous incision for flap security (Figure 6).

If operative swelling or airway patency is a concern, a #32 French nasopharyngeal airway can be trimmed to size and sutured to the nasal sill for vestibule patency and patient comfort. This additionally affords some relief in postoperative nasal congestion, a frequent complaint of patients undergoing flaps involving the nasal mucosa, although in our experience, this symptom is transient and rapidly resolves in the weeks after suture removal.

Empiric oral antibiotics are provided, and suture removal should occur within 7 postoperative days. The patient should be reevaluated 2 to 3 months postoperatively for final evaluation and assessment (Figure 7).

Conclusion

The benefits of the stair-step flap for alar revision are numerous. It replaces skin, cartilage, mucosa, and alar rim in a single step, with no distant donor sites; as a single-stage operative repair without the need for cartilage grafting, operative morbidity is dramatically less than with other reported methods of alar revision; and, in our experience, has produced uniformly reproducible results. The "stepped" z-plasties decrease linear scar contracture and help prevent further recurrence of alar notching. Tension is diminished with the interlocking nature of the flap. Using adjacent nasal skin, texture and color match are excellent. The broad lateral sidewall base ensures excellent viability of flap perfusion.[8]

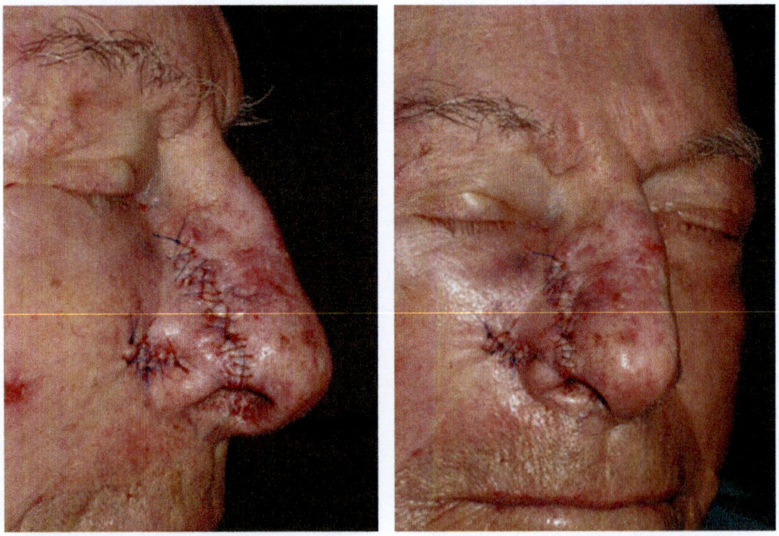

(a) (b)

Figure 6 (a) Final suture placement after removal of the recipient step on the anterior nasal rim. Note the immediate notch resolution and depression of the alar margin. (b) Oblique view of final suture placement, showing improved opening of nasal vestibule. Note the exaggerated incision eversion, especially at the nasal rim, to prevent recurrent notching.

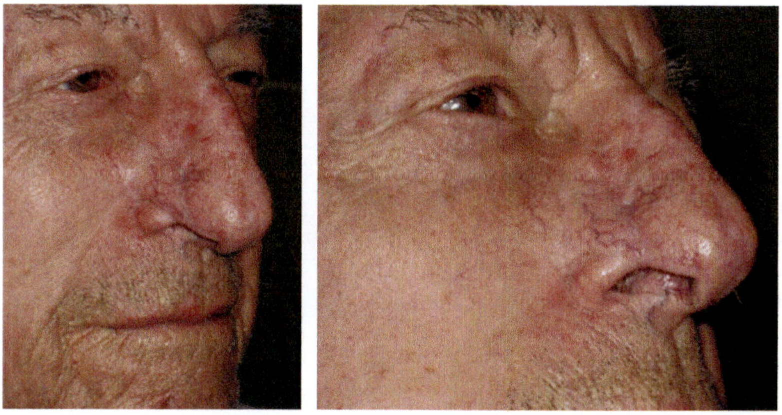

(a) (b)

Figure 7 (a) Oblique view of the revised site at 8 postoperative weeks. The patient reported the complete resolution of difficulty with nasal inspiration, mucosal sicca, and the excessive lower eyelid tension that he had experienced before revision. (b) Inferior view of the alar rim showing final correction of notching, alar rim depression, and opening of the nasal vestibule. The patient declined final focal dermabrasion or pulsed dye laser treatment for homogenization of his multiple cutaneous scars.

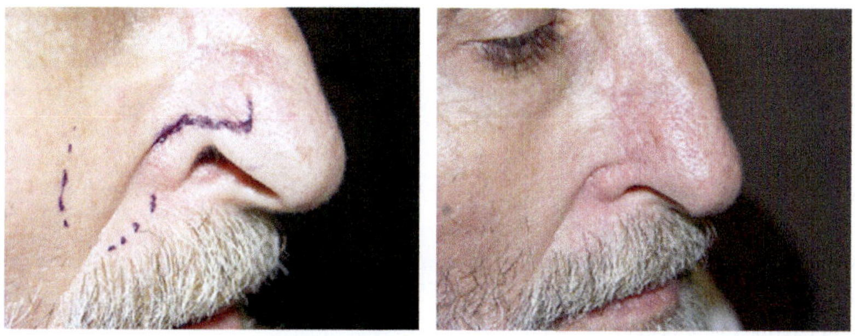

(a) (b)

Figure 8 (a) A different patient who self-referred to the Dermatologic Surgery Department for correction after a similar maldesigned repair with resultant alar notching. (b) Twelve-week postoperative view after single stair-step flap revision with good restoration of the alar rim and contour.

In our practices, we have found great utility for the stair-step flap, offering the reliable ability to revise dramatic alar rim elevation (Figure 8). Although many techniques have been described for the treatment of alar revision, the stair-step flap offers a single operative repair without the need for cartilage batten grafting. The stair-step flap should be a useful addition to the armamentarium of any dermatologic or facial reconstructive surgeon.

References

1 Hirohi T, Yoshimura K. Surgical correction of retracted nostril rim with auricular composite graft and anchoring suspension. Aesthetic Plast Surg 2003;418–22.

2 Vural E. Reconstruction of the retracted nasal alar margin. J Craniofac Surg 2007;18:442–5.

3 Tardy ME Jr,, Toriumi D. Alar retraction: composite graft correction. Facial Plast Surg 1989;6:101–7.

4 Fombeur JP, Gennevieve JP. Correction of postoperative alar retraction by sub-mucosal dissection and free cartilaginous graft. Ann Otolaryngol Chir Cervicofac 1976;93:640–3.

5 Kalan A, Kenyon GS, Seemungal TA. Treatment of external nasal valve (alar rim) collapse with an alar strut. J Laryngol Otol 2001;115:788–91.

6 Iwahira Y, Maruyama Y. Application of the two-flap method for nasal alar contracture. Plast Reconstr Surg 1990;86:133–7.

7 LaRossa DD, Rich JD, Zybyski JR. Correction of alar notches by rotation-advancement of a nostril rim segment. Plast Reconstr Surg 1977;60:267–9.

8 Dreyer TM. The stair-step flap for nasal alar reconstruction. Plast Reconstr Surg 1984;74:704–7.

Commentary on conundrum 23

The final result in this case is excellent, but the technique used is complicated and has its own issues of concern. Two parallel Z-plasties above the rim along with rim reinforcement using an auricular cartilage strut would have been another possible approach. The advantage of this strategy is that it allows the surgeon to avoid making a cut through the entire alar rim, which can lead to alar retraction in the post-revision period. The result shown here is an excellent one, but a cartilage strut would improve the chance of avoiding alar retraction.

Cartilage struts can occasionally be brittle after harvesting (Figure 23.1). In my experience, brittleness is more common with an antihelical donor site rather than the conchal bowl. Brittle cartilage also seems to pose a greater issue in elderly patients who have been on long-term oral steroids for lung or autoimmune disease, as well as in transplant patients. Use of the PDS plate (Ethicon, a J&J Company, United States) may be helpful in reinforcing brittle cartilage (Figure 23.2), thus lessening the risk of an ineffective strut and avoiding the need to go back and harvest another one.

In addition to the use of two parallel Z-plasties and cartilage strut to repair the alar notch, it is possible that a horizontal incision along the superior alar groove followed by placement of spacer cartilage or a skin graft could have been helpful in alleviating any degree of alar rim elevation. A third option is presented in Figure 23.3. An M has been drawn along the notch, which has been sewn in a V to Y fashion to lengthen the alar retraction that resulted, despite integration of cartilage into the repair of the original defect along with a full-thickness skin graft (Figure 23.3).

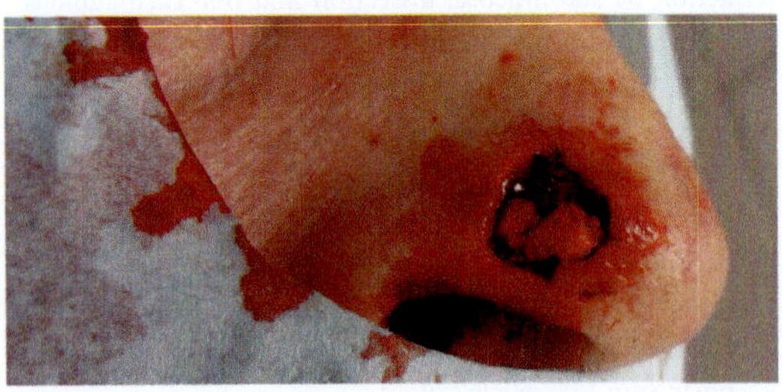

Figure 23.1 Fragile cartilage laid into alar defect. Antihelical cartilage was harvested because patient wears a hearing aid in the conchal bowl.

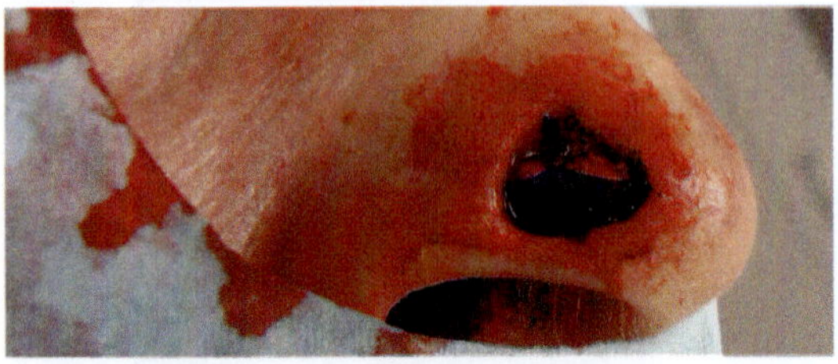

(a)

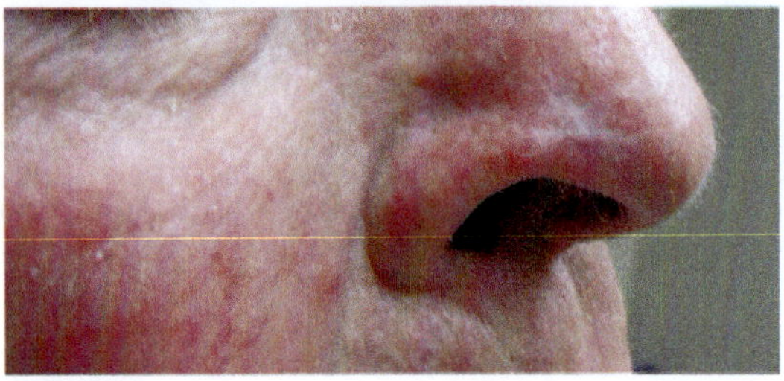

(b)

Figure 23.2 (a) PDS plate (Ethicon, a J and J Company, United States) appears purple and is attached to brittle cartilage to help preserve strut integrity. (b) Follow-up 7 months post repair with cartilage strut, PDS plate, and full-thickness skin graft harvested from right preauricular skin.

Facial plastic surgeons see alar notching commonly in the setting of revision rhinoplasty procedures (Figure 23.4). Their approach to this problem often involves making a releasing incision hidden inside the rim margin, with subsequent placement of an alar septal cartilage graft.

As an aside, the neovascularization seen in this case is quite common on the distal nose and alar subunit after reconstruction. If patients are concerned about the appearance of these vessels, there are several light-based devices or lasers that can be effective in decreasing the neovascular "blush" that can develop after facial surgical procedures (Figure 23.5). Purpuric settings have been found to be most effective in improving telangiectatic surgical scars (Figures 23.6 and 23.7).[1]

Commentary by Dr. Cohen

Reference

1 Nouri K, Vidulich K., Rivas M. Lasers for scars: a review. J Cosmetic Dermatol 2006;5(1):14–22.

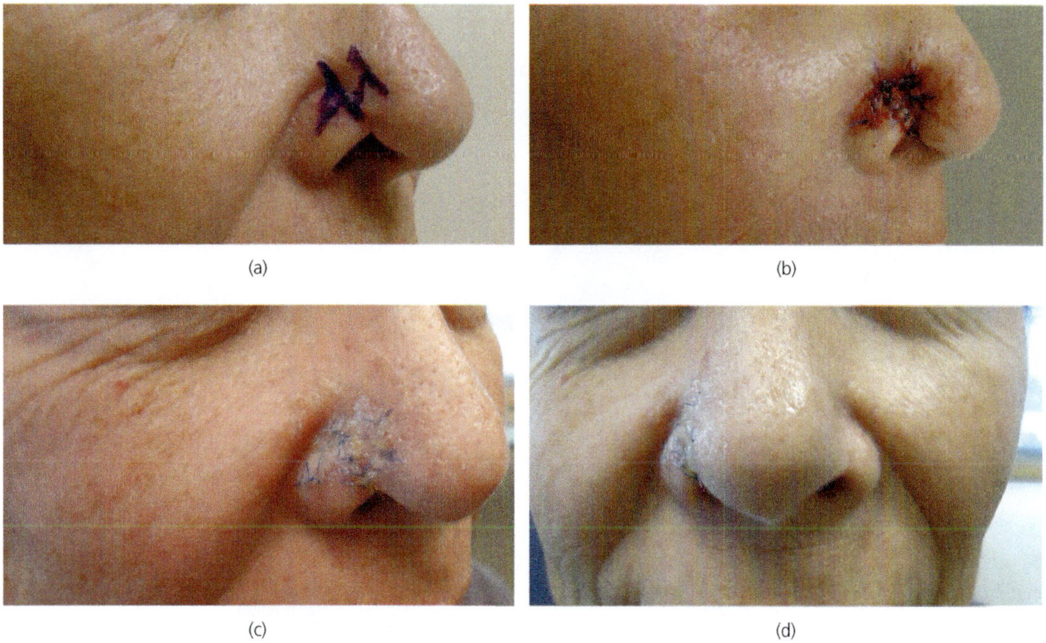

Figure 23.3 (a) Right alar notch. Proposed revision with M-plasty to lengthen scar, (b) immediately post revision with M-plasty converted to two small V to Y advancements, (c) significant improvement in notching at the time of suture removal, (d) frontal view at suture removal shows little asymmetry compared with contralateral side.

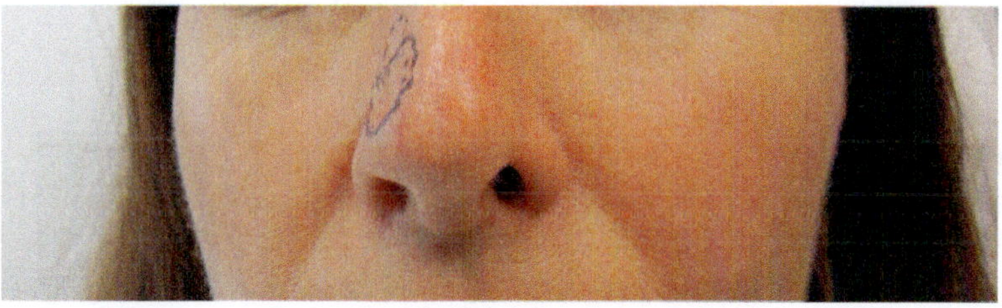

Figure 23.4 Post-rhinoplasty scars. Inferior columellar incision is visible. Left ala is notched and slightly elevated.

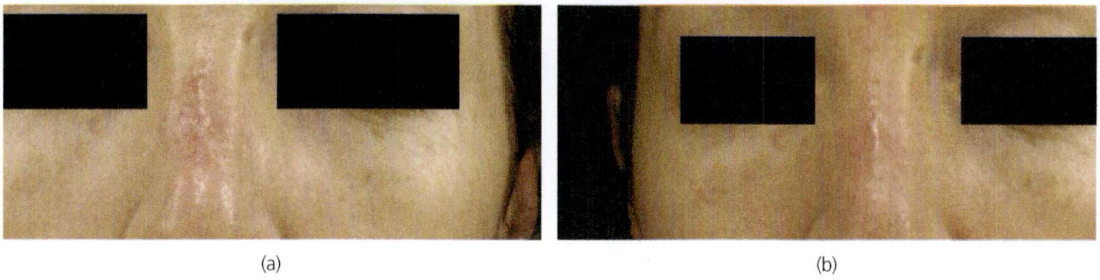

Figure 23.5 (a) Linear nasal scar 7 weeks after Mohs surgery demonstrating telangiectatic blush, (b)Four weeks after pulsed dye laser treatment.

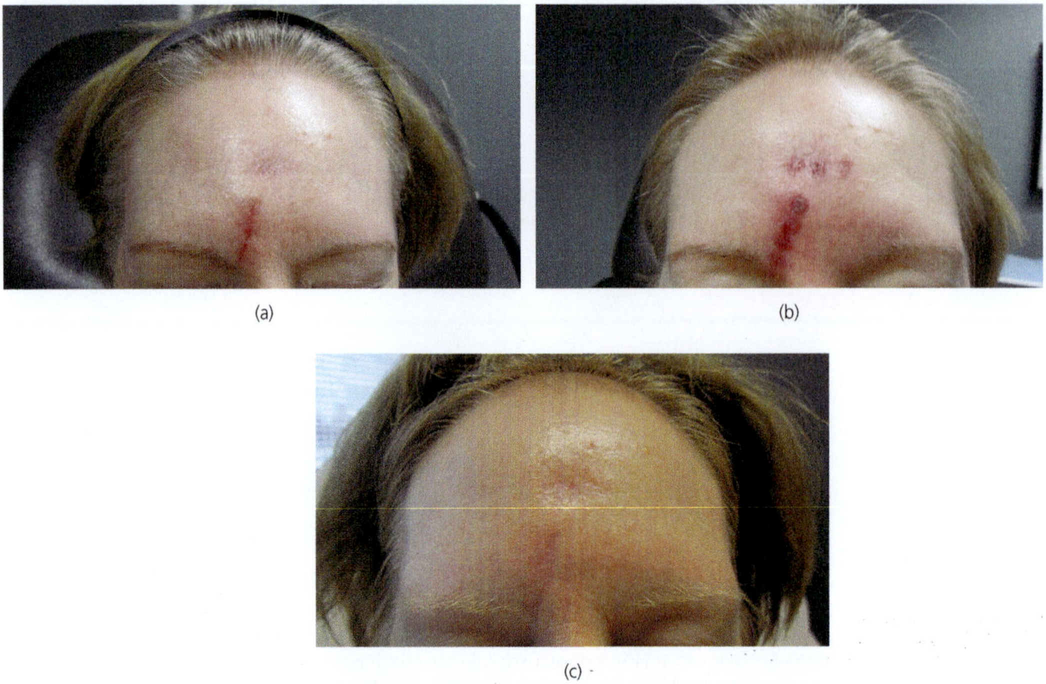

Figure 23.6 (a) Seven weeks after linear closure of a Mohs defect at the glabella, patient complained of significant scar redness that was difficult to cover with make-up. She had a history of significant type I (erythemotelangiectatic) rosacea and was famiiar with the pulsed dye laser. (b) Immediately after pulsed dye laser with purpuric settings. A linear scar on the central forehead from Mohs surgery 5 months previously was also treated. (c) At 3.5 weeks after laser treatment, much of the scars' redness has resolved, making it easier for make-up foundation to camouflage them.

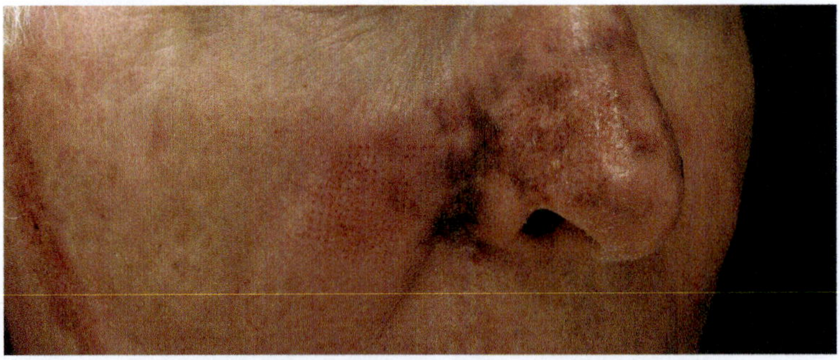

Figure 23.7 Combination of pulsed dye laser for telangiectases and fractional ablative erbium laser for hypopigmentation and palpable scar line performed on the same day.

24

CONUNDRUM 24

Reconstruction of a Surgical Defect Involving the Nasal Ala and Alar Crease

Andrew J. Kaufman
Thousand Oaks and Santa Barbara, CA

AN 80-YEAR-OLD man was referred for Mohs micrographic surgery of a squamous cell carcinoma of the left nasal ala. The lesion measured 1.0 × 0.8 cm after curettage of the bulk of the tumor and was cleared in one stage by Mohs surgery. The surgical defect measured 1.3 × 1.1 cm and involved the anterior aspect of the left nasal ala and alar crease (Figure 1). How would you reconstruct this surgical defect?

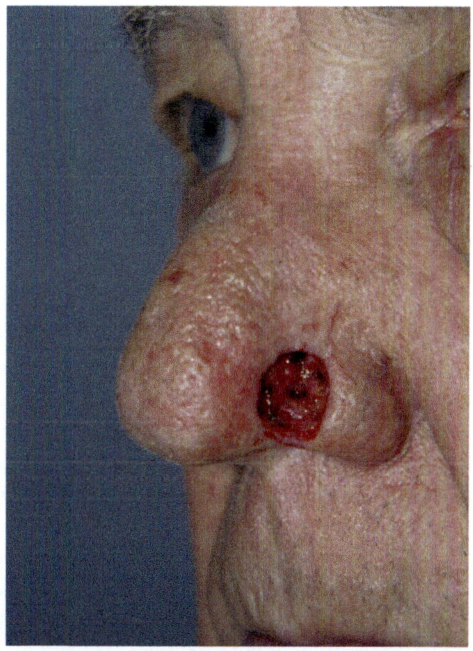

Figure 1 Postoperative view before reconstruction, oblique facial view.

Resolution

The patient presents a challenging defect of the left nasal ala and alar crease, while the alar rim, cartilaginous support, and mucosa remain intact. Points to consider in choosing a reconstructive option in this case would include the size, depth, and location of the surgical defect; the sebaceous nature of the patient's nasal skin; and the functional integrity of the nasal valve system on this side.

Proceeding from simplest to most complex alternatives, we can evaluate the alternatives that would provide the greatest aesthetic and functional result while avoiding potential complications. Secondary intention healing works well in concave surfaces such as the alar crease; however, the depth of the defect and the proximity to the alar rim in this case would risk upward deviation of the alar rim.

Side-to-side closure may be performed on small defects of the distal one third of the nose and larger defects of the proximal two thirds of the nose. Rhinophymatous nasal skin, as seen on this gentleman, may also permit

Reconstructive Conundrums in Dermatologic Surgery: The Nose, First Edition. Edited by Désirée Ratner, Joel L. Cohen and David G. Brodland.
© 2014 American Society for Dermatologic Surgery. Published 2014 by John Wiley & Sons, Ltd.

side-to-side closure for slightly larger defects; however, this defect is too large, and the location would not allow side-to-side closure without distortion of the nasal tip or ala or compromise of the nasal valve apparatus.

Grafting of the surgical defect would provide coverage of the defect but would not adequately reconstruct the soft tissue or depth of the wound. A full-thickness skin graft also would give a poor color, texture, and thickness match to the surrounding skin, especially in this patient with rhinophyma. Grafting may be an attractive alternative in a surgical defect involving all or most of a nasal subunit (e.g., dorsum, sidewall, tip) in a patient with thinner, less sebaceous skin.

Flap reconstruction allows repair with skin of similar characteristics and provides tissue for reconstruction of the depth of the wound. Regional flap choices would primarily be rotation versus transposition flaps in this location. A rotation flap would require crossing the alar crease and may affect airflow through the nasal valve apparatus. In a similar fashion, a rhombic transposition flap would reconstruct this wound, but using a donor site for direct closure so close to the nasal valve may decrease airflow by deviating medially the lateral cartilage of the nose.

A bilobed transposition flap may avoid nasal valve obstruction through two mechanisms: closure of its second lobe in an area distant to the ala and alar crease and a relative shorter angle of transposition. The first lobe of the flap reconstructs the surgical defect, whereas the second lobe of the flap reconstructs the donor site of the first lobe. Thus, there is no significant change in the area or volume of tissue near the alar crease, an area at high risk for affecting the nasal valve function. In addition, the transposition angle between the defect and the first lobe of the bilobed flap tends to be less than the angle between the defect and the rhombic flap, which also decreases the risk of external compression of the nasal valve. The choice of a medial-based pedicle also prevents dysfunction of the nasal valve through avoidance of surgically crossing the alar crease. To avoid blunting of the alar crease and to help keep patent the nasal vestibule, a single buried absorbable tacking suture holds the flap securely to the wound bed. Excision of the tricone at the point of rotation of the bilobed flap is performed near the end of reconstruction, allowing careful adjustment of the level of nasal tip and removing tissue that might externally compress the valve. After healing, the patient reported no nasal stuffiness or decrease in airflow. In fact, he reported that he is able to breathe a little better than he could before surgery, which is probably because of the correction of minimal nasal tip ptosis secondary to age and rhinophyma (Figures 2 and 3).

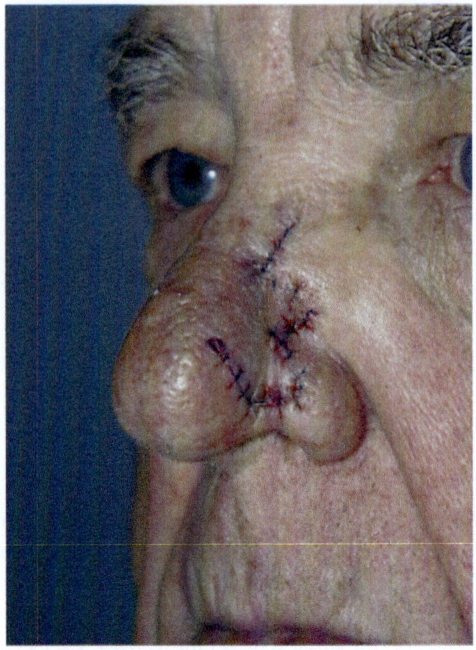

Figure 2 Postoperative view immediately after reconstruction.

Conundrum teaching points

Flap reconstruction of defects of the distal nose permits reconstruction with tissue of similar surface and thickness characteristics to the recipient area.

The nasal valve apparatus is a complex structure of soft and cartilaginous tissues that limits airflow through the nasal vestibule. In surgery, dysfunction may be secondary to external or internal factors. According to Robinson and Burget,[1] defects and reconstruction of the nasal tip, ala, or sidewall that cross or approach within 1 mm of

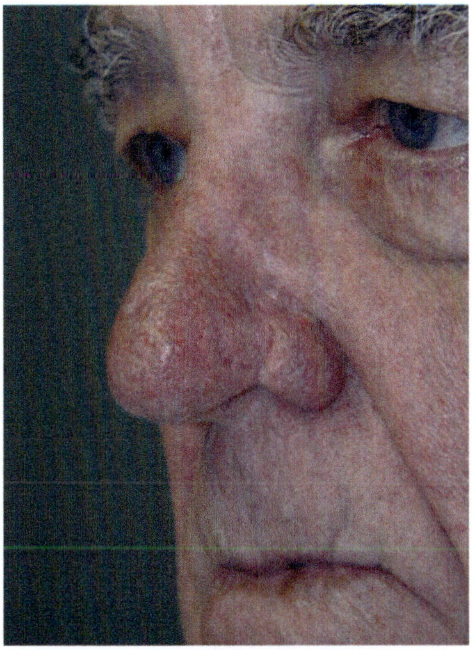

Figure 3 Healed appearance 4 months after reconstruction.

the alar crease are at risk of postoperative nasal valve obstruction.

To minimize the risk of nasal valve dysfunction in a surgical defect as presented, several factors should be considered: (1) Try to avoid crossing the alar crease with a surgical incision. (2) Avoid closures that will deviate the nasal tip or alae and thus compress the lateral or alar cartilages. (3) Borrow tissues in flap repair from areas distant to the nasal tip, ala, or alar crease (e.g., bilobed transposition or melolabial transposition flaps). (4) Carefully remove tricones to avoid external compression of the nasal valve. (5) Consider alar cartilage grafting in defects where the alar cartilage has been compromised.

Reference

1 Robinson JK, Burget GC. Nasal valve malfunction resulting from resection of cancer. Arch Otolaryngol Head Neck Surg 1990;116:1419–24.

Commentary on conundrum 24

Alar defects like this one can have many potential issues after repair, as outlined nicely in this case, including tissue mismatch, contraction of the alar rim leading to notching, and nasal valve dysfunction. Without actually taking a cotton-tipped applicator pressure to the remaining alar rim and assessing its integrity against collapse (Figures 24.1a and b), it is hard to tell whether there was a real necessity to consider cartilaginous support with an

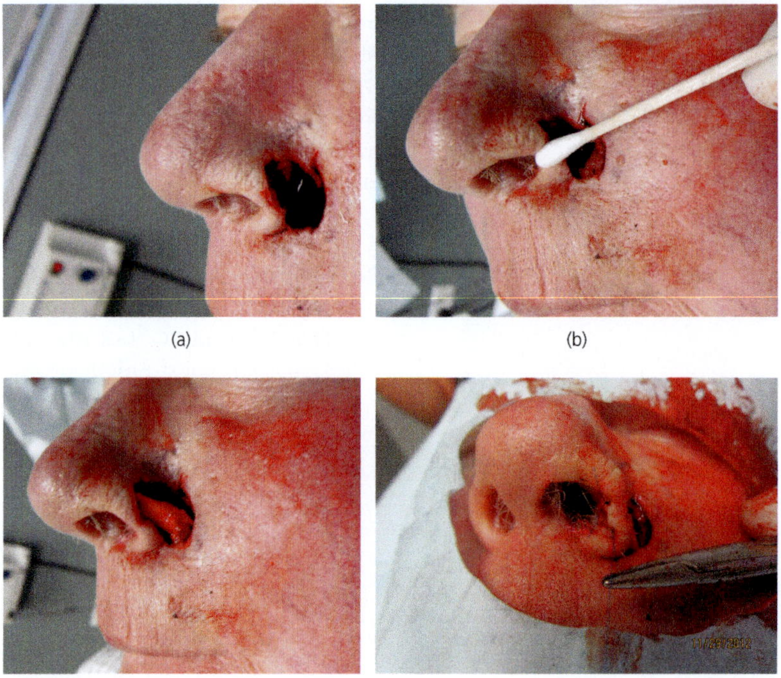

(a) (b) (c) (d)

Figure 24.1 (a) Mohs surgical defect involving the alar fim. Little structural support remains. (b) Use of cotton-tippled applicator to demonstrate buckling of remaining rim with minimal pressure. (c) Cartilage strut harvested from conchal bowl placed into soft tissue pockets undermined medially and laterally. (d) Knot placed intranasally to pull cartilage graft downward to recreate rim contour and maximize support.

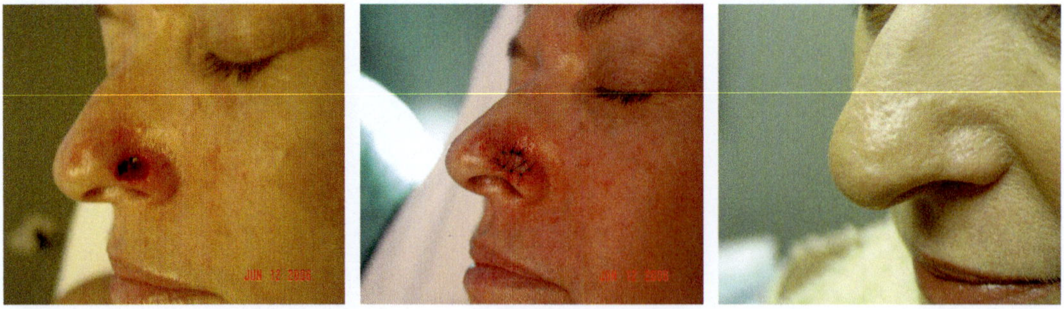

(a) (b) (c)

Figure 24.2 (a) Surgical defect after Mohs surgery. Despite close defect proximity to alar rim, remaining alar skin did not easily buckle with pressure, so cartilage strut was not placed. (b) Full-thickness skin graft harvested from conchal bowl. (c) Four-month follow-up demonstrating excellent tissue match.

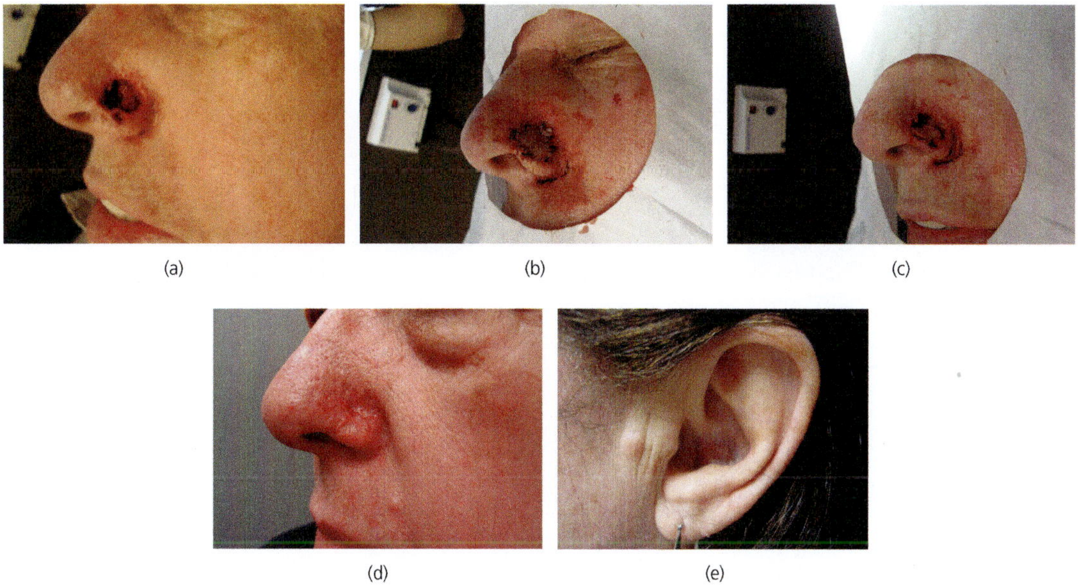

Figure 24.3 (a) Alar defect buckles to minimal external pressure with cotton-tipped applicator. (b) Conchal bowl graft placed into soft tissue pockets undermined at medial and lateral aspects of defect. (c) Full-thickness skin graft harvested from conchal bowl. (d) Three months post repair. The scar could benefit from pulsed dye laser for telangiectasias and ablative resurfacing to optimize texture. (e) Donor site at 3 months showing minimal scarring.

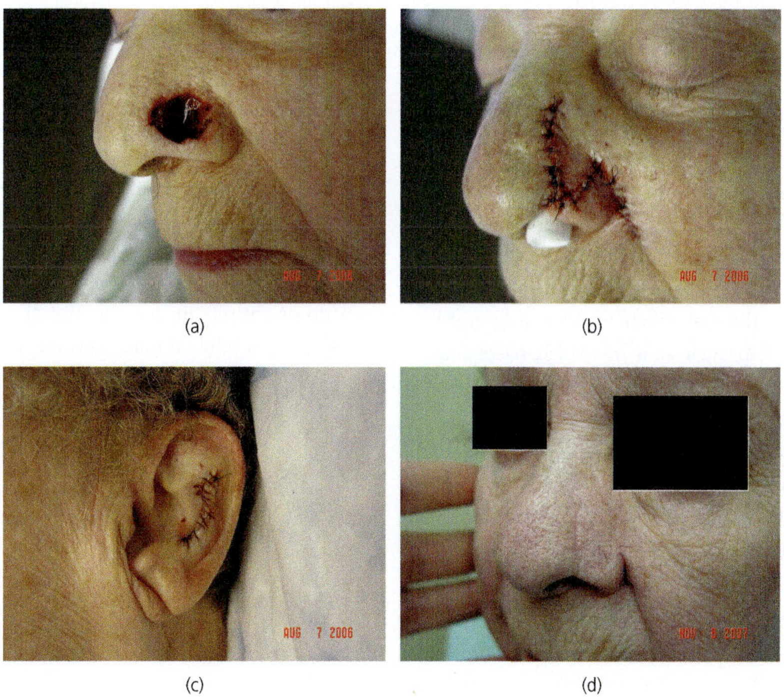

Figure 24.4 (a) Distal alar defect buckles with minimal cotton-tipped application pressure. (b) Immediately after repair with antihelical cartilage strut and one-stage nasolabial transposition flap. (c) Antihelical donor site repaired with epidermal sutures. (d) Long-term follow-up demonstrates good tissue match. Very mild superficial notching is visible, but patient declined scar revision procedures including laser resurfacing.

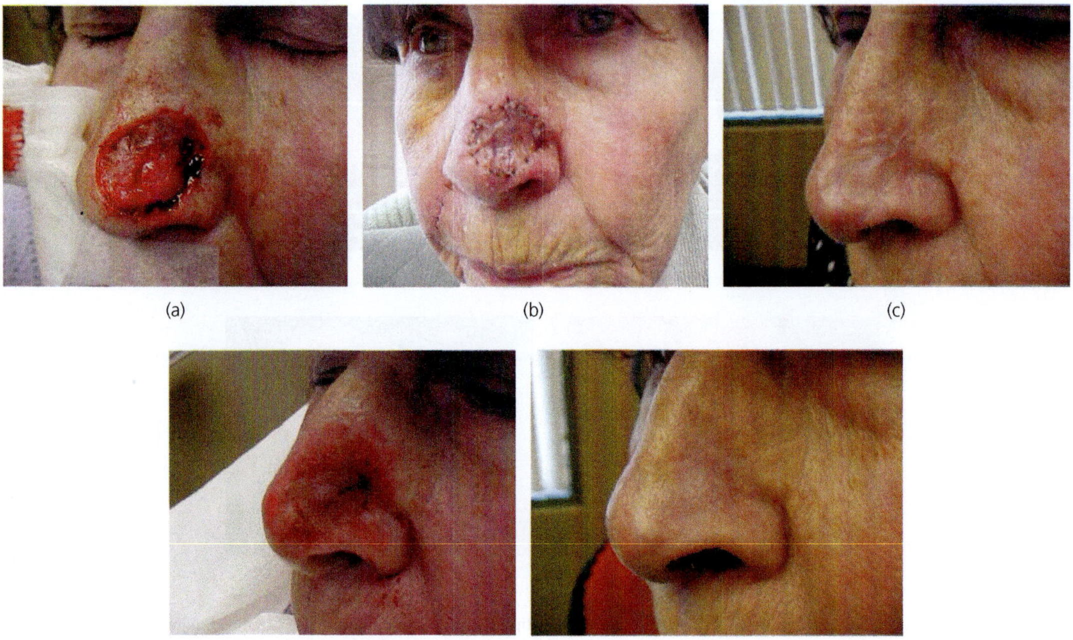

(a) (b) (c) (d) (e)

Figure 24.5 (a) Distal nasal defect after Mohs surgery. (b) Immediately post repair with preauricular full-thickness skin graft. (c) Five-month follow-up showing cigarette paper-type atrophy. (d) Immediate post-erbium resurfacing of scar. (e) Two months after resurfacing, scar texture is much improved. Subtle hypopigmentation sometimes remains after fully ablative (nonfractional) resurfacing.

auricular strut in this case (Figure 24.1c). If the alar rim is competent and resistant to cotton-tipped applicator pressure, then a simple full-thickness skin graft may suffice for repair (Figure 24.2).

However, for most defects situated this close to the rim margin, a cartilage strut is a good idea and can help give support to the rim, either under a skin graft[1] (Figure 24.3) or a flap such as a one-stage nasolabial transposition flap (Figure 24.4). The auricular cartilage strut must be secured with sutures or by interlocking it into soft tissue pockets on either side of the defect to minimize the risk of displacement. I now prefer to place the strut in pockets as well as securing it with sutures by actually pulling it down directly toward the rim by placing the sutures intranasally (as described by R. Krishnan at the American College of Mohs Surgery Meeting, 2011[2]) (Figure 24.1d). With repairs on the sebaceous skin of the distal nose, consideration may be given to blending the graft demarcation points or the flap suture line using a resurfacing device. The prominence of the pores on the adjacent skin as well as within the scar itself may also be minimized to some extent if resurfacing is performed.

If a bilobed flap is used, I find the medially based approach to be the best alternative in this instance as it preserves the alar crease, particularly for defects that are close to the alar rim and either at the extreme lateral nasal tip or entirely on the ala. The disadvantage of the medially based bilobed flap, however, is that the risk of trap-dooring is greater than with laterally based flaps. In many cases, however, these results can be improved upon with some type of ablative resurfacing procedure (Figure 24.5).

Commentary by Dr. Cohen

References

1 Ewanowski, C, Cook, J. Using cartilage and skin grafts concurrently: an alternate route to repair. Dermatol Surg (2009);35(11):1809–17.

2 Krishnan R. Presentation: American College of Mohs Surgery, Las Vegas, May 2011.

25

CONUNDRUM 25

One-Stage Reconstruction of a Full-Thickness Nasal Defect Involving the Alar Rim

Basil S. Cherpelis & J. Lauren Carls
Department of Dermatology and Cutaneous Surgery, University of South Florida, Tampa, FL

An 84-year-old male was referred for Mohs micrographic surgery of a biopsy-proven basal cell carcinoma of the right nasal ala. The primary lesion was a pearly papule measuring 0.4 × 0.4 cm (Figure 1). Mohs micrographic surgery was indicated due to the location and the ill-defined borders of the lesion. A tumor-free plane was achieved after two stages, with a resulting full-thickness defect measuring 1.4 × 0.6 cm (Figure 2). How would you reconstruct this defect?

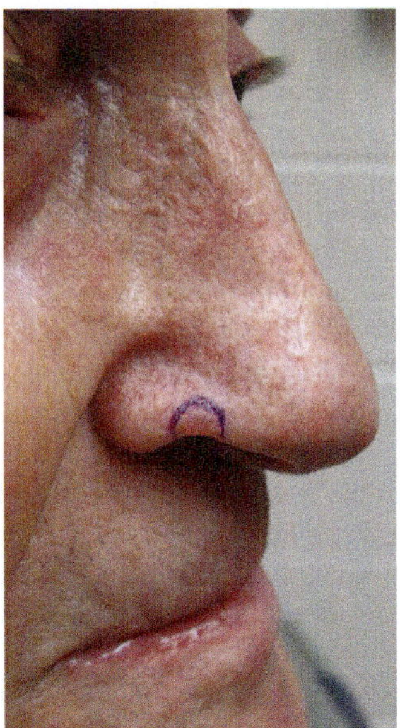

Figure 1 Basal cell carcinoma of the right alar rim.

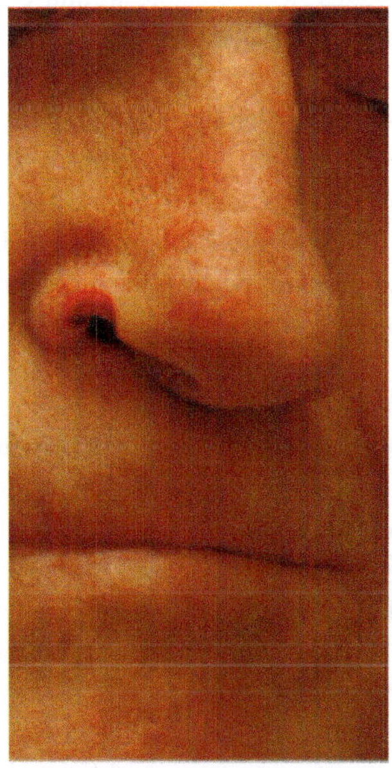

Figure 2 Full-thickness defect of the nasal ala after tumor extirpation.

Resolution

Repair of a full-thickness defect of the nasal alar rim presents challenges in restoring both appearance and

Reconstructive Conundrums in Dermatologic Surgery: The Nose, First Edition. Edited by Désirée Ratner, Joel L. Cohen and David G. Brodland.
© 2014 American Society for Dermatologic Surgery. Published 2014 by John Wiley & Sons, Ltd.

function. The ala is critical to maintaining airway patency and is of high aesthetic value. Even small degrees of asymmetry can yield unacceptable functional or aesthetic results. Points to consider in choosing a reconstructive option include size and depth of the defect, the color and texture of the patient's nasal skin, and the functional integrity of the nasal valve.

Reconstruction of this defect was performed using a composite graft of skin and cartilage harvested from the anterior helix of the ear. Various options for reconstruction were considered, including second intention healing, hinge turnover flap, turnover nasolabial flap (Spear flap), and two-stage cheek interpolation flap with free cartilage graft. In this case, second-intention healing would have resulted in predictable wound contraction, leading to alar notching and a poor cosmetic result. A hinge turnover flap was a viable option. In this patient, however, there was not enough laxity in the adjacent skin to close the secondary defect primarily. A two-stage cheek interpolation flap with free cartilage graft was an additional option. Disadvantages included multiple stages, undesirable aesthetic changes at the harvest site, and the potential for unwanted transfer of terminal hair of the cheek to the nose in men. The Spear flap would have provided a one-stage alternative but would have required a more complex reconstruction than was felt warranted for this smaller-sized defect. It also shared the other disadvantages inherent in the two-stage cheek interpolation flap as described above.

An interlocking auricular composite graft was chosen to repair this defect, as described by Ratner and colleagues.[1] This option was selected based on location of the defect, degree of tissue loss, availability of donor tissue, and patient preference for a single-stage procedure. The graft was taken from the helical crus of the right ear (Figures 3 and 4). The recipient site was measured and the

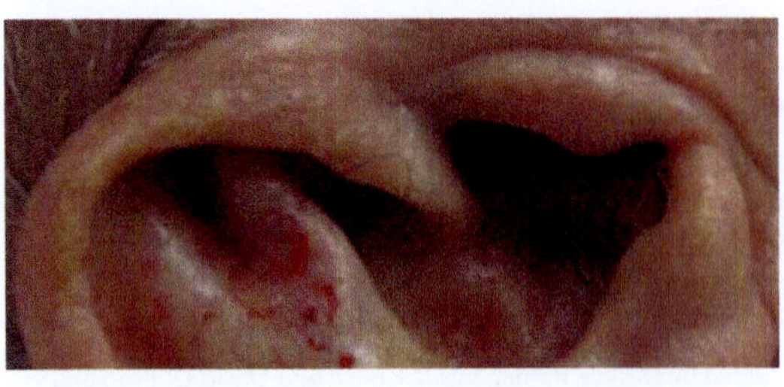

Figure 3 Composite graft design over donor site.

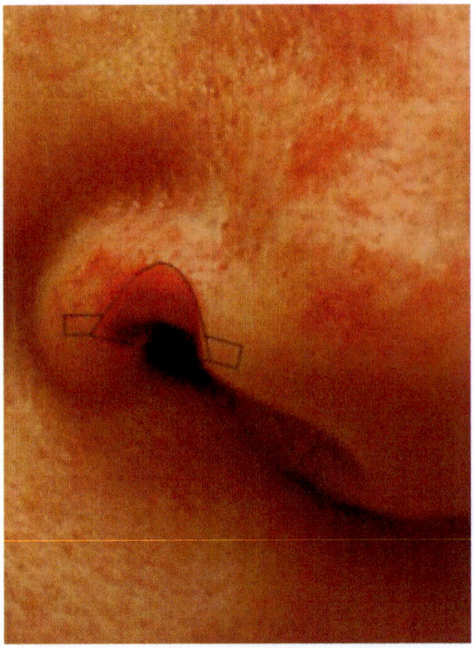

Figure 4 Composite graft design superimposed over defect.

donor site was marked such that the composite graft was approximately 1 mm larger than the defect. This oversizing was to compensate for the natural shrinkage that could occur during healing. The sites were anesthetized with 1% lidocaine with epinephrine and prepped and draped in the usual manner. A No. 15 blade was used to harvest the graft. The donor defect measured 1.5 × 0.8 cm and was closed by primary layered repair using 5-0 polyglactin 910 (Vicryl, Ethicon, Cincinnati, OH) for subcutaneous closure and 6-0 polypropylene mesh (Prolene, Ethicon) for epidermal interrupted sutures (Figure 5). The overlying skin was removed from the outer edges of the graft, leaving intact the underlying cartilage and perichondrium, thus creating cartilaginous pegs for insertion into the recipient site. The cartilaginous pegs measured 4 mm in length. The recipient site was prepared by undermining pockets in the alar tissue to receive the cartilaginous pegs. The pockets measured 4 mm in depth. Sufficient space is usually created simply by the undermining motion of the scissors. Nasal tissue does not need to be extracted unless the pegs are quite thick. The graft was then inserted into the nasal alar rim defect and secured by using 6-0 chromic gut sutures in a simple interrupted manner (Figure 6). Postoperative

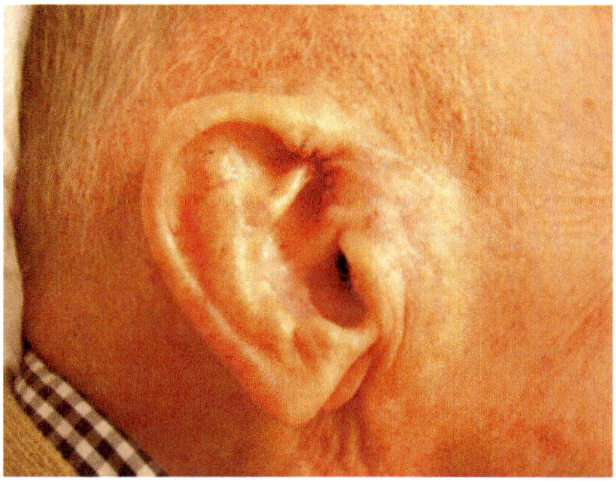

Figure 5 Donor site repair.

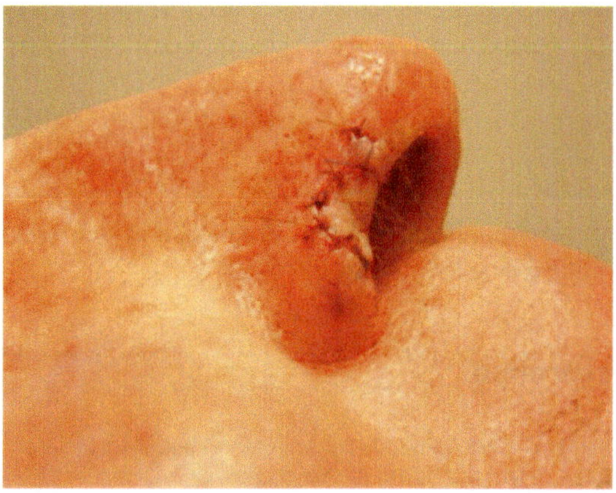

Figure 6 Immediate postoperative result.

antibiotics were given and sutures were removed 7 days later. Three-month follow-up demonstrated desirable aesthetic and functional results (Figures 7, 8 and 9). No additional surgical procedures were performed.

The interlocking auricular composite graft offers a convenient alternative for repair of small nasal alar rim full-thickness defects. Requiring only one operative visit saves time and effort and avoids potential morbidity from additional surgical procedures. The viability of composite grafts is less predictable than that of flaps. Owing to the inherent need for revascularization of all grafts, composite grafts should generally be less than 2 cm in diameter. Smaller-sized grafts will have an increased chance of survival. Smoking increases the risk of postoperative ischemia, which can lead to poor wound healing or tissue necrosis. In the case of a patient who smokes, the use of other repair methods, such as a two-staged cheek interpolation flap, should be considered. The robust blood supply of a flap would reduce the chance of necrosis as compared to a graft. Smoking should be avoided for as long as possible before and after surgery.

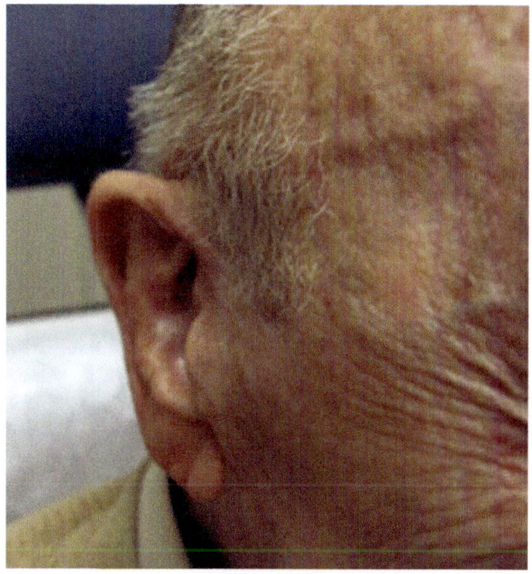

Figure 7 Donor site 3-month postoperative result.

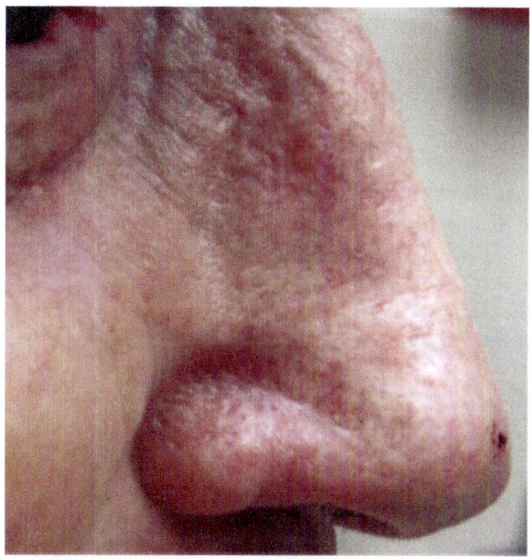

Figure 8 Three-month follow-up demonstrating intact alar rim.

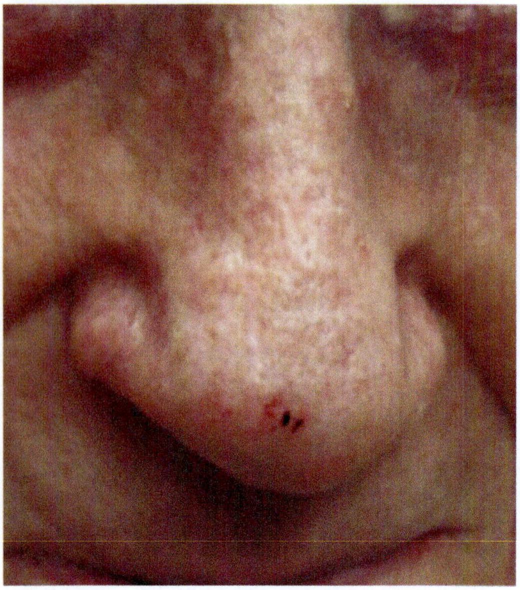

Figure 9 Three-month follow-up demonstrating pleasing alar symmetry.

It is important to handle the tissue extremely gently to avoid trauma to the graft and recipient bed. It is easier to suture the intranasal side first. Small tissue bites should be taken with the needle to avoid strangulation of the tissue. Cotton-tipped applicators are useful to stabilize the graft in place while being sutured. A dental roll may be inserted into the nostril after suturing is complete to stabilize the alar rim. Attentiveness to technique will improve the likelihood of graft survival.

The cartilage component of the graft provides critical support to prevent wound contraction and associated nasal valve compromise. It is essential to harvest a graft of enough length to comfortably span the defect. This interlocking graft provides increased graft stability, which decreases shearing forces of the graft over the recipient bed. This stability increases probability of graft survival. Appropriate selection of the donor site is vital to obtain excellent color and texture match, which is critical in obtaining an excellent aesthetic outcome.

Conundrum keys

- The interlocking auricular composite graft provides a one-stage alternative for small full-thickness nasal alar rim defects.
- The cartilaginous pegs provide graft stability, which increases survival.
- Wound retraction is minimized by use of a composite graft, resulting in preservation of function as well as a pleasing cosmetic outcome.

Reference

1 Ratner D, Katz A, Grande DJ. An interlocking auricular composite graft. Dermatol Surg 1995;21:789–92.

Commentary on conundrum 25

This defect is one that commonly occurs in the setting of skin cancer surgery. The issue, here, is that this particular defect is small as well as full thickness. The authors' choice of a composite graft is perfect for this type of defect. While we frequently read about the unreliability of composite grafts, for small defects like this one (especially in a nonsmoker) with no other simple and straightforward option, a composite graft makes sense and because it is small, the nutritional requirements are not as great as they would be for a larger graft. Composite grafts are especially appealing for similar small defects located more medially on the alar rim. As in this case, the crus/anterior helix

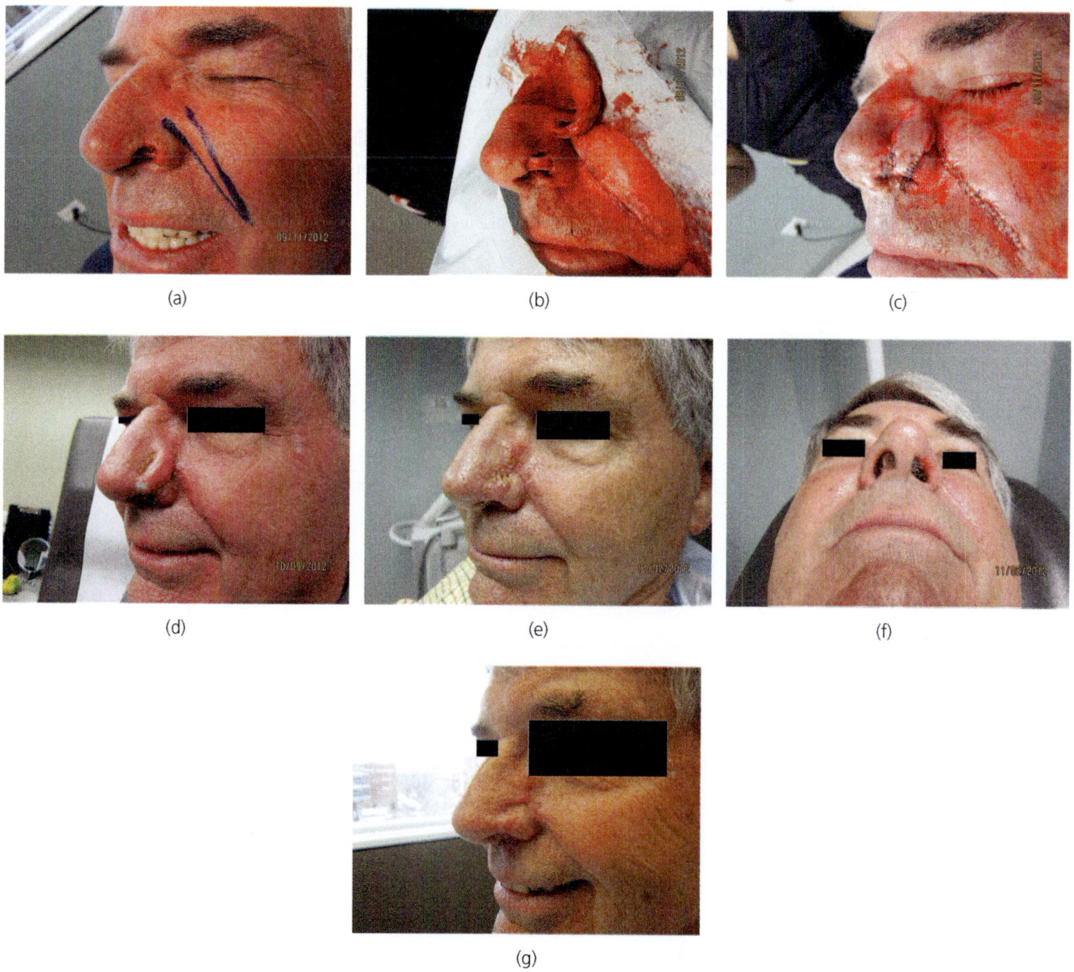

Figure 25.1 (a) Left mid-alar rim defect. Flap design is drawn on nasolabial fold. (b) Cartilage strut placed into medial and lateral subcutaneous pockets and subsequently sewn into place. Nasolabial fold flap is elevated, and the donor site reapproximated with deep sutures. (c) Pedicle transposed to the alar rim and sewn in place overlying the cartilage strut. The epidermal sutures have been placed to reapproximate the donor site carefully along the nasolabial fold. (d) Four weeks after repair, patient presents for pedicle takedown. (e) The repair has healed nicely 3 weeks after takedown. (f) Swimmer's view at 3 weeks after takedown. (g) Follow-up at 3 months showing reapproximation of nasolabial fold donor site and good tissue match.

is the typical donor site. A recent review of 25 composite grafts suggests strategies for success when performing this repair.[1]

For larger or more laterally located alar rim defects, two-stage melolabial interpolation flaps are frequently considered (Figure 25.1a–g). In this example, a cartilage strut harvested from the left conchal bowl is positioned to restore the integrity of the alar rim. Subsequently, the flap is elevated, thinned distally, and wrapped around the cartilage strut. At 4 weeks, the pedicle was taken down and reinset with careful attention to hiding the suture lines within the cosmetic subunits.

If a patient prefers to avoid the restrictions commonly associated with grafting, they may be amenable to having a smaller nostril if a simple wedge side-to-side repair can be performed. Other alternative repairs, such as an ipsilateral hinge mucoperichondrial lining flap followed by an aurticular cartilage strut and a cheek (or even a paramedian forehead) interpolation flap for skin coverage would be much larger and more complicated, carrying their own set of issues and risks.[2]

Commentary by Dr. Cohen

References

1 Zilinsky I, Farber N, Haik J, Weissman O, Israeli H, Winkler E. Nasal ala reconstruction with a crus helix composite graft: a stepladder approach. J Drugs Dermatol 2012;11(3): 376–81.

2 Baker, SR. Local flaps in facial reconstruction, 2nd Edition, Chapter 18. St Louis: Mosby, 2007: p. 464–5.

26

CONUNDRUM 26

Repair of a Defect on the Ala

Helen G. Kaporis[1] *& John A. Carucci*[2]

[1]Rockefeller University, New York, NY

[2]Weill Medical College of Cornell, New York, NY

A 71-year-old otherwise healthy woman was referred for treatment of a biopsy-proven, recurrent, aggressive-growth basal cell carcinoma on the right ala. The lesion was removed in two stages of Mohs micrographic surgery, and the resulting defect measured 2.4 × 2.1 cm and involved >70% of the right ala including the alar rim (Figure 1). How would you reconstruct this defect?

Resolution

Alar reconstruction may be challenging because of the complex topographic relationships of the nose.[1] Additionally, with the nose being a focal point on the face, even minor deformities are noticeable. Second-intention healing, while sometimes appropriate for the shallowest of nasal defects, would have resulted in severe functional compromise and deformed appearance.[2] Skin grafting in this case would have likely yielded a similar result due to loss of inferior portion of the alar rim. Single-staged melolabial flaps can be used but have been associated with blunting of the nasofacial sulcus requiring subsequent revision.[3] Zitelli's modification incorporating both advancement and transposition might have provided a good functional result;[4] however, this flap may result in blunting of the alar groove. This option may have been considered for a patient unable or unwilling to undergo a staged procedure. Paramedian forehead flaps can be used for alar replacement, but some have advocated they are best used for replacement of the nasal sidewall or tip units.[5] After consideration of all options, the decision was made to perform a staged melolabial flap with cartilage graft (Figure 2).

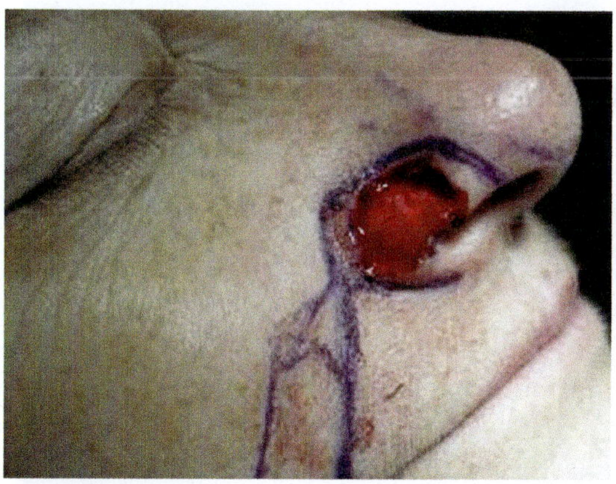

Figure 1 Defect after Mohs surgery for basal cell carcinoma on right ala.

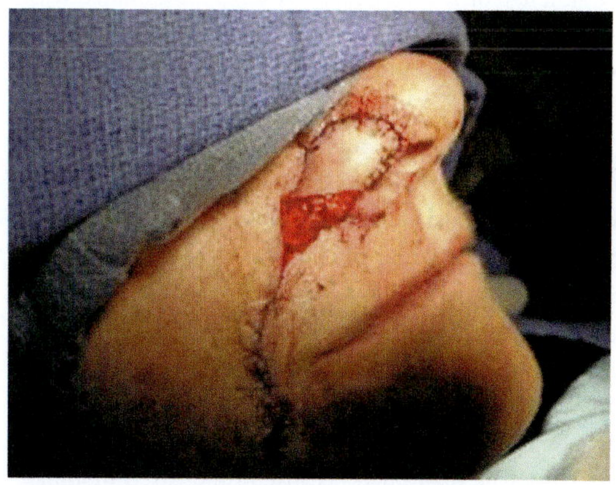

Figure 2 Staged melolabial flap in place.

Reconstructive Conundrums in Dermatologic Surgery: The Nose, First Edition. Edited by Désirée Ratner, Joel L. Cohen and David G. Brodland.
© 2014 American Society for Dermatologic Surgery. Published 2014 by John Wiley & Sons, Ltd.

Surgical technique

Staged melolabial flaps are random-pattern transposition flaps with blood supply from branches of the facial and angular arteries that perforate the levator labii muscle.[6] This particular repair is a staged procedure requiring both cartilage graft and melolabial flap at first stage followed within 2 to 3 weeks by pedicle division.

First stage: cartilage graft and melolabial flap

Consideration is given to enlarging the defect to include the entire alar subunit to facilitate best long-term healing. After determining the extent of the final alar defect, a cartilage graft is placed prior to performing the melolabial flap.

Cartilage grafting

The cartilage is harvested through an anterior approach from the conchal bowl via a U-shaped incision, allowing the development of a medially based skin flap that is easily reflected with skin hooks to reveal the conchal cartilage. The authors prefer the anterior approach since cartilage is readily accessible. In addition, the anterior approach ipsilateral to the defect requires no repositioning of the patient. Conchal cartilage is removed and trimmed as necessary and placed over the mucosal portion of the ala via stab incisions and sewn with chromic gut suture to create an outward bow to facilitate valvular competency. The skin flap on the conchal bowl is reapproximated with 5-0 fast absorbing gut.

Melolabial flap

A template is prepared from nonadherent dressing pads or foil to match the size and shape of the contralateral ala. The flap is planned to include the medial portion of the cheek donor skin to be placed at the melolabial crease. It is essential to allow for sufficient length to allow the donor site to reach the ala without tension. Redundant jowl skin allows for easy closure of the donor site. The flap may be designed as a peninsula or based strictly on a subcutaneous pedicle as a true island flap.[7] The authors prefer the true island flap because of increased mobility. The flap is developed in the subcutaneous plane excised in full-thickness fashion around its entire perimeter.[8] Deep excision around the entire perimeter of the flap allows for optimal mobility of the flap. The developed and mobile flap is transposed to reach the defect in tension-free fashion. The distal half of the flap may be thinned initially while the proximal portion is thinned after division of the pedicle. We trim the distalmost portion (~2 mm) to dermis to achieve excellent contour at completion of first stage with no effect on viability. The distal flap is sewn to the medial portion of the defect using 6-0 nylon sutures that are removed in 5 to 7 days. Layered closure of the cheek donor is then performed. The pedicle may remain attached for 2 to 3 weeks to develop collateral vascularity.

Second stage: division of the pedicle

Division of the pedicle is performed at 2 to 3 weeks under local anesthesia. We prefer pedicle division at 2 weeks rather than later since we have found it easier to

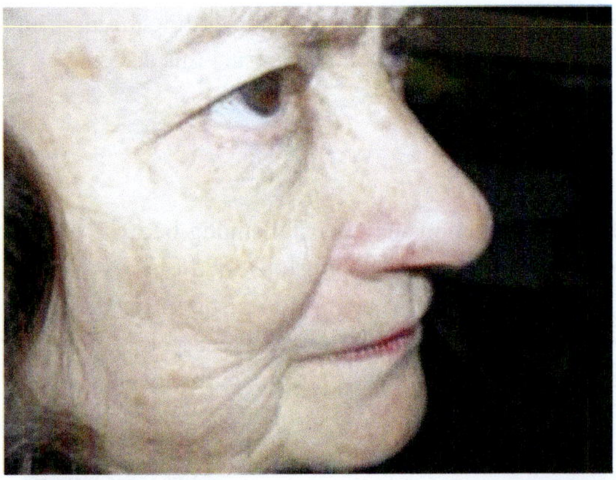

(a)

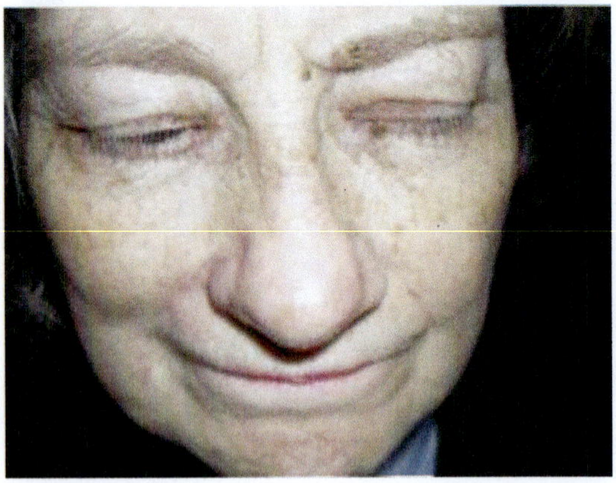

(b)

Figure 3 Three-month follow up of repair. (a) Lateral view. (b) Anterior view. Nasofacial crease, alar crease, and alar rim are preserved.

sculpt the lateral ala at this time rather than later, when scar tissue begins to compromise mobility. To divide the pedicle, the lateral aspect of the flap is amputated and the lateral portion of the alar flap is sized, thinned appropriately, and reapproximated using 6-0 nylon sutures. The cheek portion is inset by extending the incision along the melolabial fold and nasofacial sulcus as needed. The resulting cheek defect is closed in layered fashion along the melolabial crease and nasofacial sulcus while avoiding distortion of the hairless triangle. Distortion of this landmark, which represents the junction of the upper cutaneous lip, cheek, and lateral alar subunits, results in aesthetic deformity and thus must be avoided. Sutures are removed 5 to 7 days after pedicle division. Three-month follow-up is shown in Figure 3.

Conundrum keys

- A tumor-free plane must be obtained prior to considering reconstructive surgery.
- The staged melolabial flap provides both functional and aesthetic alar replacement.
- Conchal cartilage graft easily obtained via anterior approach may be necessary to assure valvular competency.
- Entire alar replacement should be considered when more than 50% is sacrificed in cancer removal.

References

1 Rohrich RJ, Griffin JR, Ansari M, et al. Nasal reconstruction–beyond aesthetic subunits: a 15-year review of 1334 cases. Plast Reconstr Surg 2004;114:1405–16; discussion 1417–9.
2 Reynolds MB, Gourdin FW. Nasal valve dysfunction after Mohs surgery for skin cancer of the nose. Dermatol Surg 1998; 24:1011–7.
3 Lindsey WH. Reliability of the melolabial flap for alar reconstruction. Arch Facial Plast Surg 2001;3:33–7.
4 Zitelli JA. The nasolabial flap as a single-stage procedure. Arch Dermatol 1990;126:1445–8.
5 Arden RL, Nawroz-Danish M, Yoo GH, et al. Nasal alar reconstruction: a critical analysis using melolabial island and paramedian forehead flaps. Laryngoscope 1999;109: 376–82.
6 Nguyen TH. Staged cheek-to-nose and auricular interpolation flaps. Dermatol Surg 2005;31(8 Pt 2):1034–45.
7 Carucci JA. Melolabial flap repair in nasal reconstruction. Dermatol Clin 2005;23:65–71, vi.
8 Fosko SW, Dzubow LM. Nasal reconstruction with the cheek island pedicle flap. J Am Acad Dermatol 1996;35: 580–7.

Commentary on conundrum 26

The key to esthetic repair of any alar rim defect is careful assessment of the free margin to determine whether cartilage is required for rim stabilization. If the individual's alar skin is relatively thick and sebaceous, with good underlying tissue support, a simple flap or FTSG may be sufficient to repair this defect without alar retraction developing later. However, should the alar rim be delicate or flimsy, cartilage grafting is nearly always required to minimize the risk of retraction. For a large lateral alar defect like the one shown in this reconstructive conundrum, comprising >70% of the nasal ala, stabilization of the rim with cartilage followed by replacement of the skin of the entire anatomic subunit is a thoughtful and well-executed reconstructive approach.

Repair of smaller partial-thickness defects involving the alar rim can pose unique reconstructive challenges. Donor tissue for local flaps is limited, and skin grafts do not always provide a good tissue match. A two-stage melolabial interpolation flap, with or without an underlying cartilage graft, can certainly be a good reconstructive alternative for a larger defect, but using this repair for a smaller alar defect may be problematic at times, as unsightly trapdooring may develop postoperatively, and the contours of the flap may be difficult to conceal.

For small, deep partial-thickness alar rim defects, a composite cartilage graft may therefore be considered as a single-stage reconstructive alternative.

A small partial-thickness defect of the ala extending onto the alar rim is shown in Figure 26.1a. It was sufficiently deep that repair with a full-thickness skin graft alone would probably have left a concavity as well as contraction of the free margin. Placement of an underlying cartilage graft would have provided alar rim support, but a skin graft on top of it would likely not have provided a suitable contour match or a desirable esthetic result. An auricular composite graft, consisting of cartilage with its overlying skin, can provide the internal support needed

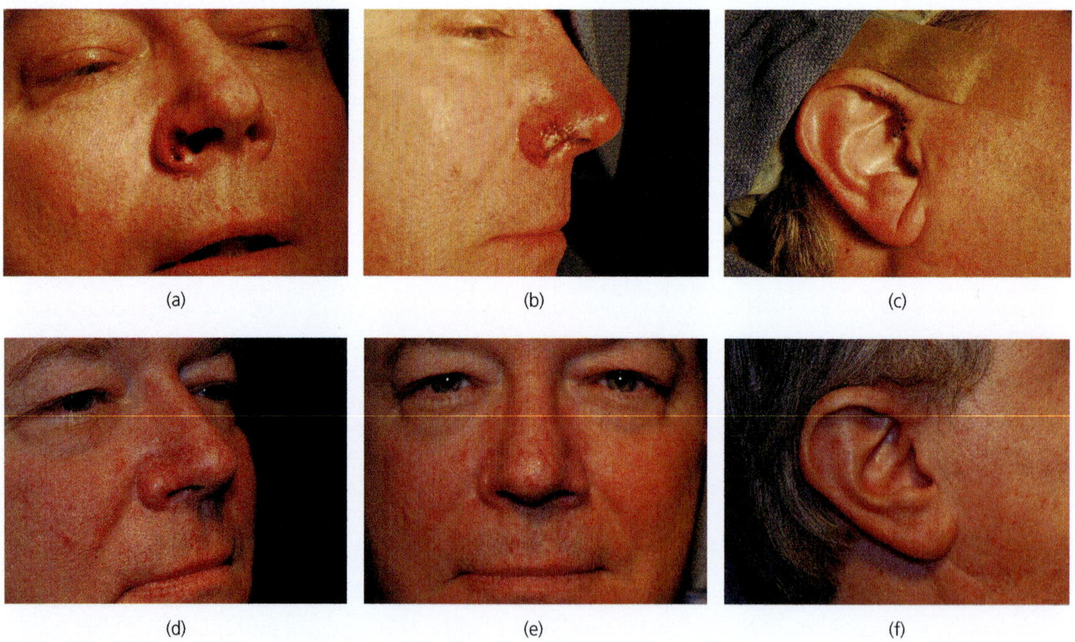

Figure 26.1 (a) Deep partial-thickness defect of right nasal ala after Mohs surgery for basal cell carcinoma. (b) Composite graft taken from right helical crus sewn into place with 6-0 fast absorbing gut sutures. (c) Right helical donor site closed primarily. (d) Follow-up view 4 years postoperatively (side view). (e) Follow-up view 4 years postoperatively (frontal view). (f) View of the donor site 4 years postoperatively.

to brace the ala against the forces of contraction due to fibrosis, while also replacing lost skin and soft tissue with a reasonable color and texture match. However, the increased metabolic needs of composite grafts put them at greater risk for necrosis; so ideally, no part of a composite graft will be more than 0.5–1.0 cm away from its recipient bed, which dictates that the graft should be less than 2 cm in greatest diameter. For this reason, larger partial-thickness alar defects are better suited for repair with other methods.

In this case, a composite graft was harvested from the helical crus, whose texture, color, and appendageal structures closely matched the alar skin. The skin overlying the cartilage on either side of the graft was removed, leaving cartilaginous "pegs" with their overlying perichondrium on either side. These pegs were interlocked with soft tissue pockets undermined on either side of the defect and the composite graft sutured into place with 6-0 absorbable sutures (Figure 26.1b). The helical donor site was closed primarily (Figure 26.1c). Front and side views taken 4 years later (Figure 26.1d and e) reveal preservation of the contour of the alar rim and a good tissue match with maintenance of facial symmetry (Figure 26.1d and e).

The decision whether to replace the entire alar subunit is dictated by the size of the defect, and may be considered when the defect comprises more than 50% of the alar area. For smaller partial-thickness alar defects, a staged melolabial flap with an underlying cartilage graft can certainly be considered. However, for small, deep defects requiring both cartilage support and skin coverage, a properly sized helical composite graft may provide a satisfactory cosmetic and functional result as well.

Commentary by Dr. Ratner

27

CONUNDRUM 27

Single-Stage Reconstruction of a Combined Upper Lip and Nasal Ala Defect

Matteo C. LoPiccolo[1] *& David J. Kouba*[1,2]
[1]Department of Dermatology, Henry Ford Health System, Detroit, Michigan
[2]Toledo Clinic Dermasurgery and Laser Center, Toledo, Ohio

A 79-year-old Caucasian woman presented with a several-month history of an enlarging mass on the right nasal ala. Physical examination revealed a 0.6-cm erythematous, friable nodule involving the right alar rim, with a portion of the tumor also present in the alar sulcus and upper lip. Biopsy revealed basal cell carcinoma. Definitive removal of the tumor using Mohs micrographic surgery required four stages and resulted in a 1.4-cm defect. This defect spanned the full thickness of the distal portion of the right nasal ala, as well as a portion of the cheek and upper cutaneous lip (Figure 1). Integrity of the distal internal alar lining was compromised, and gentle downward pressure on the nose resulted in collapse of the ala. How would you reconstruct this defect?

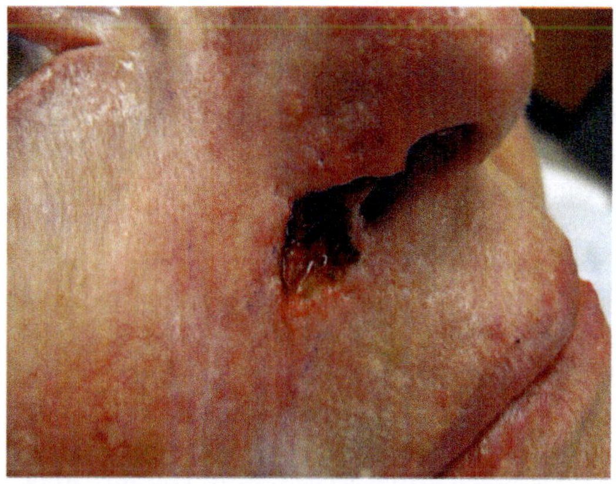

Figure 1 Resultant defect of the right nasal ala, alar sulcus, and upper cutaneous lip following Mohs micrographic surgery.

Resolution

The approach to reconstructing defects involving the ala and perialar area requires careful attention to the natural contour of the alar lobule and adjacent creases in addition to the principle of individual reconstructive subunits. Defining the extent of the defect with these principles in mind will guide your steps. Some single-stage techniques previously described to repair similar defects include use of a Spear flap, "shark" island pedicle flap, nasolabial flap, and composite cartilage and skin graft.[1–5] Others are planned two-stage procedures such as the paramedian forehead flap and other interpolated flaps.[6,7] Combining techniques is also an option for more complex defects involving multiple cosmetic subunits.[8] As deemed necessary with any of these choices, the nasal lining can be restored with a hinge or turnover flap, cartilage can be added, and all can be combined with other flap techniques to complete the reconstruction.

To preserve the integrity of both cosmetic subunits using a single-stage closure, a combination of tissue

Reconstructive Conundrums in Dermatologic Surgery: The Nose, First Edition. Edited by Désirée Ratner, Joel L. Cohen and David G. Brodland.
© 2014 American Society for Dermatologic Surgery. Published 2014 by John Wiley & Sons, Ltd.

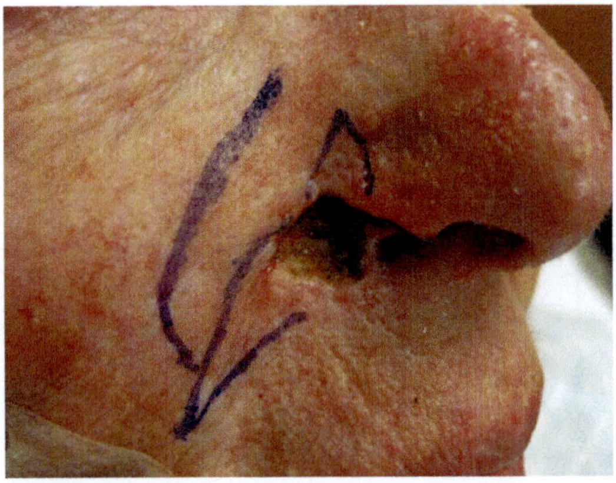

Figure 2 Incision lines for the island pedicle flap and melolabial transposition inked with sterile marking pen before beginning the repair.

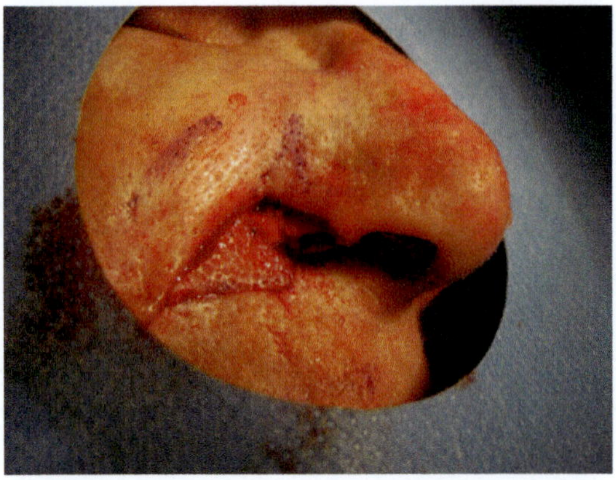

Figure 3 The island pedicle flap sutured in place after advancement.

rearrangement techniques was ultimately selected. First, an island pedicle flap was planned to close the upper lip defect. This island pedicle flap was inked extending inferiorly and laterally from the defect, with the uppermost incision line set along the melolabial fold. Next, a melolabial transposition flap was planned by inking a crescent-shape incision line extending superior-medially from the shared melolabial fold line planned to create the island pedicle flap. A Burow's triangle extending superiorly from the defect was planned to allow transposition of the melolabial flap into position for reconstruction of the nasal ala (Figure 2).

The inferior and lateral incisions to free the island pedicle were then made. The flap was advanced medially and 4-0 Vicryl buried sutures were used to secure the inferior-medial aspect of the flap in its final position on the upper cutaneous lip, juxtaposing the alar defect (Figure 3). The alar base and rim reconstruction remained. To support the compromised ala, an antihelical cartilage graft was harvested and anchored in place, as previously described.[2] A subcutaneous pocket was created superiorly to hold the cartilage graft in place. Inferiorly, no residual ala remained. The melolabial flap was then developed by incising the cheek portion and removing the alar Burow's triangle (Figure 4). After the distal portion of the melolabial flap was de-fatted, it was transposed above the island pedicle and placed over the alar cartilage graft. The donor sites for both flaps were closed using buried 4-0 Vicryl sutures, settling the incision line within the natural melolabial crease. Tacking

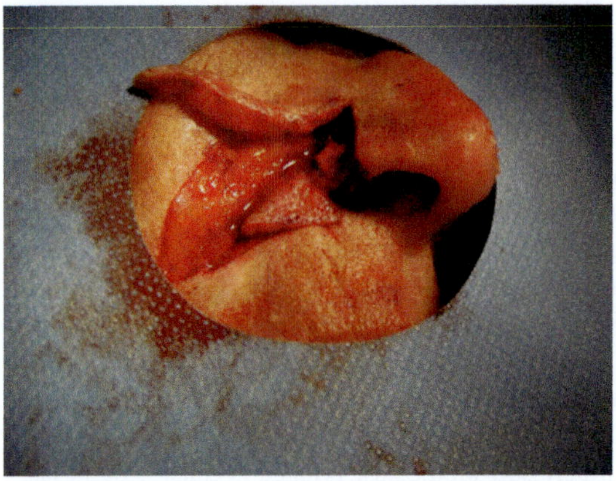

Figure 4 After incision, the melolabial flap is free for transposition into the alar defect. The cartilage strut is sutured in place.

sutures were placed on the lateral aspects of the melolabial transposition to secure its place over the cartilage strut. Tissue was then conservatively trimmed from the end of the flap, allowing room for retraction. The extirpated ala and alar lining were then recreated by turning over the distal portion of the flap and suturing it to the residual interior alar lining. Buried 4-0 Vicryl sutures were used to secure the remainder of the repair to the nasal bridge and to the medial aspect of the island pedicle advancement. Lastly, a running suture of 6-0 nylon was used to evert the wound edges of each incision (Figures 5 and 6). Three months postoperatively, the patient had healed well with no evidence of retraction and an excellent cosmetic and functional result (Figure 7).

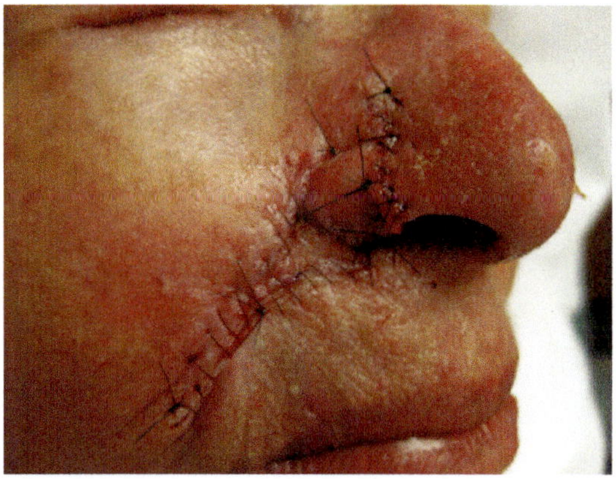

Figure 5 Postoperative repair yields reconstruction of the alar rim and preservation of the alar sulcus.

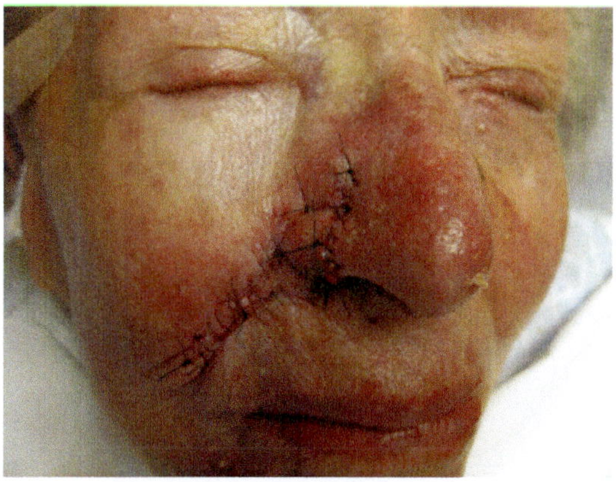

Figure 6 Frontal view immediately after operative repair.

Our approach combines two well-known tissue-rearrangement techniques – the island pedicle advancement and the melolabial transposition – to close a defect crossing two cosmetic subunits. When used to close a defect involving the nasal ala and the upper cutaneous lip, as in this case, incision along the natural melolabial fold serves to free the superior margin of the island pedicle and the inferior margin of the melolabial flap and disguises the incision along this natural skin crease. The amount of melolabial transposition flap needed to fill the alar defect should be overestimated to allow for retraction. In addition, a curved portion of antihelical cartilage provides support to recreate the contour of the alar rim. Correction of blunted alar creases and repositioning for

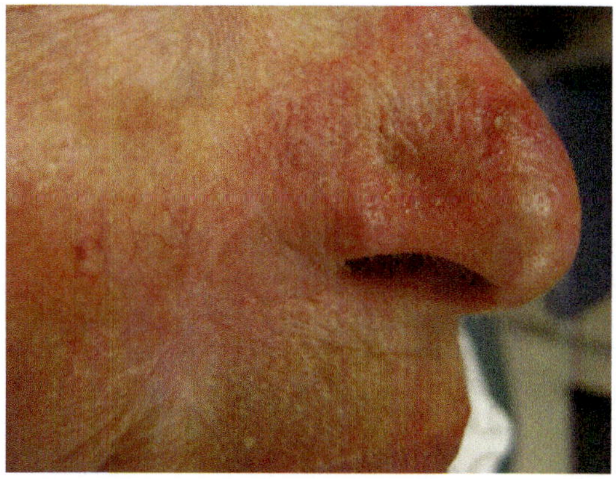

Figure 7 Excellent cosmetic results after 3 months.

precise placement of the alar base may be needed with any technique, but this technique allows for a single-stage closure of a defect involving two cosmetic subunits with excellent results.

Conundrum keys

- To allow for retraction, overestimate the amount of melolabial transposition flap needed to recreate the alar rim.
- A single curvilinear incision along the nasolabial fold serves to free the superior portion of the island pedicle and the inferior portion of the nasolabial transposition flap.
- A curved portion of antihelical cartilage can help recreate the contour of the alar rim and brace against wound contraction forces.

References

1 Spear SL, Kroll SS, Romm S. A new twist to the nasolabial flap for reconstruction of lateral alar defects. Plast Reconstr Surg 1987;79:915–20.

2 Adams DC, Ramsey ML. Grafts in dermatologic surgery: review and update on full- and split-thickness skin grafts, free cartilage grafts, and composite grafts. Dermatol Surg 2005;31: 1055–67.

3 Cvancara JL, Wentzell JM. Shark island pedicle flap for repair of combined nasal ala-perialar defects. Dermatol Surg 2006;32:726–9.

4 Zitelli JA. The nasolabial flap as a single-stage procedure. Arch Derm 1990;126:1145–8.
5 Cook JL. Reconstruction of a full-thickness alar wound with a single operative procedure. Derm Surg 2003;29:956–62.
6 Brodland DG. Paramedian forehead flap reconstruction for nasal defects. Dermatol Surg 2005;31:1046–52.
7 Mellette JR, Ho DQ. Interpolation flaps. Dermatol Clin 2005;23:87–112.
8 LeVasseur JG, Mellette JR. Techniques for reconstruction of perialar and perialar-nasal ala combined defects. Derm Surg 2000;26:1019–23.

Commentary on conundrum 27

The key to repairing defects involving the lateral ala and the apical triangle area of the cutaneous upper lip often lies in the ability to separate the defect into its individual cosmetic units. In this reconstructive conundrum, the upper lip portion of the defect requires replacement with like skin for optimal repair. Repair of the nasal portion of the defect requires attention to the lining (not removed in this case but still needing to remain intact), structural support (in the form of cartilage grafts), and skin coverage.

The island pedicle flap used to repair the lip portion of this defect is a consistently reliable reconstructive option for this area as its incision lines may be concealed along the lateral border of the nasal ala and the nasolabial fold. The transposition flap used to repair the alar portion of this defect was a less conventional choice and required an underlying cartilaginous strut for alar rim stabilization. Although the flap initially appeared to provide sufficient bulk for recreation of the alar contours as seen in the postoperative view (Figure 5), slight blunting of the lateral alar rim can be seen in the 3-month follow-up view (Figure 7). Even so, the final result is very good with imperceptible suture lines and preservation of the alar sulcus.

A similar defect is shown in Figure 27.1a, which also involves both the lateral ala and the cutaneous upper lip. It differs in that it also involves the medial cheek and apical triangle. Although an island pedicle flap could certainly have been used to repair the lateral aspect of this defect, there was a risk of lateral alar blunting and obliteration of the apical triangle had the flap been advanced to cover the entire defect. For this reason, as shown in this conundrum, repair of the cheek/lip anatomic subunits needed to be considered separately from repair of the alar subunit. Figure 27.1b shows how a lip advancement/rotation flap was used to recreate the apical triangle, with a dog-ear taken along the alar crease and onto the nasal sill to camouflage the suture line. The deep soft tissue of the flap was advanced to the lateral border of the ala to create soft tissue support for the alar base. Following this, a small Burow's graft was used to recreate the lateral portion of the ala. A cartilage graft was not required for alar stabilization as the defect was relatively superficial and did not extend medially to involve the alar rim.

Combined upper lip and alar defects frequently require combination repairs to preserve the integrity of their anatomic subunits. Analysis of the subunits involved, their adjacent tissue reservoirs, and the peripheral and deep extent of each anatomic area will help to determine the optimal reconstructive approach.

In both of these cases, taking such an approach allowed all incision lines to be disguised within the natural creases of the face, with the maintenance of the cosmetic junction lines, in a single-stage procedure.

Commentary by Dr. Ratner

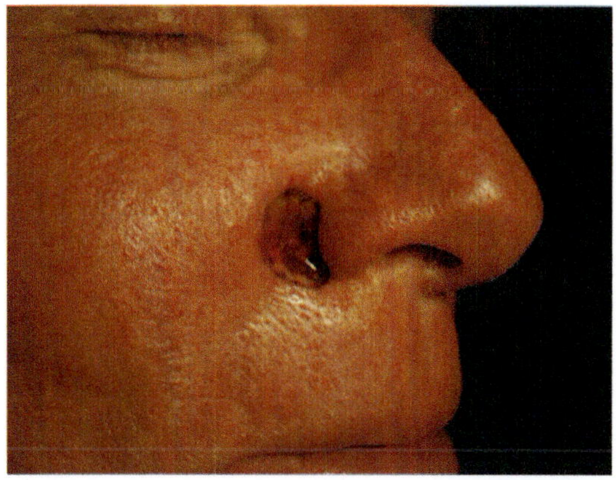

(a)

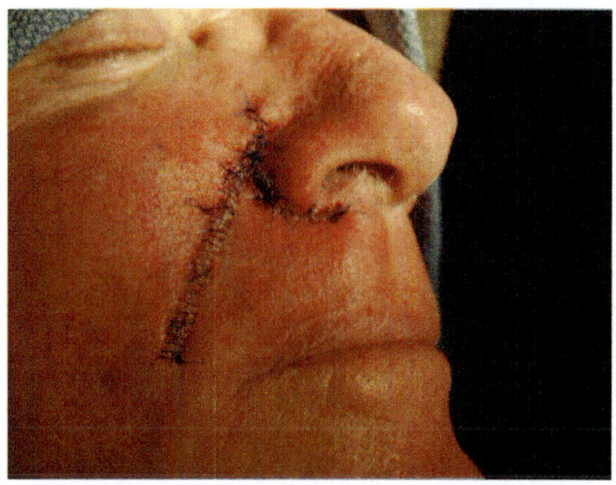

(b)

Figure 27.1 (a) Defect of the right lateral ala extending onto the medial cheek and apical triangle following Mohs surgery. (b) Lip advancement/rotation flap provided coverage for cheek and lip portions of the defect with a Burow's graft placed at the lateral aspect of the ala.

28

CONUNDRUM 28

Nasal Dorsum Transposition Flap for Closure of an Alar Rim Defect

Luciana Takata Pontes[1,2], *Leonard H. Goldberg*[2,3], *Adam J. Mamelak*[2,3], *& Arash Kimyai-Asadi*[2,3]

[1]Department of Dermatology, Hospital de Clinicas da UNICAMP, Campinas, Sao Paulo, Brazil
[2]DermSurgery Associates, Houston, Texas
[3]Department of Dermatology, Weill Cornell Medical College, Methodist Hospital, Houston, Texas

A 60-year-old Caucasian man with Fitzpatrick skin type II presented to our clinic for evaluation of a lesion on the right nasal ala. Physical examination was significant for a 1.8- × 1.2-cm nodule that was firm on palpation encompassing the majority of the right nasal ala (Figure 1). A biopsy was performed, and histologic evaluation revealed islands of atypical basaloid cells with peripheral palisading within the dermis, consistent with a basal cell carcinoma. The patient underwent Mohs micrographic surgery, and the tumor was cleared in two stages. A 2.5- × 1.5-cm surgical defect of the right nasal ala, including the nasal ala rim, resulted (Figure 2). How would you repair this defect?

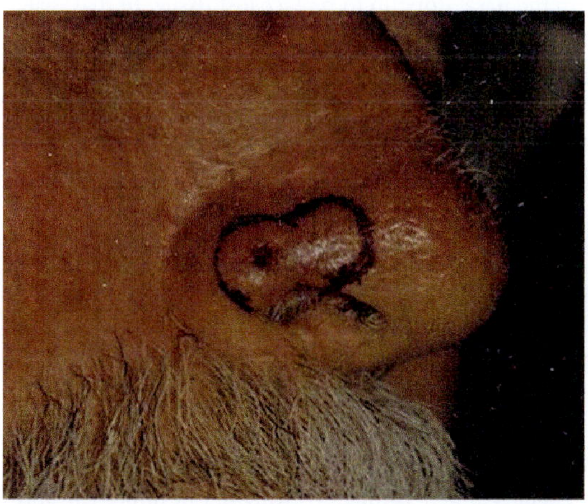

Figure 1 Basal cell carcinoma of the right nasal ala.

Resolution

Repair of defects of the nasal ala is challenging because of the complicated anatomy and the relative lack of available donor skin.[1] In our patient, the need to reconstruct a cosmetically acceptable ala and alar rim with a sufficiently patent external nostril was the main goal of the reconstruction.[2] Postsurgical problems in this location include abnormalities of the nasal contour with low, thick, or elevated alar margins; an asymmetrical alar base; an absent alar groove; and a constricted nostril.[3]

Generally, second-intention healing produces acceptable results when the wound is smaller than 1 cm in diameter and at the nose tip, dorsum, and sidewall. It may create a depressed or raised scar but rarely results in functional impairment.[4] In contrast, even small defects of the ala (1 cm) left to heal by second intention may cause notching of the nostril or partial collapse of the external nasal valve on inspiration.[1]

Primary closure of any defect is preferred if it can be accomplished without visible tissue distortion. In our

Reconstructive Conundrums in Dermatologic Surgery: The Nose, First Edition. Edited by Désirée Ratner, Joel L. Cohen and David G. Brodland.
© 2014 American Society for Dermatologic Surgery. Published 2014 by John Wiley & Sons, Ltd.

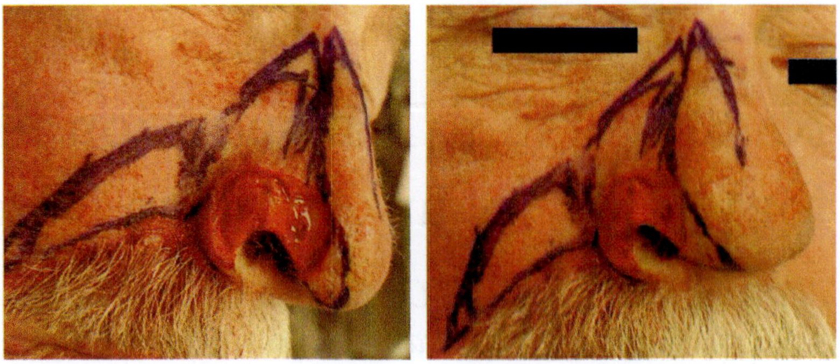

(a) (b)

Figure 2 (A and B) Full-thickness dermal surgical defect of the ala and ala rim and flap design.

patient, there was not enough adjacent skin available for a primary closure. A side-to-side closure would have resulted in loss of nasal ala structure. For this reason, we decided to close the defect by adding skin from another source.

A number of repair options were considered.

A full-thickness skin graft was a possible option. In our patient, there was not enough nasal structure left to allow for sufficient blood supply to support a full thickness skin graft. In addition, finding sufficient matching skin would be a challenge.

Advancement flaps using skin from the proximal nose to the inferior nose would have been possible in the form of a subcutaneous island pedicle flap or a bilobed flap, but we did not feel that this was possible in our patient because of the large size of the defect. A rotation flap from the nose sidewall and nose dorsum is a possibility, too, in a defect in this location, but in our case, there was not enough skin laxity to achieve this goal. Advancement and transposition flaps from the cheek skin may deform the geometry of the alar groove and cheek and would have been cosmetically unacceptable.

Another possibility considered was a paramedian forehead flap, which has an abundant blood supply, but later touch-up surgeries would have been necessary to reduce the swelling of the flap and create a cosmetically acceptable result.

A cheek-based melolabial interpolated flap preserves the aesthetically important alar facial sulcus. The major disadvantage is the need for a two- or even three-stage procedure. Another problem of the melolabial interpolated flap in men is the potential transfer of hair-bearing skin to the nose.[5]

A melolabial transposition flap is frequently used for the reconstruction of the ala and nasal sidewall because of the availability of abundant cheek skin with color, texture, sebaceous glandularity, and thickness similar to that of the natural skin of the ala, but it may deform the alar facial sulcus and the lateral portion of the alar groove.

After careful consideration, we decided to use a transposition flap from the nasal dorsum. This had the advantage of using adequate local qualitatively similar skin with a self-contained blood supply and the ability to preserve the contour and function of the nasal ala and groove. Had there been a full-thickness defect of the nasal ala, not enough tissue would have been available from the nasal dorsum to replace lost tissue. In that case, a forehead flap or an interpolation cheek flap would have been a more appropriate closure.

The Procedure

A transposition flap inferiorly based on the nasal dorsum was designed to provide skin to close the surgical defect. A template of the defect was fashioned from a telfa pad and drawn onto the proposed donor site. The ability of the donor site on the nasal dorsum to be closed was evident from the experience of the senior author, who has been able to close fairly large defects on the nasal dorsum, with excellent cosmetic results.[6] Closure of this donor site and rotation of the flap and its blood supply into the defect would shorten the length of the defect to be closed. This donor skin from the dorsum and tip of the nose is similar in quality to that of the nasal ala. Although this is a random axis type of flap, there is good blood supply to this location from the dorsal nasal artery and the external nasal artery. Having enough donor skin, we would be able to fold the flap on itself and create an adequate nasal alar rim.

Briefly, 0.5% lidocaine with 1:200,000 epinephrine was injected locally to anesthetize the prepared donor

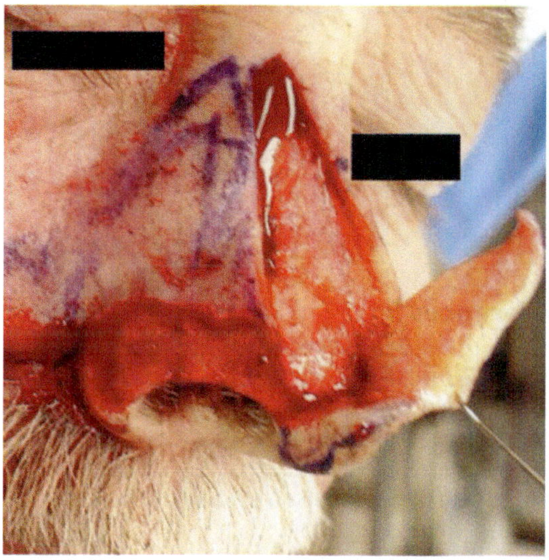

Figure 3 Incision and raising of the flap before placement.

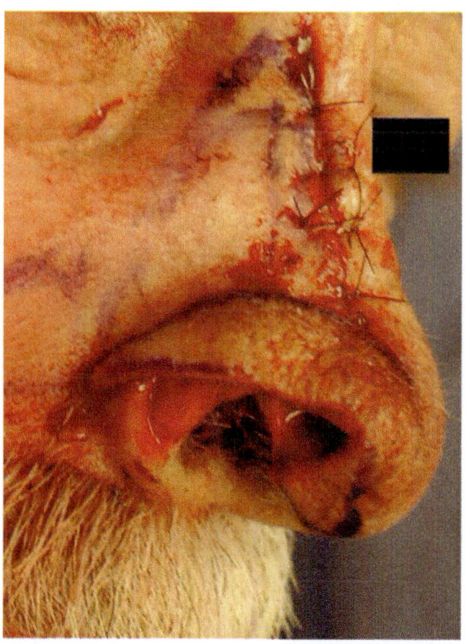

Figure 4 Initial suturing.

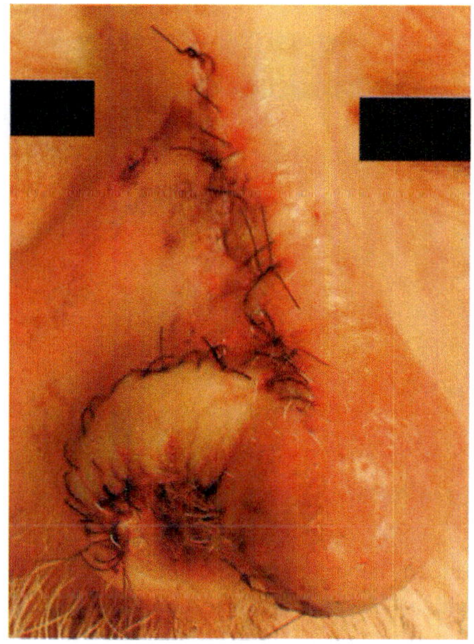

Figure 5 Final suturing.

skin area. Incisions were made around the donor tissue superior to the defect on the right nasal side-wall. The superior portion of the flap was freed, and the tissue on the nasal sidewall and dorsum was moderately undermined. The inferior medial portion of the flap was left as the pedicle, the transposed skin was sutured inferiorly to the mucosal lining of the nasal vestibule, and the superior edge was sutured to the outer skin of the nasal ala, restoring the tissue lost from the area. It remained attached to the nasal dorsum at the level of the nasal tip (Figure 3). The flap was transposed into the defect and sewn in place with 5-0 poliglecaprone 25 (Monocryl) subcutaneous suture on a P-3 needle and 6-0 nylon running cutaneous suture on a P-3 needle (Figures 4 and 5). Careful placement of the removal of the dog ear at the flap pivot point is important. If this is not done appropriately, nasal vestibule distortion will invariably occur. A pressure dressing was applied, and the patient was given oral and written standard wound care instructions. Sutures may be removed after 5 to 10 days. At 3-month follow-up, the flap had completely healed and lost its postoperative swelling and inflammation (Figure 6a and b). The ala retained its normal size, with no loss of function or deformity. No later touch-up surgeries were necessary because the transposition flap did not create any trap door deformity

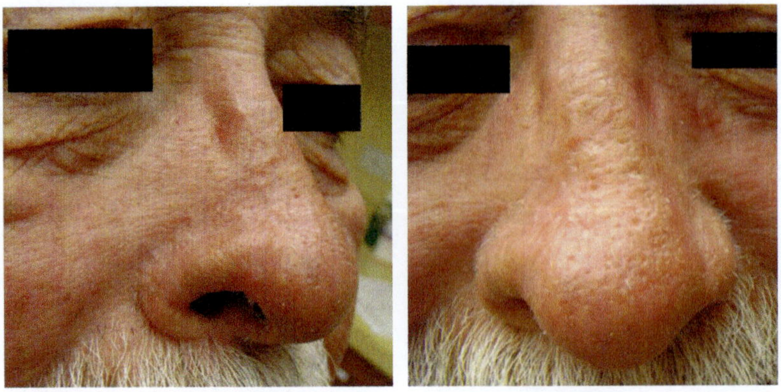

(a) (b)

Figure 6 (a and b) Final result 3 months postoperatively.

or dog ear. The donor site on the dorsum of the nose has healed with a barely perceptible scar.

Conundrum keys

- A transposition flap from the nasal dorsum and sidewall was used to repair a large defect of the right nasal ala and rim, preserving its size, contour, and function.
- This is a random axis pattern flap consisting of skin and subcutaneous tissue.
- The secondary defect was closed in a side-to-side fashion, achieving an excellent esthetic result.

References

1 Humphreys TR, Goldberg LH, Wiemer DR. Repair of defects of the nasal ala. Dermatol Surg 1997;23:335–49.
2 Tromovitch TA, Stegman SJ, Glogau RG. Flaps and Grafts for Dermatologic Surgery. St. Louis: CV Mosby Co.; 1989.
3 Burget GC, Menick FJ. Aesthetic Reconstruction of the Nose. St. Louis: CV Mosby Co.; 1994.
4 Robinson JK. Surgery of the Skin: Procedural Dermatology. Philadelphia: Elsevier Mosby; 2005.
5 Baker SR. Local Flaps in Facial Reconstruction. Philadelphia: Elsevier Mosby; 2007.
6 Mamelak AJ, Goldberg LH. Complex Linear Closure of the Nose Dorsum. Vancouver, Canada: Poster ACMS; 2008.

Commentary on conundrum 28

The repair of this defect is quite challenging given the near-total loss of the alar rim. The technique demonstrated is very creative, particularly because it uses "like" tissue exclusively while keeping all scars on the nose. The part that seems confusing is that the kink in Figure 4 seems to be dramatically minimized without any backcuts shown in Figure 5.

With this degree of volume loss as well as exposed cartilage, a more conventional repair would consist of an interpolation flap to recreate the alar rim[1]. Given that a frontal view is not shown, it is difficult to determine how much of the medial border of the alar rim is missing. To recreate the alar rim in this location, a "folded flap" is an option – either a paramedian forehead flap or a melolabial transposition flap[2]. With its robust axial blood supply, the forehead flap would likely be preferred by most surgeons. With either flap, a longer pedicle would be helpful to provide for the extra length to be folded under the alar rim. An intermediate stage could also be performed, in which a cartilage strut is inserted to stabilize the alar rim, with final pedicle takedown occurring 3–4 weeks after the initial flap repair. Other possible options include a superiorly based V to Y (island pedicle-type) advancement flap, although it is unclear whether there would be sufficient tissue available to fold distally to recreate the alar rim. With any of these extensive distal nasal flap options, it is often helpful to stent open the nasal vestibule (such as with placement of a nasopharyngeal airway) during the first 48 hours post repair. Alternatively, a gauze dental-roll gently placed in the distal vestibule (and well lubricated with ointment) can be used to prevent significant swelling and deformity of the alar rim.

Commentary by Dr. Cohen

References

1 Lee K, Swanson N, Lee H. Color atlas of cutaneous excisions and repairs. 2008: New York: Cambridge University Press. p. 150.

2 Baker SR. Local flaps in facial reconstruction, 2nd Edition. St Louis: Mosby, 2007:p. 444–7.

29

CONUNDRUM 29

Bilobed Flap for Full-Thickness Nasal Defect: A Common Flap for an Uncommon Indication

Joan-Ramon Garces[1], Alessandro Guedes[2], Marta Alegre[1], & Agustin Alomar[3]

[1]Hospital de la Santa Creu I Sant Pau, Barcelona, Spain
[2]Universitat Autonoma de Barcelona, Barcelona, Spain
[3]Department of Dermatology, Barcelona, Spain

A 60-year-old woman was referred to the Mohs surgery unit of the Sant Pau Hospital in March 2000 for the treatment of a tumor of the alar rim and tip of the nose. Histopathological examination showed a sclerodermiform basal cell carcinoma. Four stages of Mohs surgery were needed to excise the entire tumor, which involved part of the nasal cartilage and nasal mucosa, resulting in a full-thickness defect (Figure 1). How would you proceed in this case?

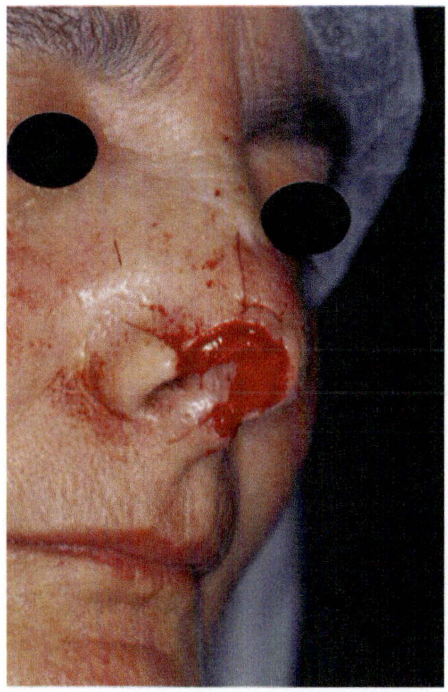

Figure 1 Nasal defect after Mohs surgery for basal cell carcinoma.

Resolution

The procedure was performed under local anesthesia with mepivacaine 2% and adrenaline 1:200,000. The bilobed flap was designed (Figure 2). The defect was measured based on the contralateral alar size, considering the inner and outer surfaces. The defect size was approximately 1.8 × 1.4 cm. Incisions were made in the primary and secondary lobes. A primary lobe of the same size as the defect was raised, and a secondary lobe was obtained from the root of the nose. The lobes were undermined above the perichondrium and periosteum. Nasal muscles were included to obtain satisfactory perfusion. The primary lobe was thinned by removing the muscle and subcutaneous tissue from the distal portion of the flap (the one that will be folded to

Reconstructive Conundrums in Dermatologic Surgery: The Nose, First Edition. Edited by Désirée Ratner, Joel L. Cohen and David G. Brodland.
© 2014 American Society for Dermatologic Surgery. Published 2014 by John Wiley & Sons, Ltd.

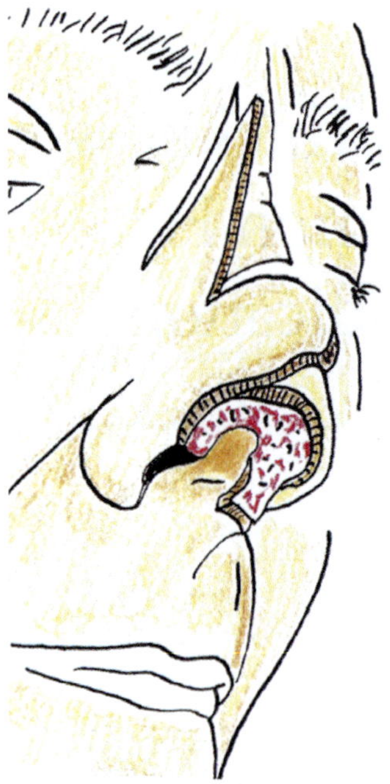

Figure 2 Schematic view of bilobed flap.

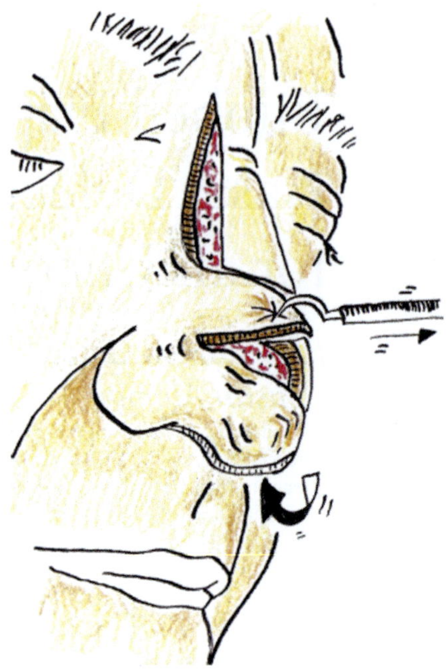

Figure 3 Schematic view of bilobed flap folded inward.

create mucosal lining). All but 1 mm of the subdermal fat was preserved to avoid alar collapse on inspiration and ensure a satisfactory functional outcome. The tertiary nasal root defect was initially closed. The primary lobe was then inserted in the site of the original defect and folded inward to restore the inner surface of the nose and the alar rim (Figure 3). Nonabsorbable sutures were placed between the primary lobe and the remaining nasal mucosa (Figure 4). Finally, nonabsorbable sutures were placed in the primary and secondary lobe with great care to promote wound-edge eversion. Postoperative antibiotics were given, and sutures were removed 7 days postoperatively. The 6-month postoperative follow-up showed a satisfactory functional and aesthetic outcome (Figures 5 and 6).

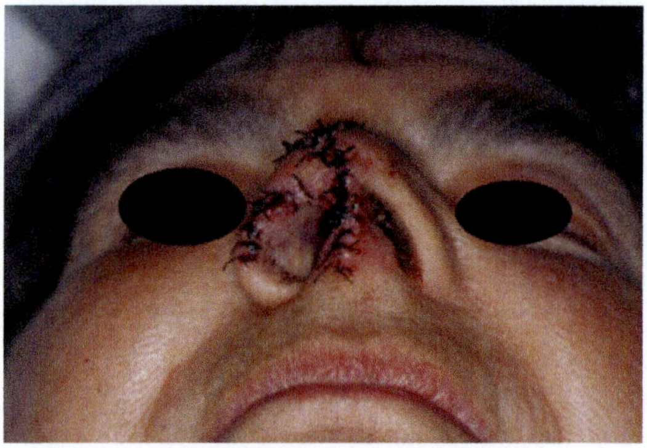

Figure 4 Bilobed flap restoring the inner surface of the nose.

Discussion

The bilobed transposition flap, initially described by Esser in 1918 and later modified by Zitelli, is a single-stage flap often used for restoring skin defects of the nasal supra-tip.[1,2] It is suitable for defects measuring up to 20 mm.[3] We used this standard procedure for an unusual indication, the reconstruction of a full-thickness nasal alar rim defect. Full-thickness nasal tip defects are a particular challenge for dermatologic reconstructive surgeons. The treatments of choice continue to be the paramedian forehead flap and the nasolabial flap.[4,5] Although they are often aesthetically and functionally successful, these procedures are often staged and complex in some aspects. Patients may refuse such treatment because of the temporary deformity, the permanent forehead scar, or the need for at least two stages to obtain satisfactory results. Procedures such as the hinge

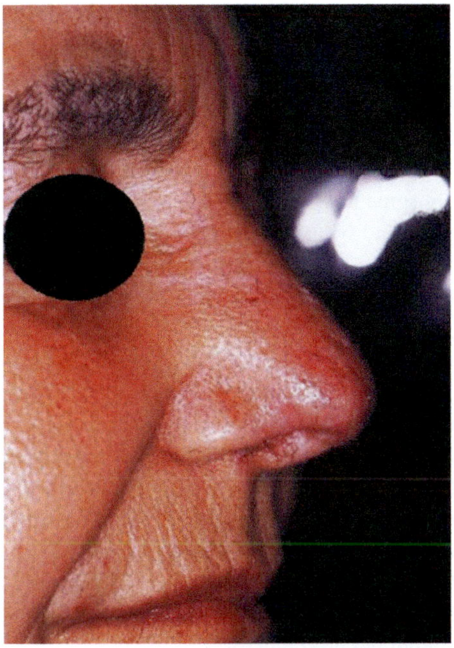

Figure 5 Lateral view: 6-month postoperative follow-up.

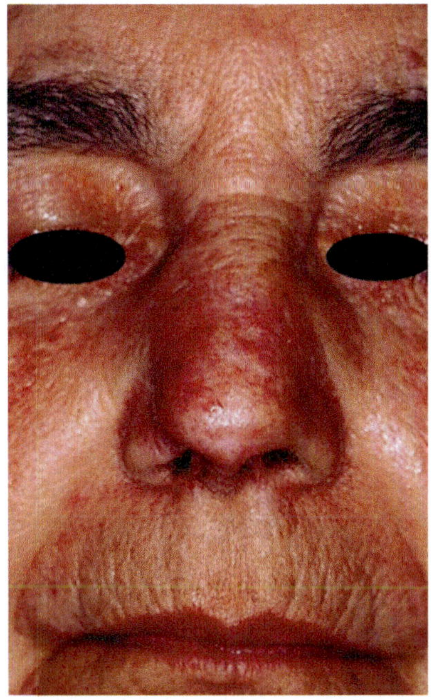

Figure 6 Frontal view: 6-month postoperative follow-up.

flap, secondary healing, and composite grafts should be considered when performing the reconstruction of full-thickness nose defects.[6]

Although it is not commonly used in full-thickness nasal rim defects, the bilobed flap has several advantages. First, it is a one-stage procedure. Second, the tissue transferred to the defect is closest in color and texture. Third, it is a more conservative procedure than the paramedian flap, and it is less technically complex and has lower morbidity.

The bilobed flap cannot be used to reconstruct defects larger than 20 mm. In our case, we calculated the defect area as the sum of the outer (skin) and inner (mucosa) surfaces, based on the size of the contralateral nose ala. If the measurement of the outer part only is used, the flap will be too small to allow for folding and covering of the inner surface of the defect.

Sometimes a chondral graft may be needed as a structural support to prevent alar collapse and notching due to scar contracture. Other than having a slight distortion of the nostril shape on frontal view, our patient did not have any airway compromise, and no alar retraction or notching was present. Several aspects should be considered when performing this type of bilobed flap. The diameter of the primary lobe of the bilobed flap needs to be equivalent to the nasal defect. If the primary lobe is undersized, the nasal ala can be displaced upward. In the case of full-thickness defects, a short primary lobe may result in failure to cover the inner part of the defect. The size of the secondary lobe is variable. Its purpose is to allow closure of the secondary defect without tension, but if it is overestimated, the tertiary defect cannot be sutured. If possible, the secondary lobe should be placed perpendicular to the nasal ala to prevent ala displacement.[7] Wide undermining of the flaps and the recipient areas is advised to achieve extensive flap motion.

Conclusion

Although the bilobed flap procedure is routinely performed in the reconstruction of defects located on the lower third of the nose, it is not often used to restore full-thickness nasal alar rim defects. It should be considered an option in these cases because it is a one-stage, low-complexity flap that provides aesthetic and functional results rivalling those of the routinely used pedicle flap when correctly indicated and performed.

References

1 McGregor JC, Soutar DS. A critical assessment of bilobed flap. Br J Plast Surg 1981;34:197–205.
2 Alam M, Goldberg LH. Two-lobed advancement flap for cutaneous helical rim defects. Dermatol Surg 2003;29:1044–9.
3 Fujiwara M. One-stage reconstruction of an alar defect using a bilobed nasolabial-nasal tip flap based on the aesthetic subunits in Orientals: case report. Aesth Plast Surg 2004;28: 13–6.
4 Boyd CM, Baker SR. The forehead flap for nasal reconstruction. Arch Dermatol 2000;136:1365–70.
5 Iwao F. Alar reconstruction with subcutaneous pedicled nasolabial flap: difficulties, considerations, and conclusions for this procedure. Dermatol Surg 2005;31:1351–4.
6 Cherpelis BS, Carls JL. One-stage reconstruction of a full-thickness nasal defect involving the alar rim. Dermatol Surg 2007;33:1361–4.
7 Cook JL. A review of the bilobed flap's design with particular emphasis on the minimization of alar displacement. Dermatol Surg 2000;26:354–62.

Commentary

The authors are faced with a challenging defect involving multiple cosmetic subunits of the nose with partial full-thickness loss and have achieved acceptable cosmetic results with an unconventional use of the Zitelli modification of the bilobed flap. The authors acknowledge the resultant alar deformity due to the inevitable flap contraction but report that no airway obstruction results. If this is the case when the patient is upright, there is almost certainly some airway obstruction when the patient is recumbent and lying on her left side. This airway collapse is likely to be distressing to the more-demanding patient and would probably have been eliminated by using a small cartilage graft to maintain the patent airway seen immediately after repair. A second procedure could be performed at this time to insert a batten of cartilage along the alar rim in an attempt to reopen the constricted airway, but scar contraction may prevent significant improvement at this point. Nonetheless, the authors have provided an example of a single-stage procedure that provides acceptable results in a setting where two-stage procedures are usually required to achieve superior results.

The author has no conflicts.

David B. Pharis, MD
Atlanta, GA

Commentary on conundrum 29

This case illustrates an unconventional use of a bilobed flap. Under proper circumstances, there is no reason why this flap cannot be considered in the reconstruction of difficult defects such as the one presented here. However, several conditions must be present in order to achieve a good functional and cosmetic result with this closure. The first condition is adequate laxity of skin within the donor site on the nasal dorsum. Secondly, the skin on the nose must be flexible and mobile enough for the primary flap to reach the defect without distortion and, more importantly, to fold upon itself to recreate the soft triangle and alar rim. There are many skin types that are unable to accommodate this movement because they do not have sufficient flexibility or elasticity. Lastly, the structure of the remaining ala must be sturdy enough to withstand the rotational movement of this large flap. Some noses with the virtue of flexible skin may have similarly flexible alar skin, which lacks the firm structure necessary to support the flap rotation forces which are concentrated on the mid ala. The strain of having the rotation point located on the alar rim is evident in Figure 6, where partial collapse of the left ala is shown.

Given these requirements, the bilobed flap is certainly robust enough to accomplish closure of this defect, as is nicely illustrated in this case. The authors mention the inclusion of the nasalis muscle in the design of the flap to ensure sufficient blood flow. Excellent vascularity is particularly important due to the crimping effect of folding the distal tip of the flap upon itself. Care must be taken to minimize damage to the vasculature and injury to the tissue in the process of developing this flap. Likewise, when thinning the flap the surgeon must strike a balance between improving the "foldability" of the flap and maintaining adequate vascularity.

The authors advocate closure of the dorsal donor site first. In general, a good rule of thumb for transposition flaps is to close the donor defect with the first suture. The second suture is best placed at the pivot point of the flap, at which a Burow's triangle is removed to accommodate the tissue redundancy generated from the flap's rotation. The third key suture is placed to suspend and precisely position the primary lobe, setting up easy placement of the remaining sutures. Dermal absorbable suture has the advantage of accommodating the tension of flap movement below the skin surface, thus avoiding surface suture marks. Furthermore, when properly placed, dermal sutures can diminish the chance of wound dehiscence should a complication occur within the first two weeks after surgery. Once these key sutures are placed, if there is significant distortion of adjacent structures, further mobilization of the flap may be needed.

When considering all the pros and cons of various closures, including the inconvenience a patient will experience after a two-stage reconstruction, one must also consider whether these inconveniences are outweighed by a substantially higher chance of success in flap execution. Many times, we have patients who, either because of inconvenience or medical issues, seem to be less than optimal candidates for two-stage procedures. In trying to circumvent these more complex procedures, closure with a single-stage local flap can sometimes have such a high risk of failure or adjacent structure distortion, or have such high prospects of requiring a second-stage revision, that the two-stage option becomes the more practical one. That being said, the feasibility of a single-stage reconstruction should always be evaluated when considering more involved two-stage procedures.

Other considerations for closure would include the placement of a cartilage graft for structural support along the alar rim. In my opinion, the thickness of a cartilage graft in addition to the double thickness of the flap folded upon itself would probably result in an unacceptably bulky alar rim. Placement of a cartilage graft would likely be best done as a second stage if necessary. A bucket handle mucosal advancement flap could also be considered, which is executed with a parallel incision made 6 mm cephalad to the mucosal defect. This mucosal strip becomes a bipedicled flap, which is then advanced inferiorly to replace the lost mucosa. If this alternative can be accomplished, it may obviate the need to fold the flap upon itself.

Another repair option for this defect would be a cheek interpolation flap. Despite being a two-stage flap, this is a somewhat smaller procedure than a forehead flap and, in my experience, provides excellent tissue match and structure in recreating the alar rim. In men, the presence of facial hair is a complicating factor that would need to be considered in the decision for closure. A forehead flap would be another excellent alternative in many patients with this type of defect.

Thinking outside of the box and extending the use of traditional reconstruction techniques for patient's benefit are standard aspects of a creative reconstructive surgeon's daily routine. Knowing when these creative variations will succeed is the true test of a good surgeon.

Commentary by Dr. Brodland

30

CONUNDRUM 30

One-Stage Reconstruction Following Complete Alar Loss

Glenn D. Goldman

Fletcher Allen Health Care, University of Vermont College of Medicine, Burlington, VT

An 80-year-old man was presented with a longstanding recurrent basal cell carcinoma of the right alar crease. The lesion was excised in three stages of Mohs surgery, leading to full-thickness loss of the entire right nasal ala and a cutaneous defect bridging the right upper lip apical triangle and right medial cheek. How would you manage this wound?

Resolution

The patient required reconstruction for a complete loss of the nasal ala, partial loss of the tip subunit, loss of the apical triangle of the lip, and a partial loss of the medial cheek (Figure 1). A standard approach that was considered consisted of a cheek advancement, a large septal mucosal flap, a cartilage graft, and a paramedian forehead pedicle flap. Such an approach repairs the nasal mucosa with septal mucosa, stabilizes the ala with a cartilage graft, advances the cheek, and recreates the nose with a forehead pedicle.

Single-stage repair of full-thickness wounds of the lateral nose and ala can be accomplished with a "turnover" nasolabial flap, as elegantly described by Spear and colleagues.[1,2] The patient desired a 1-day procedure, and fortunately, the adjacent cheek skin was ample, lax, and contained only vellus hair. In planning an appropriate single turnover flap (Figure 2), it was felt that the alar loss was too extensive for this procedure alone. Specifically

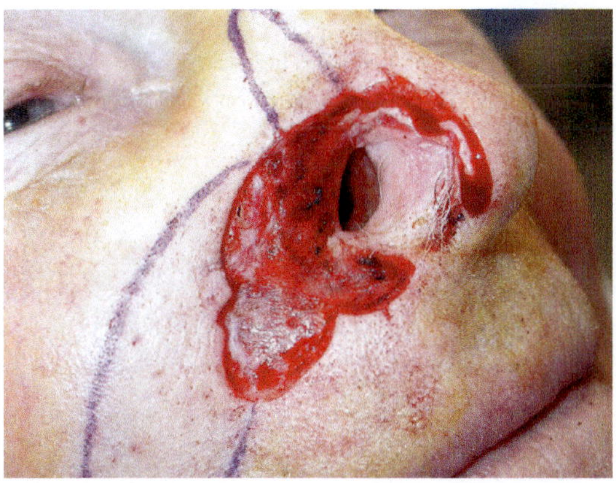

Figure 1 Defect following tumor removal involves entire right ala, a portion of the right medial cheek, and the apical triangle of the right upper lip.

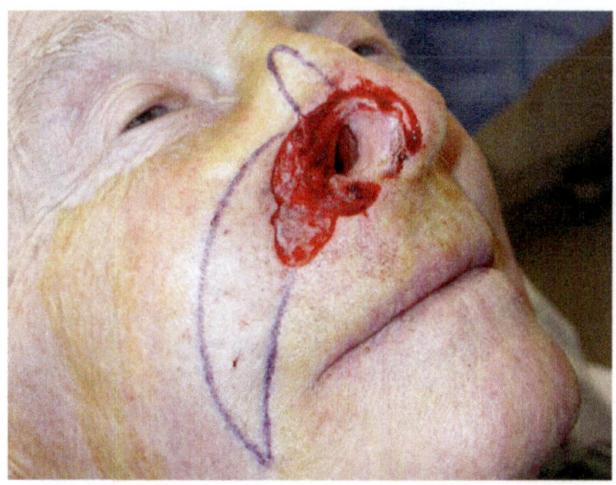

Figure 2 Planned operative repair delineating turnover hinge flap on nasal sidewall and turnover nasolabial flap on right cheek.

Reconstructive Conundrums in Dermatologic Surgery: The Nose, First Edition. Edited by Désirée Ratner, Joel L. Cohen and David G. Brodland.
© 2014 American Society for Dermatologic Surgery. Published 2014 by John Wiley & Sons, Ltd.

given the width of the alar wound, execution of this flap alone would have placed considerable horizontal tension on the proximal portion (lining side) of the flap. Consideration was given to a repair that incorporated two simultaneous tissue transfers in order to alleviate lateral to medial tension on the more proximal portion of the Spear flap, thus improving the chance for survival of the distal flap.

In order to line the medial third of the right nose, a triangular hinge flap was elevated just above the nasalis with its base at the pyriform aperture and its tip just medial to the medial canthus. The base of the flap was left attached to the inferior nasalis, and the flap was turned over the pyriform aperture and sewn into place along the nasal septum with 5.0 chromic gut (Figure 3). This flap has been described elsewhere.[3,4] The adjacent medial cheek was undermined and advanced to close the nasal sidewall defect resulting from the turnover hinge flap (Figure 4).

On the right cheek a broad flap was designed to course along and lateral to the right nasolabial fold. The flap was elevated above musculature as a banner and was left attached to a narrow pedicle that contained several visible arterial and venous perforators (Figure 5). The entire length of the flap was thinned to the superficial subcutaneous plexus and remained pink and viable. To recreate the lateral nasal lining, the flap was transposed, inverted, and sewn to the turnover hinge flap with several 5.0 Vicryl® (Ethicon, Somerville, NJ, USA) sutures and multiple simple interrupted 5.0 chromic sutures (Figure 6). The fact that a portion of lip and cheek medial

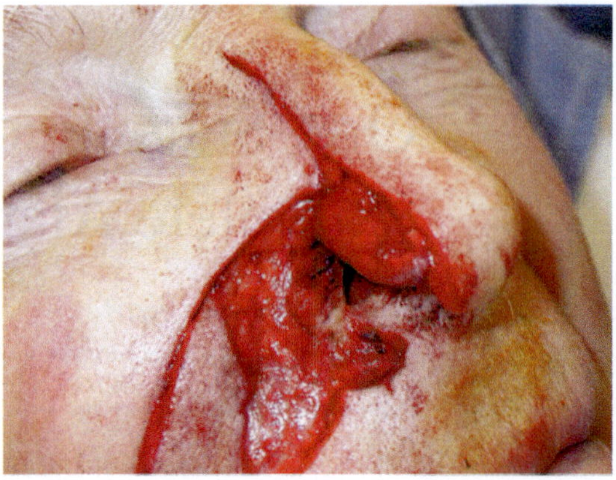

Figure 4 Medial cheek advanced to close nasal sidewall defect.

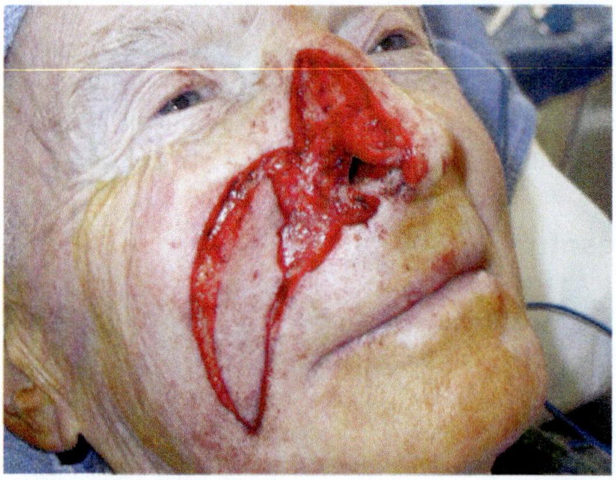

Figure 5 Spear flap has been incised and elevated. The entire flap has been undermined up to the medial edge. In this photo the nasal sidewall has not yet been closed.

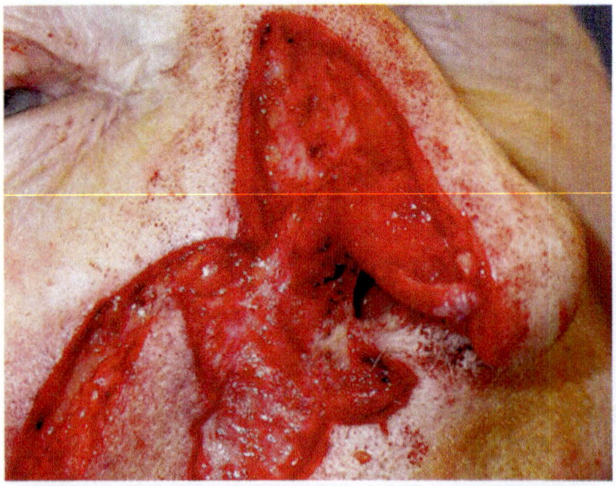

Figure 3 Hinge flap turned down to line medial ala. Flap hinges on nasalis muscle which provides vascular pedicle.

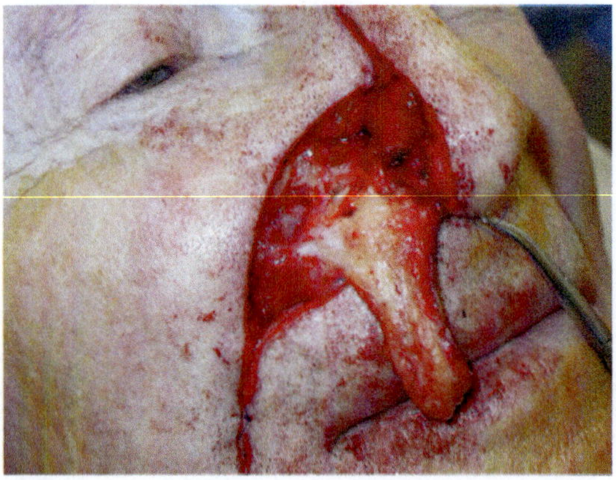

Figure 6 Spear flap turned over to line the lateral two thirds of the ala. nasolabial fold is in process of being sutured closed.

to the flap had been deepithelialized at tumor removal was actually beneficial in allowing the flap to transpose and invert. In order to stabilize the ala, a broad cartilage graft was harvested from the right pinna between the upper antihelix and helix (Figure 7) and fastened medially and laterally with four 5.0 Vicryl® sutures. The Spear flap was then turned over the cartilage brace and sewn into place with several buried 5.0 Vicryl® sutures and simple interrupted 5.0 Prolene® (Ethicon) surface sutures. The right nasolabial fold was reapproximated linearly.

The apical triangle of the right upper lip was repaired with a small skin graft obtained by amputating the tip of the Spear flap. A small area of the nasal sill was allowed to heal secondarily, and a drain was placed in the wound (Figure 8).

At 1 week the flap was fully viable, and only minor surface slough compromised the small apical lip graft. Over the next 4 months the repair matured, recreating an aesthetic and functional right ala, a proper alar crease, and a suitable apical lip triangle (Figure 9). The nasolabial fold on the right was dimished but visible. Air movement through the right nare was normal and unimpeded (Figure 10).

Discussion

Repair of full-thickness nasal wounds is usually a two-session process. The Spear flap is an elegant and aesthetic one-step repair for full-thickness lateral alar

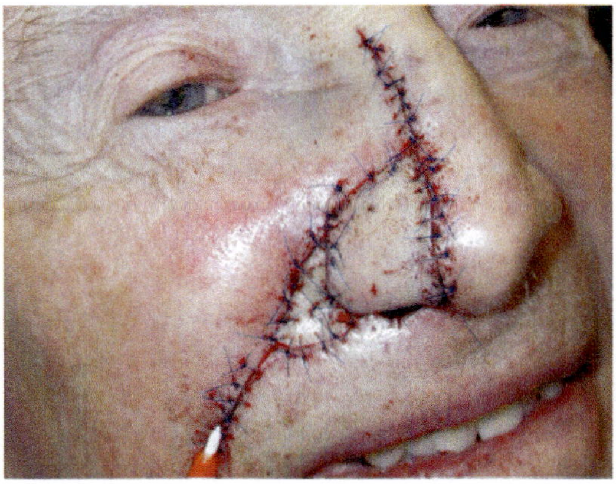

Figure 8 Completed repair. The cartilage graft has been inserted to brace the ala and the nasolabial turnover flap has been folded over onto itself. The tip of the flap has been amputated and used for a skin graft to repair the apical triangle of the lip.

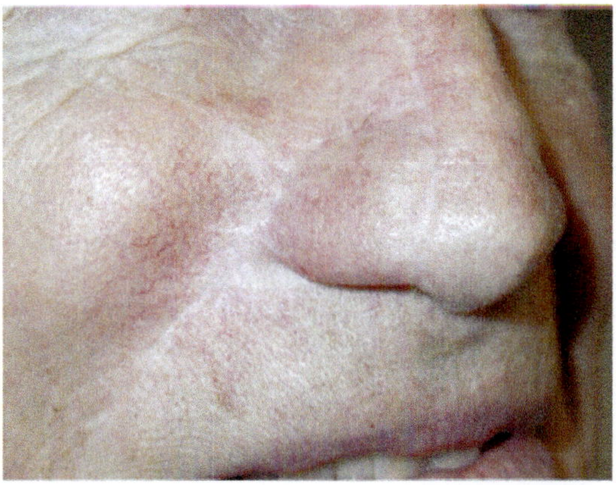

Figure 9 Final result oblique view. Nare is widely patent.

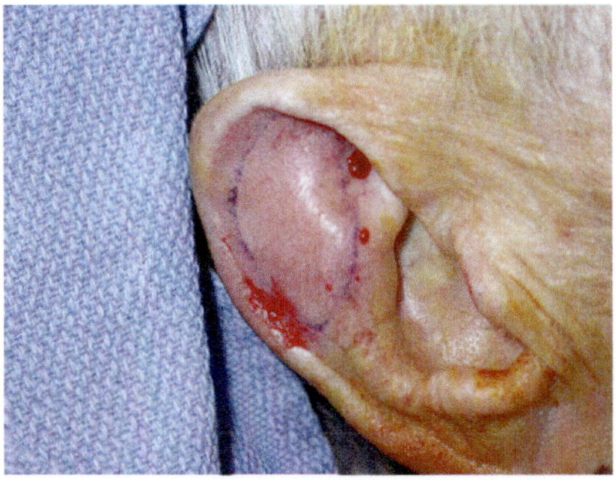

Figure 7 Cartilage graft harvest site. The skin is to be reflected anteriorly and the graft harvested from the upper pinna lateral to the antihelix.

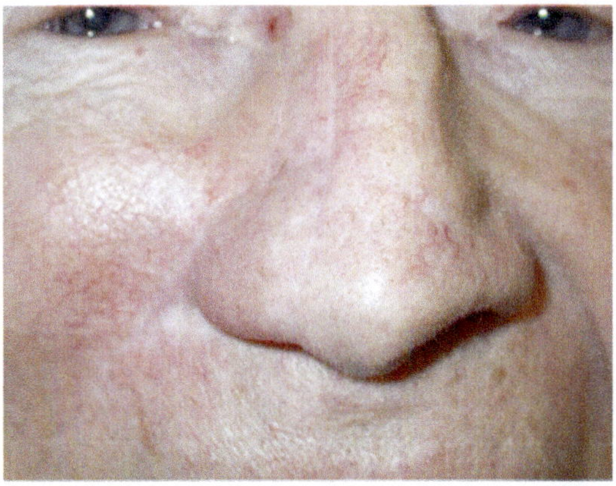

Figure 10 Final result face on with recreation of ala, alar crease, apical triangle, and nasolabial fold.

wounds. This flap is a subunit repair, which hides the harvest scar within a recreated nasolabial fold. In our case, the alar defect was extensive, and a septal mucosal flap and forehead flap would have been large and technically challenging. In addition, while our patient had an abundant reservoir of tissue just lateral to the nasolabial fold, he did not have enough tissue to repair the defect with a single flap. For that reason, a turnover hinge flap was added to the reconstruction to diminish the tension on the proximal portion of the turnover flap.

In many cases, a turnover nasolabial flap can be completed successfully without the use of a cartilaginous support. In our case, as the flap was folded on itself, there was partial collapse of the nare. We chose to utilize a cartilage graft from the pinna, an ideal area for the donation of large pieces of ear cartilage. As long as a 3 or 4 mm peripheral rim of cartilage is left in place, the effect on ear stability and integrity is minimal, and this site is much less painful postoperatively than the conchal bowl. The cartilage graft harvested in this case was a broad wafer, and the graft was gently scored and sewn into place bowed outward to avoid alar collapse.

While the Spear flap is based on the perialar musculature and receives perforators from the angular artery, the majority of the flap is elevated within the subcutis.

The more that the flap can be thinned, the more easily the flap may be folded on itself and the more likely that an aesthetic result can be achieved.

In this case, by utilizing all adjacent reservoirs of tissue, a successful and aesthetic single-stage repair was effected for a very large defect. One disadvantage of this repair is that the ala is lined internally by skin rather than mucosa, however, with a small amount of Vaseline applied daily this has not been problematic. In addition, the area is sensate, as opposed to the usual sensory loss that commonly accompanies a two-stage pedicle flap repair.

Additional readings

1 Spear SL, Kroll SS, Romm S. A new twist to the nasolabial flap for reconstruction of lateral alar defects. Plast Reconstr Surg 1987;79:915–20.
2 Cook JL. Reconstruction of a full-thickness alar wound with a single operative procedure. Dermatol Surg 2003;29:956–62.
3 Fader DJ, Wang TS, Johnson TM. Nasal reconstruction utilizing a muscle hinge flap with overlying full-thickness skin graft. J Am Acad Dermatol 2000;43:837–40.
4 Lee KK, Gorman AK, Swanson NA. Hinged turnover flap: a one-stage reconstruction of a full-thickness nasal ala defect. Dermatol Surg 2004;30:479–81.

Commentary on conundrum 30

This conundrum was solved with the Spear flap to restore complete lateral loss of the nasal ala. Closure of the nasal lining was augmented in this case by the use of a turn-down flap, which ultimately allowed the superior portion of the flap to be slightly narrower than the rest of the flap. The Spear flap facilitates repair of the nasal lining and the external nasal surface by folding upon itself while simultaneously recreating the junction between the alar base and the apical triangle of the lip. Although this flap addresses only very specific defects involving the base of the ala, it is a workhorse for solving a conundrum that has very few other viable solutions.

As mentioned by the authors, the vascular plexus at the junction between the cheek, lip, and nose is a rich blood supply upon which lengthy flaps can be based. The vascularity of this area rivals that of the glabella and medial brow plexus upon which the forehead flap is based.

One technique which is helpful in maximizing flap mobility while preserving the pedicle's vasculature is "vertical spreading." With this technique, an iris scissors is inserted with closed tips, which are carefully spread in the direction of expected vascular flow. The pedicle can thus be loosened and mobilized without compromising blood supply.

A cartilage graft was used in this case to ensure the structural integrity of the ala and nasal valve. Although cartilage grafts are not always necessary with the Spear flap, when in doubt, their use can help to assure a well-formed and functioning ala. The authors propose an interesting donor site using cartilage from the pinna of the ear. The advantage of cartilage from this location is that it tends to be thinner and more flexible than conchal cartilage. Initially, one might think that more flexible cartilage would be less structurally competent. However, as long as the cartilage is correctly positioned and maintained in this position for the first 2–4 weeks postoperatively, even very thin struts of cartilage become rigid and dependably maintain the shape of the ala.

A technique to maintain and protect a well-positioned cartilage graft for the alar rim is intranasal bolstering. The insertion of a "foam nasal cannula" (e.g., Merocel Laminated Nasal Dressing) or the fashioning of an intranasal cast using Thermoplast (Aquaplast PS Thermoplastic Nasal Splints, WFR/Aquaplast Corporation, Avondale, PA 19311, United States) can safeguard the shape and position of the cartilage in the critical early phases of healing. If those products are not available, simple nasal packing with petroleum jelly gauze or a petroleum jelly-impregnated dental roll can serve the same purpose.

The final photos show the excellent result of this single-stage closure that rivals any two-staged procedure. Illustrated in the long-term follow-up photos is the tendency for the lateral base of the ala to be displaced laterally. This is a difficult phenomenon to avoid while attempting to preserve the blood supply to the distal tip of this flap. However, a tacking suture from the would-be alar base medially to the underlying bone of the maxilla can optimize alar position. This refining touch can obviate the need for a second stage to reposition the alar base. When this technique cannot be accomplished without compromising blood supply, a delayed repositioning procedure can be performed. This is best accomplished with a Z-plasty transposition of the new alar base over an intranasal flap, which is designed with the middle limb of the flap passing vertically and slightly obliquely along the medial aspect of the alar base. The lateral limb of the Z-plasty is located on the lateral aspect of the alar base while the medial limb is located intranasally and oriented vertically.

In summary, the Spear flap is the "go to" flap for reconstructing lateral alar base defects. This island flap effectively resurfaces both the intranasal and extranasal surfaces of the lateral ala and can provide excellent cosmetic and functional results.

Commentary by Dr. Brodland

Index

Reconstructive Conundrums in Dermatologic Surgery: The Nose, First Edition. Edited by Désirée Ratner, Joel L. Cohen and David G. Brodland.
© 2014 American Society for Dermatologic Surgery. Published 2014 by John Wiley & Sons, Ltd.

Printed and bound by CPI Group (UK) Ltd, Croydon, CR0 4YY
16/09/2026
14963474-0008